T0210159

ANTI-INFECTION HANDBOOK

ANTI-INFECTION HANDBOOK

Frank Zhu
BMed, MMed, FRACGP

ELSEVIER

ELSEVIER

Elsevier Australia. ACN 001 002 357
(a division of Reed International Books Australia Pty Ltd)
Tower 1, 475 Victoria Avenue, Chatswood, NSW 2067

International Standard Book Number: 978-0-7295-4294-4

Cataloging-in-Publication Data

A catalogue record for this
book is available from the
National Library of Australia

NATIONAL
LIBRARY
OF AUSTRALIA

Senior Content Strategist: Larissa Norrie
Content Development Specialist: Rochelle Deighton
Senior Project Manager: Anitha Rajarathnam
Edited by Caroline Hunter, Burrumundi Pty Ltd
Proofread by Melissa Faulkner
Cover Designer: Lisa Petroff
Index by Innodata Indexing
Typeset by Toppan Best-set Premedia Limited
Printed in China by 1010

Contents

Preface

Anti-infection Handbook presents a comprehensive view of various infectious diseases and provides a compact guide for the diagnosis and management of infections. Although most of the infectious diseases included in the book are seen worldwide, it is written from an Australian perspective and does not contain a comprehensive list of all infectious pathogens worldwide. The antibiotic and immunisation policies are also Australian-based and may be different from policies in other countries.

The book is designed to serve the needs of busy hospital doctors, general practitioners, microbiology laboratory staff, infection control staff and nurses who require a quick, concise and up-to-date guide for diagnosis and treatment of infections. It also provides a broad-based overview of infectious diseases for medical students.

The handbook layout makes it easy to find an infection or a pathogen and to check what tests are needed for diagnosis or what antimicrobials should be chosen for the treatment, placing this information right at your fingertips. The information is very useful, practical and convenient.

FEATURES

- **All-in-one:** contains most infections found in Australia and other countries, with more than 275 infectious diseases and conditions related to bacteria, viruses, fungi, protozoa, parasites and insects.
- **A to Z:** infections are arranged in alphabetical order for easy searching.
- **Immunisation** (including travel vaccination): integrated in the relevant diseases and appendices.
- **Pocketbook size:** easy to carry.

How to use this book

To find information on an infectious disease (e.g. pertussis):

- Turn the page directly to Pertussis alphabetically OR
- Find Pertussis from the contents page or the index

To find information on a pathogen (e.g. *Helicobacter pylori*):

- Turn the page directly to *Helicobacter pylori* alphabetically OR
- Find *Helicobacter pylori* from the contents page or index

To find what tests can be ordered for diagnosis of an infectious disease (e.g. malaria):

- Turn the page directly to Malaria alphabetically and look in the laboratory section OR
- Find Malaria from the contents page or index and look in the laboratory section

To find what antimicrobials can be chosen for an infectious disease (e.g. pelvic inflammatory disease):

- Turn the page directly to Pelvic inflammatory disease alphabetically and look in the treatment section OR
- Find Pelvic inflammatory disease from the contents page or index and look in the treatment section

To find alternative antibiotics that are not listed on the sensitivity report of an isolated bacterium (e.g. *Enterobacter* spp):

- Go to Appendix 6 and follow the instructions there

To find vaccination information on a particular infection (e.g. yellow fever):

- Turn the page directly to Yellow fever alphabetically and look in the vaccination section OR
- Find Yellow fever from the contents page or index and look in the vaccination section OR
- Go to Appendix 5 and find Yellow fever alphabetically

To order a vaccine for a traveller (e.g. rabies):

- Turn the page directly to Rabies alphabetically and look in the vaccination section OR
- Find Rabies from the contents page or index and look in the vaccination section OR
- Go to Appendix 5 and find Rabies alphabetically

To find the duration of school exclusion for an infectious disease (e.g. chickenpox):

- Go to Appendix 7

About the author

Dr Frank Zhu is a general practitioner (family doctor) at the Sydney Medical Centre, Sydney.

He graduated from the Second Military Medical University in Shanghai, China in 1983 and became a Master of Medicine in 1989, and a Physician and Associate Professor in 1992. He was a member of the Hospital Infection Control Committee in China.

He is also the author of the *Handbook of Practical Anti-infection Therapy* and *New Concepts in Antibiotic Treatment*.

ACNE

Causes

- Increased sebum production—secondary to increased androgen production
- Abnormal follicular keratinisation
- Overgrowth of *Propionibacterium acnes*
- Inflammation

Treatment

Mild acne (comedones with some papules and pustules)

Start with one of topical retinoids

- Option 1: adapalene (e.g. Differin) gel/cream top nocte
- Option 2: tretinoin (e.g. Retrieve, Stieva-A) gel/cream top nocte
- Option 3: isotretinoin (e.g. Isotrex) gel top nocte
- Option 4: tazarotene (e.g. Zorac) cream top nocte

If inadequate control after 6 weeks, add benzoyl peroxide or topical antibiotics

- Option 1: adapalene + benzoyl peroxide (e.g. Epiduo) gel top nocte
- Option 2: benzoyl peroxide (e.g. Benzac, Brevoxyl, Oxy) gel/cream top mane
- Option 3: clindamycin (e.g. ClindaTech, Zindaclin, Dalacin T) lotion/gel top mane
- Option 4: benzoyl peroxide + clindamycin (e.g. Duac) top mane
- Stop topical antibiotics once papular inflammation settled
- Use retinoids or benzoyl peroxide for long-term maintenance

For mild truncal acne (large area) use keratolytic

- Salicylic acid 3–5% solution/gel/cream top nocte

Moderate acne (widespread papules and pustules +/– mild scarring)

Any topical agents + oral antibiotics

- Option 1: doxycycline 50–100 mg PO daily for 3–6 months
- Option 2: minocycline 50–100 mg PO daily for 3–6 months (if cannot tolerate doxycycline)
- Option 3: erythromycin 250–500 mg PO bid for 3–6 months (if pregnant)

If no response after 6 weeks

- Increase the dose of oral antibiotic or change to another antibiotic
- Add OCP with anti-androgen (for girls):
  - OCP with cyproterone (e.g. Brenda-35 ED, Diane-35 ED) 1 tab PO daily

Severe acne (nodular abscesses and cysts + extensive scarring)
Any topical agents + high-dose oral antibiotic

- Doxycycline 100 mg **or** minocycline 100 mg PO q12h for up to 6 weeks

If no improvement after 6 weeks refer to a dermatologist
Any topical agents + oral retinoid

- Isotretinoin 0.5 mg/kg PO daily for 2–4 weeks, continue for 16 weeks

Maintenance

- Topical retinoid **or** topical benzoyl peroxide

(Use a gel for oily skin and a cream for dry or sensitive skin)

Co-care of the skin

- Cleanse face with a cleanser for sensitive skin type
- Moisturise face with oil-free lotion

ACTINOMYCETOMA

Actinomycetoma is a mycetomal disease affecting skin and connective tissue. It is the bacterial form of mycetoma (eumycetoma is the fungal form of mycetoma).

Pathogens

- *Actinomadura madurae*
- *Actinomadura pelletieri*
- *Streptomyces somaliensis*
- *Nocardia brasiliensis*

Distribution

- Mainly in tropical areas, India, Africa, South America, Central America and Southeast Asia

Clinical

- A slowly progressive, destructive infection of the cutaneous and subcutaneous tissues, fascia and bone
- Starts as a painless nodule, suppurates, spreads along fascial plains and drains through chronic fistulas

Diagnosis

- Presence of tumour, sinuses and grain-flecked discharge
- Gram stain and microscopic examination of the discharge
- Biopsy may be necessary—can reduce the chances of a re-established infection prior to sinus formation

Treatment

- Surgery—remove the tumour and a portion of surrounding tissue
- Antibiotic therapy can reduce the chances of a re-established infection
  - Benzylpenicillin (IV)

After improvement, switch to oral
  * Penicillin V (PO) for 8–12 months
If penicillin allergy
  * Rifampicin (PO) **plus** cotrimoxazole (PO) for 8–12 months

Dosage of above agents
  * Benzylpenicillin 0.6–1.2 g (child: 30–60 mg/kg up to 1.2 g) IV q6h
  * Penicillin V 500 mg (child: 10 mg/kg up to 500 mg) PO q6h
  * Rifampicin 600 mg (neonate: 10 mg/kg; child: 20 mg/kg up to 600 mg) PO daily
  * Cotrimoxazole 160/800 mg (child: 4/20 mg/kg up to 160/800 mg) PO q12h

Prognosis
* Recovery from mycetoma may take months or years
* Recurrence after surgery in at least 20% of cases

ACTINOMYCOSIS

Pathogens
* *Actinomyces* spp (particularly *A. israelii*)—gram-positive, anaerobic-to-microaerophilic filamentous bacteria, normally found in mouth and bowel

Distribution
* Occurs worldwide, including in Australia, with a higher prevalence rate in people with low socioeconomic status and poor dental hygiene

Clinical
Painful abscesses in four common sites:

* Pelvic actinomycosis (IUCD user)
* Cervicofacial actinomycosis (poor dental conditions or trauma to mouth)
* Thoracic actinomycosis (history of aspiration)
* Abdominal actinomycosis (post-abdominal surgery or perforated viscus)

The abscesses grow larger over a period of months and may penetrate surrounding tissue to skin, resulting in leakage of large amounts of pus.

Laboratory
* Sulfur granules (yellowish particles) may be seen in the pus
* Gram stain of pus—beaded and branched gram-positive filamentous rods
* Culture from draining sinuses, deep needle aspirate or biopsy specimens (promptly transport the specimens in an anaerobic transport device)
* PCR testing for *Actinomyces*—rapid and more accurate
* Pelvic ultrasound shows abscesses

Treatment

- Removal of IUCD may lead to complete resolution
- Surgical intervention can be an adjunct treatment in selected cases
- Antibiotic therapy (some bacteria may have penicillin resistance) (seek expert advice)

Mild infection

- Option 1: benzylpenicillin (IV), **then** penicillin V (PO) for 6–12 months
- Option 2: amoxicillin/clavulanate (PO) for 6–12 months

If penicillin allergy or no response

- Option 1: doxycycline (PO)
- Option 2: clindamycin (IV, then PO)

Moderate to severe cervicofacial and thoracic actinomycosis

- Ceftriaxone (IV, then oral [above choices])

Moderate to severe abdominal and pelvic actinomycosis

- Imipenem/cilastatin (IV, then oral [above choices])

Dosage of above agents

- Benzylpenicillin 1.2–2.4 g (child: 30–60 mg/kg up to 2.4 g) IV q4h
- Penicillin V 500 mg (child 10 mg/kg up to 500 mg) PO q6h
- Amoxicillin/clavulanate 875 mg (child: 20 mg/kg up to 875 mg) PO q12h
- Doxycycline 100 mg (child >8 years: 2 mg/kg up to 100 mg) PO or IV q12h
- Clindamycin 600 mg (child: 10 mg/kg up to 600 mg) IV q8h, then 300 mg (child: 7.5 mg/kg up to 300 mg) PO q8h
- Ceftriaxone 2 g (child: 50 mg/kg up to 2 g) IV daily
- Imipenem/cilastatin 1 g (child: 15–25 mg/kg up to 1 g) IV q6h

ADENOVIRUS

Pathogens

- Human adenovirus (HAdV): 6 species (A–F) and 51 serotypes
- Different serotypes are associated with different infections:
  - Respiratory disease—HadV-B and C
  - Conjunctivitis—HAdV-B and D
  - Gastroenteritis—HAdV-F serotypes 40 and 41

Transmission

- Respiratory tract—through droplets
- GI tract—faecal–oral route
- Direct contact—hand-to-eye transfer
- Venereal

Incubation

- 5–8 days

Adenovirus-associated human diseases

- Adenovirus is responsible for 5% of acute childhood respiratory illness and 10% of infantile gastroenteritis
- **Respiratory tract infection**—pharyngitis, croup, bronchiolitis, bronchitis or pneumonia
- **Gastroenteritis**—may cause intussusception as a complication in babies
- **Conjunctivitis**—pharyngoconjunctival fever and epidemic keratoconjunctivitis
- **Genitourinary infections**—cervicitis, urethritis and haemorrhagic cystitis
- **Meningoencephalitis**—a complication of respiratory adenovirus infection
- **Generalised infection**—can occur in immunocompromised patients and can be chronically debilitating and life-threatening

Laboratory

- Adenovirus antigen detection (from respiratory secretions or faeces)
- Adenovirus culture (from respiratory secretions or faeces)
- Adenovirus PCR assay
- Adenovirus serology

Treatment

- Supportive and rehydration
- Antivirals have generally been ineffective
- Intravenous ribavirin—a potential treatment for severe adenovirus infection in immunocompromised patients

Immunity

- Adenovirus infection results in long-lasting immunity against the specific serotype
- Maternal antibody is protective
- No vaccine available

Prevention

- Chlorination of swimming pools for preventing adenovirus conjunctivitis
- Hand-washing
- Measures to prevent hospital transmission

AMOEBIASIS

Other names: amoebic dysentery, amoebic liver abscess

Pathogens

- *Entamoeba histolytica*

Transmission

- Faecal–oral route (contamination of food or water)

Incubation

- 2–4 weeks—during this period the infected person will excrete cysts

Clinical

- Most commonly occurs after travel to an endemic country
- Mild infection—may be asymptomatic or have mild diarrhoea
- Severe infection—may cause amoebic dysentery, amoebic colonic abscesses, amoebic liver abscesses or peritonitis from bowel perforation

Laboratory

- Faeces OCP microscopy—find trophozoites and cysts
- Faecal multiplex PCR testing—sensitivity 98–100%, result available in 24 hours
- Amoeba antibodies (*Entamoeba histolytica* serology)

Treatment

For amoebic colitis (dysentery)

- Option 1: tinidazole (PO) for 3 days (for 10 days if no response)
- Option 2: metronidazole (PO) for 7–10 days (can be repeated after 2 weeks)
- Option 3: diloxanide* + secnidazole* (PO) for 10 days (if above treatment fails)

Followed by eradicating cysts (prevent relapse)

- Paromomycin* (PO) for 7 days

For extra-intestinal amoebiasis (e.g. amoebic liver abscess)

- Option 1: metronidazole (IV or PO) for 7 days
- Option 2: tinidazole (PO) for 5 days

Followed by eradicating cysts (prevent relapse)

- Paromomycin* (PO) for 7 days

If no improvement after 3–5 days, aspiration of abscess

Asymptomatic carrier

- Paromomycin* (PO) for 7 days

Dosage of above agents

- Tinidazole 2 g (child: 50 mg/kg up to 2 g) PO daily
- Metronidazole 600 mg (child: 15 mg/kg up to 600 mg) PO q8h
- Diloxanide 500 mg PO q8h
- Secnidazole 400 mg PO q8h
- Paromomycin 500 mg (child: 10 mg/kg up to 500 mg) PO q8h (with meals)
- Metronidazole 750 mg (child: 15 mg/kg up to 750 mg) IV q8h
- Metronidazole 800 mg (child: 15 mg/kg up to 800 mg) PO q8h

*Available via Special Access Scheme <www.tga.gov.au/hp/access-sas.htm> or from compounding chemist

- *Entamoeba dispar*, *Entamoeba moshkovskii*, *Entamoeba hartmanni*, *Entamoeba coli*, *Iodamoeba bütschlii*
- May be found in faeces samples
- Considered to be commensals and antimicrobial treatment is not required

AMOEBIC MENINGITIS

Other name: primary amoebic meningoencephalitis (PAM)

Amoebic meningitis was first documented in Australia in 1965. It is a rare but fatal infection. Early diagnosis and treatment are vital.

Pathogens

- *Naegleria fowleri* (also known as brain-eating amoeba)—a unicellular organism found in warm fresh water
- *Balamuthia mandrillaris*—unrelated to *Naegleria fowleri*, but also causes brain damage known as granulomatous amoebic encephalitis in people with immunosuppression

Distribution

- Usually found in tropical countries where the fresh-water temperature exceeds 30°C, such as ponds, lakes, rivers and hot springs; it is also found in poorly chlorinated or unchlorinated swimming pools
- The organism can remain dormant in soil for long periods and reactivate in fresh water

Transmission

- History of exposure to fresh water during summer months
- The only way it enters the body is through the nose/sinuses
- The contaminated water must be insufflated into the nose and sinus cavities for transmission
- The organism attaches to the olfactory nerve and migrates through the cribriform plate into olfactory bulbs of the forebrain

Incubation

- 3–7 days

Clinical

- Most victims have been children unaware of the dangers of swimming in or playing with contaminated water
- Early symptoms: parosmia, rapidly progress to anosmia (with ageusia)
- After the organism has multiplied and consumed the olfactory bulbs, the infection rapidly spreads through the mitral cell axons to the rest of the cerebrum, resulting in severe headache, nausea and vomiting, high fever, rigidity of neck, delirium, seizures and eventually coma

- Death usually occurs within 14 days of exposure as a result of respiratory failure; the fatality rate is about 97%

Treatment

Seek expert advice

- By the time definitive diagnosis is made, most patients will have already manifested signs of terminal cerebral necrosis
- Treatment includes prompt amphotericin B (IV + intrathecal) or rifampicin (IV)
  - Option 1: amphotericin B 1–1.5 mg/kg IV daily
  Intrathecal amphotericin B: 25–100 mcg (up to 500 mcg) q48–72h
  - Option 2: rifampicin 600 mg (child: 10–20 mg/kg up to 600 mg) IV daily

Prevention

- Swim/play in safe water only
- Do not allow untreated water to go into the nose
- Wear nose-clips to prevent insufflation of contaminated water
- Do not play with garden hoses

ANTHRAX

Pathogens

- *Bacillus anthracis*—a large gram-positive spore-forming bacillus

Transmission

- Cutaneous—broken skin in contact with infected animals or spores
- Inhalational—aerosol (from possible biological warfare)

Incubation

- Cutaneous: 1–6 days
- Inhalation: 1–60 days

Clinical

- **Cutaneous anthrax**—a boil-like skin lesion develops into eschar (a large, painless necrotic ulcer with a black centre)—rarely fatal if treated
- **Inhalational anthrax**—initial flu-like symptoms for several days, followed by severe (and often fatal) respiratory collapse—mortality is nearly 100%
- **Gastroenteric anthrax**—vomiting of blood, severe diarrhoea

Laboratory

- Gram stain—smears of skin vesicular fluid, eschar, blood or CSF
- PCR for *Bacillus anthracis*
- *Bacillus anthracis* serology

Treatment

For cutaneous anthrax

- Option 1: ciprofloxacin (PO)
- Option 2: doxycycline (PO)

After improvement and if bacteria are susceptible, change to:

- Amoxicillin (PO) for total of 60 days

For inhalational anthrax

- Ciprofloxacin (IV) **plus** clindamycin (IV) **plus** 1 or 2 additional antibiotics (if bacteria are susceptible): ampicillin (IV), benzylpenicillin (IV), meropenem (IV), rifampicin (PO) or vancomycin (IV)

After improvement, switch to oral:

- Ciprofloxacin (**or** doxycycline) (PO)

Children may switch to amoxicillin (PO) (if bacteria are susceptible)

Duration of treatment

- For total of 60 days

Dosage of above antibiotics

- Ciprofloxacin 500 mg (child: 15 mg/kg up to 500 mg) PO q12h
- Doxycycline 100 mg (child >8 years: 2.5 mg/kg up to 100 mg) PO q12h
- Amoxicillin 500 mg (child: 25 mg/kg up to 500 mg) PO q8h
- Ciprofloxacin 400 mg (child: 10 mg/kg up to 400 mg) IV q12h
- Clindamycin 600 mg (child: 15 mg/kg up to 600 mg) IV q8h

Post-exposure prophylaxis

- Option 1: ciprofloxacin 500 mg (child: 15 mg/kg up to 500 mg) PO q12h for 60 days
- Option 2: doxycycline 100 mg (child >8 years: 2 mg/kg up to 100 mg) PO q12h for 60 days

For children, if bacteria are susceptible

- Amoxicillin 25 mg/kg up to 500 mg PO q8h for 60 days

APHTHOUS ULCERS

Aphthous ulcers are very common and affect at least 1 in 10 people.

Causes and risk factors

- The causes are not precisely known
- Most often in adolescents and young adults
- More often in women before menstruation and with premenstrual tension
- Trauma to mouth mucosa from tooth brushing, self-biting, rough dentures, dental work or hot food
- Iron, folate or vitamin B_{12} deficiency, or coeliac disease

- Emotional or physical stress
- Can be associated with coeliac disease or ulcerative colitis
- Behcet's syndrome (aphthous ulcers with genital ulcers and eye disease)
- PFAPA syndrome (child with periodic fever, aphthous stomatitis, pharyngitis and cervical adenitis)

Clinical

- The ulcers are small, shallow, yellow or grey in colour, surrounded by a bright-red halo
- Generally occur on cheek, inside of lip and floor of mouth rather than mucosa of gingivae and hard palate
- There are three forms:
    1. **Minor aphthous ulcers**—ulcers 2–4 mm in diameter, heal in 7–10 days
    2. **Major aphthous ulcers**—ulcers ≥10 mm in diameter, last up to 6 weeks, heal with scarring
    3. **Herpetiform aphthous ulcers**—ulcers 1–2 mm in diameter, recurrent, heal within 1–2 weeks
- The ulcers may be very painful for the first 3 days and interfere with eating
- Recurrent attacks of ulcers are quite common in some people

Laboratory

- Full blood count, iron studies, and serum vitamin B_{12} and folate

Treatment

- Treat underlying causes
- In most cases the ulcer will heal without any treatment
- Any ulcer that lasts beyond 6 weeks should have a biopsy
- Analgesia
- Apply a wet, squeezed-out black teabag directly to the ulcer 3–4 times daily

For mild ulcers

- Lidocaine (lignocaine) gel or paint 2% (e.g. SM-33) top q3h
- Chlorhexidine 0.2% mouthwash (e.g. Difflam-C, Savacol) 10 mL rinse mouth tds
- Triamcinolone acetonide 0.1% paste (e.g. Kenalog) top tds
- Betamethasone valerate 0.05% oint (e.g. Cortival) top tds

For more severe ulcers

- Betamethasone dipropionate 0.05% oint (e.g. Diprosne) top tds

For major aphthous ulceration (only)

- Prednisolone 25 mg PO daily for 5 days

For severe ulceration in immunocompromised patient

- Seek expert advice

ASPERGILLOSIS

Pathogens

- *Aspergillus fumigatus*
- *Aspergillus niger*
- *Aspergillus flavus*

It may cause

- Allergic bronchopulmonary aspergillosis (ABPA)
- Invasive pulmonary aspergillosis
- Aspergilloma (mycetoma)
- Otitis externa
- Corneal infection
- Brain abscess
- Disseminated infection

1. ALLERGIC BRONCHOPULMONARY ASPERGILLOSIS

- An allergic reaction to *A. fumigatus*
- It is not a fungal infection

Clinical

- Bronchial asthma (wheeze)
- Black-coloured sputum, brownish plugs in sputum
- Fleeting pulmonary infiltration and lobar/segmental collapse on chest x-ray
- Central bronchiectasis, with haemoptysis (late disease)

Diagnosis

- Eosinophilia
- Serum IgE—elevation
- Sputum culture—growth of *A. fumigatus*
- Aspergillus serology—elevated anti-*A. fumigatus* IgE/IgG
- Skin-prick test—immediate wheal-flare response to *A. fumigatus* extract

Treatment

- Prednisolone 25–50 mg PO daily until improvement, titrate to maintain
- May need bronchoscopic aspiration of mucus plugs to treat lobar collapse

2. INVASIVE PULMONARY ASPERGILLOSIS

Fungal pneumonia caused by infection of *A. fumigatus*

Clinical

- Occurs in immunocompromised patients (e.g. neutropenia)
- Rapidly progressive pneumonia with consolidation, necrosis and cavitation

Diagnosis

- Suspect the infection in immunocompromised patient with severe suppurative pneumonia and unresponsive to antibiotic therapy
- Sputum—microscopy and culture for fungus (*A. fumigatus*)
- Biopsy (transbronchial or open lung biopsy)—microscopy and fungal culture

Treatment

Seek expert advice

Mild disease (non-neutropenic)

- Option 1: voriconazole (PO)
- Option 2: itraconazole (PO)

Severe disease (often neutropenic)

- Option 1: voriconazole (IV then PO)
- Option 2: amphotericin B liposomal (IV)
- Option 3: caspofungin (IV) (for salvage treatment)

Dosage of above agents

Mild disease

- Voriconazole 200–300 mg (child >2 years: 4 mg/kg up to 200 mg) PO q12h
- Itraconazole 300 mg (child: 7.5 mg/kg up to 300 mg) PO q12h for 3 days, then 200 mg (child: 5 mg/kg up to 200 mg) PO q12h (monitor plasma concentration)

Severe disease

- Voriconazole 6 mg/kg IV q12h for 2 doses, then 4 mg/kg IV q12h, then 4 mg/kg PO q12h (child <50 kg: 9 mg/kg IV q12h for 2 doses, then 8 mg/kg IV q12h or 9 mg/kg up to 350 mg PO q12h)
- Amphotericin B *liposomal (AmBisome)* 3 mg/kg IV daily

3. ASPERGILLOMA (MYCETOMA)

A. fumigatus fungal ball is formed in pre-existing lung cavity (e.g. cavity caused by tuberculosis)

Clinical

- Usually asymptomatic—often incidentally detected on chest x-ray or CT
- Haemoptysis—small percentage of aspergillomas may invade into the wall of the cavity and cause bleeding (occasionally life-threatening)

Diagnosis

- Chest x-ray or chest CT—fungal ball
- Sputum—microscopy and culture for fungus (*A. fumigatus*)
- Biopsy (transbronchial)—with fungal culture

Treatment

- Most cases of aspergilloma do not require treatment
- Surgical excision if massive haemoptysis occurs

AVIAN INFLUENZA

Other names: bird flu, influenza H5N1

Pathogens

- A subtype of influenza A viruses, which have 16 H and 9 N subtypes
- Only some of H5 and H7 subtypes are highly pathogenic and cause severe disease in poultry
- H5 and H7 viruses are usually introduced to poultry flocks in their low pathogenic form; after circulating in poultry populations, the viruses can mutate into highly pathogenic forms
- H5N1 is one of the highly pathogenic avian influenza viruses (HPAIV)
- New highly pathogenic H7N9 infection was reported in 2013

Transmission

- Direct contact with infected poultry (birds, including chickens, ducks and geese), or surfaces and objects contaminated by their faeces (main route)
- Human-to-human transmission has been reported

Clinical

- Widespread persistence of avian influenza virus in birds poses following risks for human health:
  - direct infection when the virus passes from poultry to humans, resulting in very severe disease. The disease caused by H5N1 and H7N9 follows an unusually aggressive clinical course, with rapid deterioration and high fatality. Primary viral pneumonia and multi-organ failure are the common cause of death
  - the virus—if given enough opportunities—may change into a form that is highly infectious for humans and will spread easily from person-to-person. Such a change could mark the start of a global outbreak (a pandemic)

The most important warning signals that a pandemic is about to start

- Clusters of patients with symptoms of influenza, closely related in time and place—suggests that human-to-human transmission is taking place
- Detection of cases in healthcare workers caring for avian influenza patients—suggests that human-to-human transmission has occurred

Laboratory

- Nasal pharyngeal/throat viral swabs—for avian influenza virus PCR

Treatment

- Isolate patients—in negative-pressure room, wearing N95 mask
- Supportive treatment
- Antiviral therapy
  - Option 1: oseltamivir (Tamiflu) (PO) for 5 days (category B1)
  - Option 2: zanamivir (Relenza) (inh) for 5 days (category B1)

Dosage of above agents

- Oseltamivir (Tamiflu) 75 mg (child >1 year and <15 kg: 30 mg; 15–23 kg: 45 mg; 23–40 kg: 60 mg; >40 kg: 70 mg) PO q12h
- Zanamivir (Relenza) (adult and child >5 years) 10 mg inh using Diskhaler q12h

Vaccination

- *Panvax H5N1* vaccine is available for use when the Australian government declares an avian influenza pandemic

BABESIOSIS

Babesia infection, a tick-borne zoonosis, has been reported in Australia.

Pathogens

- *Babesia microti*—a tick-borne microscopic parasite

Transmission

- Babesiosis is well documented in local cattle, dogs and rodents
- Tick-borne—bite of an infected tick overseas or in Australia
- Transfusion of blood products—from an infected donor
- Congenital transmission—from an infected mother to her baby

Incubation

- 5 to 33 days

Clinical

- Range from asymptomatic to life-threatening
- Asymptomatic—many people infected with *Babesia* do not have symptoms
- Mild infection—flu-like symptoms (fever, chills, sweats, headache, body aches, loss of appetite, nausea or fatigue)
- Severe infection—marked haemolytic anaemia, thrombocytopenia, DIC, haemodynamic instability, acute respiratory distress, myocardial infarction, multi-organ failure, altered mental status and death

High risk

- Asplenia
- Advanced age
- Impaired immunity (e.g. HIV, malignancy and corticosteroid therapy)

Laboratory

- Blood film microscopy—3 sets of thick and thin blood films, taken 8–12 h apart—to find *Babesia* parasites inside red blood cells (may be difficult to distinguish from malaria); examination by a reference laboratory should be considered for confirmation of the diagnosis
- PCR for *Babesia microti*—can detect low levels of parasites
- *Babesia* serology—does not reliably distinguish active from prior infection

Treatment

- Severe case requires ICU admission and supportive treatment
  - Option 1: atovaquone (PO) **plus** azithromycin (PO or IV)
  - Option 2: quinine (PO) **plus** clindamycin (IV or PO)

Duration of treatment

- At least 7–10 days

Dosage of above agents

- Atovaquone 750 mg (child: reduced dose) PO bid **or** 1.5 g PO daily with fatty food
- Azithromycin 500 mg–1 g (child >6 months: 10–20 mg/kg up to 500 mg–1 g) PO or IV daily
- Quinine 600 mg (child: 10 mg/kg up to 600 mg) PO tds
- Clindamycin 450–600 mg (child: 5–10 mg/kg up to 600 mg) IV or PO q8h

Prevention

- Prevent tick bite

BALANITIS AND BALANOPOSTHITIS

Balanitis—inflamed glans penis
Balanoposthitis—inflamed glans penis and foreskin
- Need to exclude diabetes and Reiter's disease

1. BACTERIAL INFECTION

- More common in pre-pubertal boys
- Can cause swollen foreskin and glans penis and painful urination
- Rash may involve perianal skin

Pathogen

- *Streptococcus pyogenes*

Treatment

- Swab for culture
- Carefully wash behind the foreskin—often effective
- If paraphimosis complicates balanoposthitis, may need urgent surgical treatment
- Antibiotic treatment (if unresponsive to washing or *S. pyogenes* cultured)
  - Penicillin V (PO) for 5–10 days
For non-adherent patients
  - Benzathine penicillin (IM) as a single dose
If allergic to penicillin
  - Cefalexin (PO) for 5–10 days
If immediate penicillin allergy
  - Azithromycin (PO) for 5 days

Dosage of above antibiotics

- Penicillin V 500 mg (child: 15 mg/kg up to 500 mg) PO q12h
- Benzathine penicillin 900 mg (child 3–6 kg: 225 mg; 6–10 kg: 337.5 mg; 10–15 kg: 450 mg; 15–20 kg: 675 mg; >20 kg: 900 mg) IM as a single dose
- Cefalexin 1 g (child: 25 mg/kg up to 1 g) PO q12h
- Azithromycin 500 mg (child 12 mg/kg up to 500 mg) PO daily

2. *CANDIDA* INFECTION

- More common in uncircumcised male adults

Pathogen

- *Candida albicans*

Clinical

- Red, scaly maculopapular lesions on glans penis or the foreskin, with severe itching and/or burning sensation; may have white discharge

Treatment

- Swab for microscopy and culture
- Carefully wash under the foreskin—often effective
- Dry under the foreskin after washing
- Antifungal treatment
  - Option 1: clotrimazole 1% + hydrocortisone 1% cream (e.g. Hydrozole) top bid, until 2 weeks after lesions resolve
  - Option 2: miconazole 2% + hydrocortisone 1% cream (e.g. Resolve Plus 1.0) top bid, until 2 weeks after lesions resolve

If prefer oral therapy
  - Fluconazole 150 mg PO as a single dose
- For recurrent candida balanoposthitis—check female partner with a vaginal swab; if she has positive vaginal *Candida*, treat her as for *Candida vaginitis* (p. 37)
- For recurrent relapsing candida balanitis, consider circumcision
- If unresponsive to antibiotic or antifungal treatment, consider non-infectious balanitis; a skin biopsy may be required; referral to a dermatologist is recommended

BARMAH FOREST VIRUS

Barmah Forest virus (BFV), a common and widespread arbovirus, has been detected in most parts of mainland Australia.

Transmission

- Mosquitoes transmit the virus between animals and humans
- Infection does not occur directly from person-to-person contact

Incubation

- 7–10 days

Clinical

- Most BFV infections have mild or no symptoms
- Flu-like symptoms—some patients develop rash, fever, chills, headache and photophobia

- Joint and muscle symptoms—pain, tenderness, stiffness of joints and muscles, swollen joints with decrease in mobility; the rheumatic symptoms can manifest suddenly or may be felt initially in only a few joints and then develop gradually or explosively over the following weeks
- Tiredness is common and can persist or recur later

Laboratory

- BFV serology (positive BFV IgM or four-fold rise of BFV IgG) (all family members should be asked about symptoms and checked for BFV serology if necessary)
- PCR for BFV

Treatment

- Symptomatic treatment
- Non-steroidal anti-inflammatory drugs can give dramatic symptomatic relief

Progress

- The severity and extent of symptoms gradually diminish
- Some patients will recover fully in 3 months and most within a year
- Infection with BFV probably confers life-long immunity

Prevention

Mosquito reduction and avoidance:

- Wear loose-fitting light-coloured clothing, especially at dusk and dawn
- Add insect screens around the home or use a mosquito net
- Use insecticides and insect repellent

BARTHOLINITIS AND BARTHOLIN ABSCESS

Causes

Obstruction of Bartholin duct → painless **Bartholin cyst** → becomes infected → **bartholinitis** → progresses into **Bartholin abscess**

Pathogens

- Anaerobes
- Aerobes (e.g. *E. coli*, *Staphylococci*)
- *Neisseria gonorrhoeae* (10–15% of cases)
- *Chlamydia trachomatis* (much less frequent than gonorrhoea)
- Rare pathogens (e.g. *S. pneumonia*, *Haemophilus* spp)

Clinical

- Swollen, hot and red labium (usually one side only) with extreme pain; patient may be unable to sit down

Laboratory

- Pus from abscess—Gram stain and culture (including *N. gonorrhoeae*)
- Urine or cervical (or high vaginal) swab—for gonorrhoea and *Chlamydia* PCR

Treatment

Bartholinitis

- Sitz baths 2–3 times a day to promote healing and provide comfort
- Amoxicillin/clavulanate 875 mg PO q12h

If allergic to penicillin

- Clindamycin 300–450 mg PO q6–8h

Modify antibiotics based on culture and susceptibility

Bartholin abscess

- Refer for abscess incision and drainage (pus for culture)

If problem recurs

- Refer to a gynaecologist for permanent drainage by marsupialisation of the cyst
- If gonococcal or *Chlamydia* infection is confirmed—antibiotic treatment for gonorrhoea and *Chlamydia*, see Urethritis (p. 419)
- Postmenopausal women—need to evaluate for malignancy after acute problem has resolved

BITES

All human and animal bite wounds are contaminated, with high risk of infection

Pathogens and risk factors

- **Human bites**—*Staphylococcus aureus*, *Eikenella corrodens*, *Streptococcus* spp and anaerobic bacteria
- **Animal bites**—*Pasteurella multocida*, *Staphylococcus aureus*, *Capnocytophaga canimorsus*, *Streptococcus* spp and anaerobes; cat bites are worse than dog bites and cat claw injuries are equivalent to cat bites
- **Bat bites**—rabies or lyssavirus, see Rabies and Australian bat lyssavirus (p. 345)

Management

1. Wound management

- Thoroughly cleanse, irrigate and debride
- Avoid suturing unless cosmetically essential (e.g. on face)

2. Tetanus prophylaxis (see Table 2.1)

Adults who have not received primary course of tetanus vaccination need

- dTpa (e.g. Adacel, Boostrix) **or** dT (e.g. ADT) 0.5 mL IM, followed by 2 doses of dT 0.5 mL IM, at least 4 weeks apart

TABLE 2.1

TETANUS PROPHYLAXIS

Tetanus prophylaxis	Last tetanus vaccine (≥3 doses)		Had <3 doses of tetanus vaccine*
	>5 years but ≤10 years	*>10 years*	
Tetanus booster[1]	Dirty wounds	All wounds	All wounds
Tetanus Ig[2]	No need	No need	Dirty wounds

*Includes those with uncertain tetanus vaccination history

[1]**Tetanus booster:** dTpa is preferred to dT as it also boosts pertussis
- dTpa (e.g. Adacel, Boostrix) or dT (e.g. ADT) 0.5 mL IM st

[2]**Tetanus immunoglobulin (TIG):**
- Tetanus immunoglobulin-VF (TIG) 250 IU (500 IU if injury >24 hours) IM as soon as practicable after injury

Tetanus booster and TIG should be given in opposite limbs

3. Antibiotic prophylaxis

Antibiotic prophylaxis is not indicated for uninfected low-risk wounds:

- Wounds not involving bones, joints or tendons
- Wounds presented within 8 hours post-injury

Antibiotic prophylaxis is indicated for the following high-risk wounds:

- Wounds presented ≥8 hours post-injury
- Wounds on face, hands or feet
- Puncture wounds
- Wounds involving bones, joints or tendons
- Wounds in immunocompromised patients

4. Antibiotic treatment

Prophylactic antibiotics or treatment for mild to moderate infections
- Amoxicillin/clavulanate (PO) for 5 days

If penicillin allergy
- Option 1: ciprofloxacin (PO) **plus** clindamycin (PO) for 5 days
- Option 2: doxycycline (PO) **plus** metronidazole (PO) for 5 days
- Option 3: cotrimoxazole (PO) **plus** metronidazole (PO) for 5 days

More severe infections (with systemic symptoms)
- Option 1: piperacillin/tazobactam (**or** ticarcillin/clavulanate) (IV)
- Option 2: ceftriaxone (**or** cefotaxime) (IV) **plus** metronidazole (PO)

If immediate penicillin allergy
- Seek expert advice

Once improved, change to oral therapy according to susceptibility **or**, if the pathogen is uncertain, use above oral regimens

Duration of treatment

- Total of 14 days (IV + PO), longer if injuries involve bones, joints or tendons

Dosage of above antibiotics

- Amoxicillin/clavulanate 875 mg (child: 22.5 mg/kg up to 875 mg) PO q12h

- Ciprofloxacin 500 mg (child: 12.5 mg/kg up to 500 mg) PO q12h
- Clindamycin 450 mg (child: 10 mg/kg up to 450 mg) PO q8h
- Doxycycline 200 mg (child >8 years: 4 mg/kg up to 200 mg) PO on day 1, then 100 mg (child >8 years: 2 mg/kg up to 100 mg) PO daily
- Metronidazole 400 mg (child: 10 mg/kg up to 400 mg) PO q12h
- Cotrimoxazole 160/800 mg (child: 4/20 mg/kg up to 160/800 mg) PO q12h
- Piperacillin/tazobactam 4 g (child: 100 mg/kg up to 4 g) IV q8h
- Ticarcillin/clavulanate 3 g (child: 50 mg/kg up to 3 g) IV q6h
- Ceftriaxone 1 g (child >1 month: 50 mg/kg up to 1 g) IV daily
- Cefotaxime 1 g (child: 50 mg/kg up to 1 g) IV q8h
- Metronidazole 400 mg (child: 10 mg/kg up to 400 mg) PO q12h

BLASTOCYSTIS HOMINIS

Other names: Blastocystosis
Blastocystis hominis is one of the most common parasites found in the human digestive tract. It was previously classified as a non-pathogenic organism. It is a potential pathogen causing diarrhoea in day-care centres, travellers and people who are debilitated or immunocompromised.

Pathogen

- *Blastocystis hominis*—an intestinal protozoon

Transmission

- Faecal–oral route
- Animals may be a risk factor for human infection

Clinical

- Many of those infected are asymptomatic carriers
- Symptoms—diarrhoea, abdominal pain, anorexia, bloating, flatulence, loss of appetite, loss of weight and chronic fatigue; often misdiagnosed with irritable bowel syndrome

Laboratory

- **Faecal microscopy**—presence of *B. hominis* (vacuolar form)
    - If *B. hominis* is found along with other pathogens, other pathogens are more likely to be the cause of the infection
    - If *B. hominis* is found in faecal samples and no other causes are identified, *B. hominis* infection is most likely the cause of diarrhoea
    - In outbreak situations, laboratories should routinely search for and report this parasite in faecal samples
- **Faecal multiplex PCR testing**—sensitivity 98–100%, result available in 24 hours

Treatment

- Asymptomatic carrier—no treatment is required
- If *B. hominis* is found with other known causes, treat other causes
- If no other causes found and diarrhoea is persistent, antibiotic therapy
  - Option 1: metronidazole (PO) for 7 days (**or** nitazoxanide* (PO) for 3 days)
  - Option 2: cotrimoxazole (PO) for 7 days (14 days for the immunocompromised)

If no response, use either of following combination therapy

- Secnidazole* + diloxanide* + cotrimoxazole (PO) for 10 days
- Secnidazole* + diloxanide* + norfloxacin (PO) for 10 days (if sulfur allergy)
- Nilazoxanide* + secnidazole* + furazolidone* + doxycyclin (PO) for 10 days

Note

- Take medicine with food and avoid drinking alcohol
- Repeat stool test 4–6 weeks after treatment to determine the eradication

Dosage of above antibiotics

- Metronidazole 400 mg (child: 10 mg/kg up to 400 mg) PO tds
- Nitazoxanide 500 mg (child 1–3 years: 100 mg; 4–11 years: 200 mg) PO bid
- Cotrimoxazole 160/800 mg (child: 4/20 mg/kg up to 160/800 mg) PO bid
- Secnidazole 400 mg PO tds
- Diloxanide furoate 500 mg PO tds
- Norfloxacin 400 mg op bid
- Furazolidone 100 mg PO tds
- Doxycyclin 50 mg PO bid

BLEPHARITIS

Blepharitis is an inflammation of the eyelid margins. It is often associated with seborrhoeic dermatitis, rosacea or eczema.

1. SEBORRHOEIC BLEPHARITIS (ANTERIOR BLEPHARITIS)

Daily routine of lid margin hygiene to avoid relapse:

- Lid margin cleaning—warm wet compression (such as a face washer with hot water) to the lids for 2 minutes, gently and repeatedly scrub along the lid margins (with eyes closed) with non-irritating baby shampoo to remove crusted debris and scales

---

*Available via Special Access Scheme <www.tga.gov.au/access-sas.htm> or from a compounding chemist

- Topical anti-inflammatory medication
  - Sulfacetamide 10% eye drops: 2 drops, massage into lid margins bid

2. STAPHYLOCOCCAL BLEPHARITIS (ANTERIOR BLEPHARITIS)

- Can sometimes lead to a chalazion or stye
- Lid margin cleaning—gently scrub along the lid margins (with eyes closed) with non-irritating baby shampoo to remove crusted debris and scales
- Antibiotic eye ointment (with eyes closed)
  - Chloramphenicol 1% eye ointment to lid margins bid until resolved

3. CHRONIC BLEPHARITIS (POSTERIOR BLEPHARITIS)

- Associated with rosacea (ocular rosacea)—common
- Associated with keratoconjunctivitis and meibomianitis—less common
- Artificial tears may provide symptomatic relief
- Short-term mild topical corticosteroids may be helpful
- Oral doxycycline or erythromycin has an anti-inflammatory effect
- For severe cases and child ocular rosacea—ophthalmologist referral
  - Doxycycline PO for 1–2 months or longer

For pregnant or breastfeeding women
  - Erythromycin PO for 1–2 months or longer

Dosage of above antibiotics

  - Doxycycline 50 (child >8 years: 1 mg/kg up to 50 mg) PO daily (if no improvement after 1 month—may increase the dose to 100 mg [child >8 years: 2 mg/kg up to 100 mg])
  - Erythromycin 250 mg (or erythromycin ethylsuccinate 400 mg) PO daily

BOILS, FURUNCLES AND CARBUNCLES

Boils/furuncles—abscesses involving a hair follicle and associated glands
Carbuncles—boils with multiple heads, most often on back of neck

Pathogens

- *Staphylococcus aureus* (may be MRSA)
- *Streptococcus pyogenes* (occasionally in combination with *S. aureus*)

Treatment

- Swab for culture (to detect MRSA)
- Small lesions—incisional drainage alone
- Large lesions with cellulitis or with systemic symptoms—incision and drainage (send pus for culture) + antibiotic therapy

1. Empirical therapy

  - Option 1: cefalexin (PO) (preferred in children)
  - Option 2: flucloxacillin (PO)

If immediate penicillin allergy
- Option 1: clindamycin (PO)
- Option 2: cotrimoxazole (PO)

Duration of treatment

- Usually 5 days or until the swab/pus culture is available, adjust accordingly
- Longer therapy for more severe infection

Dosage of above antibiotics

- Cefalexin 500 mg (child: 12.5 mg/kg up to 500 mg) PO q6h **or** 1 g (child: 25 mg/kg up to 1 g) PO q12h
- Flucloxacillin 500 mg (child: 12.5 mg/kg up to 500 mg) PO q6h
- Clindamycin 450 mg (child: 10 mg/kg up to 450 mg) PO q8h
- Cotrimoxazole 160/800 mg (child: 4/20 mg/kg up to 160/800 mg) PO q12h

2. MRSA treatment (guided by susceptibility results)

Non–multi-resistant MRSA (CA-MRSA)
- Option 1: clindamycin (IV then PO **or** PO) for 7 days
- Option 2: cotrimoxazole (PO) for 7 days
- Option 3: doxycycline (PO) for 7 days

Multi-resistant MRSA—seek expert advice
- Option 1: vancomycin (IV)
- Option 2: rifampicin (PO) **plus** fusidate sodium (**or** fusidic acid) (PO)
- Option 3: linezolid (PO)
- Option 4: pristinamycin (PO)

Dosage of above antibiotics

- Clindamycin 450 mg (child: 10 mg/kg up to 450 mg) IV q8h, then same dose PO q8h
- Cotrimoxazole 160/800 mg (child: 4/20 mg/kg up to 160/800 mg) PO q12h
- Doxycycline 200 mg (child >8 years: 4 mg/kg up to 200 mg) PO on day 1, then 100 mg (child >8 years: 2 mg/kg up to 100 mg) PO daily
- Vancomycin 25–30 mg/kg IV for the 1st dose (further dosing see p. 462)
- Rifampicin 300 mg (child: 5–10 mg/kg up to 300 mg) PO q12h
- Fusidate sodium 500 mg (child: 12 mg/kg up to 500 mg) PO q12h
- Fusidic acid suspension 500 mg (child: 18 mg/kg up to 750 mg) PO q12h
- Linezolid 400–600 mg (child: 10 mg/kg up to 600 mg) PO q12h
- Pristinamycin (Pyostacine) 2 g PO q12h (Available via Special Access Scheme <www.tga.gov.au/hp/access-sas>)

3. Recurrent boils, furuncles and carbuncles

- Take nasal and/or perineal swabs for culture
- If swabs are positive for *Staphylococcus aureus*:
  - **total body eradication** for patient, family members and close contacts

See Recurrent staphylococcal skin infection (p. 383)

BOTULISM

Pathogens

- *Clostridium botulinum*—an anaerobic bacterium producing spores that can survive heating to 100°C

Transmission and incubation

- **Food-borne botulism**—ingestion of toxin-containing food contaminated with *C. botulinum*; incubation 6 hours to 10 days after ingestion of toxin
- **Wound botulism**—caused by contaminated soil or gravel invading a wound; *C. botulinum* produces toxin in the wound; incubation 4 days to 2 weeks
- **Infant botulism**—consuming food (e.g. honey), dust or soil that contains *C. botulinum* spores; incubation period varies from 3 to 30 days

Clinical

- **Food-borne botulism**—cranial nerve signs: diplopia, blurred vision, dilated pupils, dysarthria, dysphagia and progressive symmetrical descending paralysis (sensation is intact), leading to respiratory muscle paralysis and death
- **Wound botulism**—similar to food-borne botulism, but GI symptoms are absent; wounds generally appear benign, without typical signs of infection
- **Infant botulism**—constipation, floppy baby, hypotonia, weak cry, poor feeding, progressive weakness, impaired respiration and death

Diagnosis

Suspect botulism if cranial nerve weakness with normal sensation

- **Food-borne botulism**—detection of botulinum toxin from blood, faeces, suspect food or ingested material
- **Wound botulism**—wound swab for anaerobic culture; isolation of *C. botulinum* is suggestive of the infection
- **Infant botulism**—faeces culture for *C. botulinum*; provides presumptive evidence of infection

Treatment

Do not use antibiotics: antibiotics (especially aminoglycosides or clindamycin) may paradoxically cause dramatic acceleration of paralysis as the affected bacteria release toxin

- Early induction of vomiting, stomach pumping and enema after ingestion
- Thorough wound debridement, even if appearing to heal well, followed by injection of 3% hydrogen peroxide or antitoxin directly into the wound site
- Hyperbaric oxygen therapy if available
- Supportive, with mechanical ventilation when needed
- Botulism antitoxin should be given as soon as clinical diagnosis is established
  - Botulism antitoxin (botulinum immune globulin, BIG)*—a skin test followed by IV or IM dose (high anaphylaxis risk)

BRAIN ABSCESS

1. BRAIN ABSCESS AND SUBDURAL EMPYEMA

Pathogens

- Most brain abscesses—mixed aerobic (e.g. *Streptococcus anginosus/milleri* group) and anaerobic bacteria infection
- Ear-origin brain abscess—enteric Gram-negative bacilli are common
- Post trauma or surgery—*Staphylococcus aureus* is the predominant cause
- In immunosuppressed patients—*Nocardia* spp, *Toxoplasma* and fungi (e.g. *Aspergillus* or *Scedosporium*) are more likely to be the cause

Laboratory

- Aspiration or biopsy—Gram stain, microscopy and culture
- Culture-negative brain abscess—16s rRNA gene sequencing (pus or biopsy)

Treatment

- Subdural empyema requires urgent surgical drainage
Empirical therapy (according to Gram stain)
  - Ceftriaxone (**or** cefotaxime) (IV) **plus** metronidazole (IV)

Modify therapy according to Gram stain, culture and susceptibility results

Duration of treatment

- 2–6 weeks

Dosage of above antibiotics

- Ceftriaxone 4 g (child >1 month: 100 mg/kg up to 4 g) IV daily **or** 2 g (child >1 month: 50 mg/kg up to 2 g) IV q12h
- Cefotaxime 2 g (child: 50 mg/kg up to 2 g) IV q6h
- Metronidazole 500 mg (child: 12.5 mg/kg up to 500 mg) IV q8h

---

*BIG is available via Special Access Scheme <www.tga.gov.au/hp/access-sas.htm>

2. BRAIN ABSCESS POST-NEUROSURGERY OR TRAUMA

Pathogens

• Staphylococci (predominant)

Treatment

Empirical therapy
  • Ceftazidime (**or** meropenem) (IV) **plus** vancomycin (IV)

Modify therapy according to Gram stain, culture and susceptibility results

Duration of treatment

• 2–6 weeks

Dosage of above antibiotics

  • Ceftazidime 2 g (child: 50 mg/kg up to 2 g) IV q8h
  • Meropenem 2 g (child: 40 mg/kg up to 2 g) IV q8h
  • Vancomycin 25–30 mg/kg IV for the 1st dose (further dosing see
    p. 462)

3. BRAIN ABSCESS IN THE IMMUNOCOMPROMISED

Pathogens

• *Toxoplasma gondii* (p. 400)
• *Nocardia* spp (see Nocardiosis, p. 251)
• *Aspergillus* (see Aspergillosis, p. 11)
• *Scedosporium* spp

Treatment

• According to the pathogens (see individual infection)

BRONCHIECTASIS

Pathogens

• *Haemophilus influenzae* (the most common)
• *Streptococcus pneumoniae*
• *Moraxella catarrhalis*
• *Pseudomonas aeruginosa*
• *Staphylococcus aureus*
• *Mycobacterium avium* complex (rare)

Clinical

• Chronic cough with purulent sputum
• Haemoptysis, from intermittent blood stain to life-threatening
  haemoptysis
• Crackles, wheezing and SOB during exacerbations
• Clubbing of the fingers (<5%)

Diagnosis

- Suspected—if persistent symptoms not responding to standard treatment
- Suspected—if sputum culture showed *P. aeruginosa*
- Chest CT (high-resolution)—confirm the diagnosis
- Diagnostic testing for some of the specific conditions associated with bronchiectasis (e.g. immune deficiencies, ciliary dyskinesia, cystic fibrosis, fibrotic lung diseases, etc)—refer to expert

Treatment

- Postural drainage and chest percussion
- Nebulised mucolytics, inhaled corticosteroids (may reduce sputum production)
- Influenza vaccination (annually) and pneumococcus vaccination (every 5 years)
- Sometimes surgical resection for localised bronchiectasis or severe haemoptysis
- Antibiotics for infection

1. Infrequent exacerbations

- Increase in volume and purulence of sputum
- Antibiotics are indicated only during acute episodes
- If sputum culture shows mixed flora, antibiotic choice will be empirical
- If sputum culture shows a specific pathogen, use it to guide the therapy

Empirical antibiotic therapy (to cover H. influenzae *and* S. pneumoniae*)*

  - Option 1: amoxicillin (PO) for 2 weeks
  - Option 2: amoxicillin/clavulanate (PO) for 2 weeks
  - Option 3: doxycycline (PO) for 2 weeks
  - Option 4: clarithromycin (PO) for 2 weeks
  - Option 5: azithromycin (PO) for 6 days
  - Option 6: cefuroxime (PO) for 2 weeks
  - Option 7: cefaclor (PO) for 2 weeks
  - Option 8: cotrimoxazole (PO) for 2 weeks

Dosage of above antibiotics

  - Amoxicillin 500 mg (child: 15 mg/kg up to 500 mg) PO q8h
  - Amoxicillin/clavulanate 875 mg (child: 22.5 mg/kg up to 875 mg) PO q12h
  - Doxycycline 200 mg (child >8 years: 4 mg/kg up to 200 mg) PO on day 1, then 100 mg (child >8 years: 2 mg/kg up to 100 mg) PO daily
  - Clarithromycin 500 mg (child >1 month: 7.5 mg/kg up to 500 mg) PO q12h
  - Azithromycin 500 mg (child >6 months: 10 mg/kg up to 500 mg) PO daily
  - Cefuroxime 500 mg (child 3 months–2 years: 10 mg/kg up to 125 mg; >2 years: 15 mg/kg up to 500 mg) PO q12h

- Cefaclor 500 mg (child: 10 mg/kg up to 500 mg) PO q8h
- Cotrimoxazole 160/800 mg (child: 4/20 mg/kg up to 160/800 mg) PO q12h

2. Frequent acute exacerbations or constant copious purulent sputum

- Sputum culture to exclude *P. aeruginosa* infection
- Rotating use of above antibiotics (to reduce the risk of bacterial resistance)
- Long-term low-dose macrolides may be tried

3. *P. aeruginosa* infection

- *P. aeruginosa* infection causes greater rate of deterioration of lung function and quality of life
- Only treat infective exacerbations (do not treat otherwise well patients with *Pseudomonas* colonisation)
- Antibiotic choice based on sensitivity (choose from following antibiotics)
  - Option 1: ciprofloxacin (IV or PO) **plus** gentamicin (IV)
  - Option 2: piperacillin (IV) **plus** gentamicin (IV)
  - Option 3: ticarcillin/clavulanate (IV) **plus** gentamicin (IV)
  - Option 4: cefepime (IV) **plus** gentamicin (IV)
  - Option 5: ceftazidime (IV) **plus** gentamicin (IV)
  - Option 6: imipenem/cilastatin (IV) **plus** gentamicin (IV)

Duration of therapy

- 10–14 days or longer

Inhalation of nebulised antibiotics may be used

  - Option 1: tobramycin 300 mg + normal saline to 4 mL neb bid
  - Option 2: gentamicin 80 mg + normal saline to 4 mL neb bid
  - Option 3: ceftazidime 1 g + normal saline to 4 mL neb bid
  - Option 4: colistin 150 mg + normal saline to 4 mL neb bid

Dosage of above antibiotics

  - Ciprofloxacin 400 mg (child: 10 mg/kg up to 400 mg) IV q12h
  - Ciprofloxacin 750 mg (child: 15 mg/kg up to 750 mg) PO q12h
  - Gentamicin 4–7 mg/kg (child: 7.5 mg/kg up to 320 mg) IV for the 1st dose (further dosing see p. 459)
  - Piperacillin 4 g (child: 75 mg/kg up to 4 g) IV q4–6h
  - Piperacillin/tazobactam 4 g (child: 100 mg/kg up to 4 g) IV q6–8h
  - Ticarcillin/clavulanate 3 g (child: 50 mg/kg up to 3 g) IV q4–6h
  - Cefepime 1–2 g (child: 50 mg/kg up to 2 g) IV q8–12h
  - Ceftazidime 2 g (child: 50 mg/kg up to 2 g) IV q8h
  - Imipenem/cilastatin 1 g (child: 25 mg/kg up to 1 g) IV q6h

BRONCHIOLITIS

Bronchiolitis is a common upper and lower respiratory tract infection in infants and young children up to the age of 2 years.

Pathogens

- Respiratory syncytial virus (RSV) (accounts for 90% of cases)
- Parainfluenza
- Influenza
- Human metapneumovirus (hMPV)
- Adenoviruses

High-risk age groups

- Infants <6 months, preterm babies and babies with heart or chronic lung diseases

Clinical

- Asthma-like presentation with cough, tachypnoea, intercostal and subcostal recession, generalised wheeze and crepitations; cyanosis and apnoea may occur
- Usually afebrile or low fever; if high fever, complications (e.g. RSV pneumonia) or other infections should be considered
- Illness lasts for approximately 10 days and the mortality is around 1–2%

Laboratory

- Nasopharyngeal aspirate (NPA) or swab—for RSV antigen and bacterial culture

Treatment

- Symptomatic treatment, minimal handling and frequent observation
- Hospital admission if severe, oxygen and tube feeding may be required.
  Indication for hospital admission:
    - SpO_2 <94%
    - Difficulty feeding
    - Moderate to severe SOB
    - Increased respiratory rate (RR)—RR >60/min if age <3 months; RR >50/min if age >3 months
- Nebulising 3% hypertonic saline may reduce the length of hospital stay
- Steroids and bronchodilator are ineffective
- **Ribavirin** nebulising for RSV infection: seek expert advice
    - Restricted to infants and children <2 years with serious underlying problems (e.g. congenital heart disease, cystic fibrosis or bronchopulmonary dysplasia)
    - Start treatment within first 3 days of infection
  - Ribavirin solution (20 mg/mL) inh for 12–18h/d for 3–7 days
    - Reconstitute and dilute powder 6 g with water to 300 mL to get final 20 mg/mL
    - Use SPAG-2 inhalation unit to minimise environmental exposure to aerosolised ribavirin

- **Antibiotic therapy** is only indicated for very ill hospitalised infants, especially if there is associated consolidation on chest x-ray (possible secondary bacterial infection)
  - Option 1: ceftriaxone 25 mg/kg IV daily for 3–5 days
  - Option 2: cefotaxime 25 mg/kg IV q8h for 3–5 days

Prevention

RSV immunoglobulin (RSVIG)

- Prevent RSV infection in high-risk babies (e.g. congenital heart disease, cystic fibrosis or bronchopulmonary dysplasia)
  - Palivizumab (Synagis) 15 mg/kg IM monthly, start before RSV season (autumn and winter) for up to 6 months

BRONCHITIS

1. ACUTE BRONCHITIS

Pathogens

- Viral infection—about 90% of all cases
- Bacterial infection (*Mycoplasma pneumoniae*, *Chlamydia pneumoniae*, *Streptococcus pneumoniae* or *Bordetella pertussis*)—only 10% of cases

Clinical

- Purulent sputum can result from either a viral or a bacterial infection
- Prolonged dry cough, especially with wheeze or with family history of asthma (so called 'post-viral cough') does not require antibiotic; it may respond to inhaled bronchodilators and/or inhaled steroids

Treatment

Antibiotic therapy is not usually indicated in the first 2 weeks of disease

Antibiotic may be considered in following conditions:

- Purulent productive cough lasts for more than 10–14 days with toxic symptoms, elevated WBC and neutrophils, particularly if patient is a smoker
- Prolonged dry cough with no nasal symptoms—mycoplasma or *Chlamydia* infection is suspected
- Persistent paroxysmal cough (>2 weeks) with or without whoop (a deep gasp after coughing bouts) or vomiting (post-tussive vomiting)— pertussis is suspected (see Pertussis, p. 282)

Antibiotic choice
  - Option 1: azithromycin (PO) for 3–5 days (also covers pertussis)
  - Option 2: clarithromycin (PO) for 5–7 days (also covers pertussis)
  - Option 3: doxycycline (PO) for 5 days

Dosage of above antibiotics

- Azithromycin 500 mg (child ≥6 months: 10 mg/kg up to 500 mg) PO daily
- Clarithromycin 500 mg (child >1 month: 7.5 mg/kg up to 500 mg) PO q12h
- Doxycycline 100 mg (child >8 years: 2 mg/kg up to 100 mg) PO q12h

2.   CHRONIC BRONCHITIS

For exacerbation of chronic bronchitis, see COPD—exacerbation (p. 66)

BRUCELLOSIS

Other names: undulant fever, Malta fever

Pathogens

- *Brucella* spp—a Gram-negative intracellular coccobacillus (a zoonosis)
- Four *Brucella* spp can cause human infection: *B. melitensis*, *B. abortus*, *B. suis* and *B. canis*
- The disease exists worldwide

Transmission

- Mainly via mouth—ingestion of raw milk from infected cattle or goats
- Less frequently via respiratory tract, genital tract, cuts or abrasions on skin
- Animal exposure—common in abattoir workers, butchers and farmers (animals that can be infected: goats, sheep, cattle, camels, pigs, dogs and other wild animals)
- Vets may be accidentally inoculated from administering animal *Brucella* vaccine
- Person-to-person transmission—very rare

Incubation

- 1–3 weeks

Clinical

- Undulant or intermittent fever, malaise, headache, weakness, myalgia night sweats, lymphadenopathy and hepatosplenomegaly

Complications

- Osteomyelitis, orchitis, epididymitis, pneumonia and endocarditis

Chronic disease

- Bouts of fever, fatigue, myalgia, depression and splenomegaly

Laboratory

- *Brucella* serology (agglutination test)—a single titre >1 : 160 or four-fold rise over 4 weeks
- *Brucella* PCR testing—very sensitive, specific and rapid diagnostic
- *Brucella* cultures—blood, bone marrow or CSF (take up to 2 weeks to grow)

Treatment

Adults and children ≥8 years
- Doxycycline (PO) for 6 weeks **plus** gentamicin (IV) for 7 days

If gentamicin is contraindicated
- Doxycycline (PO) **plus** rifampicin (PO) for 6 weeks

Children 1 month to 8 years or pregnant women use either
- Cotrimoxazole (PO) **plus** rifampicin (PO) for 6 weeks
- Cotrimoxazole (PO) for 6 weeks **plus** gentamicin (IM or IV) for 1 week

  If relapse after above therapy, *prolonged therapy is required*

Dosage of above antibiotics

Adults and children ≥8 years
- Doxycycline 100 mg (child >8 years: 2 mg/kg up to 100 mg) PO q12h
- Gentamicin 5 mg/kg (child: 7.5 mg/kg up to 320 mg) IV daily (monitor blood levels, p. 462)
- Rifampicin 600 mg (child: 15 mg/kg up to 600 mg) PO daily

Children 1 month to 8 years or pregnant women
- Cotrimoxazole 160/800 mg (child: 6/30 mg/kg up to 160/800 mg) PO q12h
- Gentamicin child: 7.5 mg/kg up to 320 mg; pregnant woman: 5 mg/kg IM or IV daily (monitor blood levels, p. 462)

C

CAMPYLOBACTER ENTERITIS

Other names: campylobacteriosis
Campylobacter is one of the most common causes of diarrhoeal illness in many developed countries and an important cause of traveller's diarrhoea.

Pathogens

Campylobacter spp—gram-negative, spiral- and comma-shaped bacteria, including:

- *Campylobacter jejuni* and *Campylobacter coli*—the most common
- *Campylobacter fetus*—an opportunistic pathogen

Transmission

- More frequently occurs in the summer months
- Faecal–oral—ingestion of contaminated food, raw meat or water
- Person-to-person sexual contact

Incubation

- 2–5 days

Clinical

- Diarrhoea (may be bloody), nausea and vomiting, abdominal cramping and fever
- The illness typically lasts one week
- Bacteraemia may occur
- It usually occurs sporadically, but can also occur in outbreaks

Laboratory

- Faeces microscopy and culture (asymptomatic contacts do not require faeces culture)
- Faecal multiplex PCR testing—sensitivity 98–100%, result available in 24 hours

Treatment

- Usually self-limiting
- Asymptomatic contacts do not require treatment
- Symptomatic treatment and rehydration
- Antibiotics are indicated for:
    - Severe or prolonged diarrhoea
    - Pregnant women in 3rd trimester
    - Immunocompromised people, infants or frail elderly people
    - Food handlers and childcare assistants

- Antibiotics can shorten the duration of symptoms if given early in the illness
  - Option 1: azithromycin (PO) for 3 days
  - Option 2: ciprofloxacin (PO) for 3 days
  - Option 3: norfloxacin (PO) for 5 days

For bacteraemia

- Gentamicin (IV) **or** ciprofloxacin (IV)

Dosage of above antibiotics

- Azithromycin 500 mg (child: 10 mg/kg up to 500 mg) PO daily
- Ciprofloxacin 500 mg (child: 12.5 mg/kg up to 500 mg) PO q12h
- Norfloxacin 400 mg (child: 10 mg/kg up to 400 mg) PO q12h
- Gentamicin 5–7 mg/kg (child <10 years: 7.5 mg/kg; ≥10 years: 6 mg/kg) IV daily
- Ciprofloxacin 400 mg (child: 10 mg/kg, up to 400 mg) IV q12h

CANDIDA OESOPHAGITIS

Other names: oesophageal candidiasis

Pathogen

- *Candida albicans*

Risk factors

- Usually occurs in the immunocompromised individual (e.g. HIV infection, cancer, post-chemotherapy, poorly controlled diabetes, inadequate nutrition, chronic illness and drug or alcohol abuser)

Clinical

- Difficulty in swallowing with pain and oral lesions
- Oral candidiasis is a predisposing factor but oesophageal involvement can occur without evidence of oral lesion

Laboratory

- Endoscopy should be ordered in patients with swallowing symptoms, particularly in the immunocompromised with oral candidiasis
- Oral lesion swab for fungal culture and susceptibility testing

Treatment

- Antifungal therapy

For susceptible strains

- Fluconazole (PO or IV) daily for 2–3 weeks

If no response to fluconazole

- Itraconazole (PO) daily for 2 weeks

For itraconazole-resistant *Candida* spp

- Option 1: posaconazole (PO) for 2 weeks
- Option 2: voriconazole (PO) for 2 weeks

For azole-resistant *Candida* spp

- Option 1: caspofungin (IV) for 2 weeks
- Option 2: amphotericin B (IV) for 2 weeks

For immunocompromised patients

- May need long-term suppressive therapy with one of the above agents

Dosage of above agents

- Fluconazole 200 mg (child: 6 mg/kg up to 200 mg) PO for day 1, then 100 mg (child: 3 mg/kg up to 100 mg) PO daily
- Itraconazole 200 mg (child: 5 mg/kg up to 200 mg) PO daily
- Posaconazole 300 mg PO q12h (for 1st day, then 300 mg daily)
- Voriconazole 200 mg (child 2–12 years: 6 mg/kg up to 400 mg) PO q12h for day 1, then 200 mg (child 2–12 years: 4 mg/kg up to 200 mg) PO q12h
- Caspofungin 50 mg IV daily
- Amphotericin B lipid complex (Abelcet) 5 mg/kg IV at 2.5 mg/kg/h daily
- Amphotericin B liposomal (AmBisome) 1–3 mg/kg IV daily

CANDIDA SEPSIS

Other names: candidaemia

Pathogens

- *Candida albicans*
- Non-albicans spp: *Candida glabrata*, *Candida krusei*

Risk factors

- Intravascular lines
- Urinary catheter
- Prolonged ventilation
- Broad-spectrum antibiotics
- Immunosuppression
- IV nutrition

Laboratory

- Blood fungal culture and susceptibility test
- The tip of the IV line for fungal culture

Treatment

- If candida sepsis is related to an intravascular line or urinary catheter—remove
- Antifungal therapy

Empirical treatment (to cover fluconazole-resistant spp)

- Option 1: anidulafungin (IV)
- Option 2: caspofungin (IV)
- Option 3: amphotericin B liposomal (IV)

For *C. albicans* and other susceptible strains

- Fluconazole (IV then PO) for total 2–3 weeks

For fluconazole-resistant *Candida* spp (e.g. *C. krusei*, *C. glabrata*)

- Option 1: voriconazole (IV then PO) for total 2–3 weeks
- Option 2: caspofungin (IV) for 2–3 weeks

For neutropenic patients with hepatosplenic candidiasis or eye infection

- Prolonged antifungal therapy—seek expert advice

Dosage of above agents

- Anidulafungin 200 mg IV for the 1st dose, then 100 mg IV daily
- Caspofungin 70 mg (child <3 months: 25 mg/m^2; ≥3 months: 70 mg/m^2 up to 70 mg) IV st for day 1, then 50 mg (child <3 months: 25 mg/m^2; ≥3 months: 50 mg/m^2 up to 50 mg) IV daily
- Amphotericin B liposomal (AmBisome) 1–3 mg/kg IV daily
- Fluconazole 800 mg (child: 12 mg/kg up to 800 mg) IV for the first dose, then 400 mg (child: 6 mg/kg up to 400 mg) IV daily, after improvement change to oral: 400 mg (child: 6 mg/kg up to 400 mg) PO daily

CANDIDA VAGINITIS

Other names: vaginal thrush, vulvovaginal candidiasis (VVC)

1. ACUTE *ALBICANS* VULVOVAGINAL CANDIDIASIS

Pathogen

- *Candida albicans*

Clinical

- Itching, soreness and/or burning discomfort in the vagina and vulva
- Heavy white curd-like vaginal discharge
- Bright-red rash affecting inner and outer parts of the vulva, sometimes spreading widely to the groin, pubic areas, inguinal areas and thighs

Treatment

Antifungal intravaginal preparations (choose one of the following)

- Clotrimazole 1% vaginal cream intravaginally for 6 nights
- Clotrimazole 100 mg pessary intravaginally for 6 nights

- Clotrimazole 2% vaginal cream intravaginally for 3 nights
- Clotrimazole 10% vaginal cream intravaginally st at night
- Clotrimazole 500 mg pessary intravaginally st at night, with or without use of clotrimazole 1% cream topically to vulvovaginal and perianal areas q8–12h
- Miconazole 2% vaginal cream intravaginally for 7 nights
- Nystatin* 100 000 units/5 g vaginal cream intravaginally q12h for 14 days
- Nystatin* 100 000 units pessary intravaginally q12h for 7 days

If prefer oral therapy or intolerant of topical therapy

- Fluconazole 150 mg PO st

Note

- Most infections in healthy people are uncomplicated, sporadic
- Treatment of asymptomatic vaginal candidiasis is unnecessary
- Treatment of sexual partners is not required
- The overuse of over-the-counter azole antifungal agents increases the incidence of infection of resistant *Candida* spp.

2. NON-*ALBICANS* (ATYPICAL) VULVOVAGINAL CANDIDIASIS

Pathogens

- *C. glabrata* (5% of cases)
- *C. parapsilosis*
- *C. tropicalis*

Clinical

- Accounts for 5–10% of recurrent vulvovaginal candidiasis
- Postmenopausal women and immunocompromised people are more likely to be infected with non-*albicans* spp
- Reduced susceptibility to topical azoles and oral fluconazole

Treatment

Nystatin remains significantly more effective than azoles for non-albicans spp

- Nystatin 100 000 units/5 g vaginal cream intravaginally q12h for 7 days
- Nystatin 100 000 units pessary intravaginally q12h for 7 day

If fail to respond

- Boric acid** 600 mg intravaginally daily for 10–14 days

May need repeated treatment or long-term maintenance (see below)
Seek specialist advice

---

*Nystatin is less effective for *Candida albicans*, but better tolerated than clotrimazole
**Extemporaneous preparation as gelatin capsule, available from compounding chemist

3. RECURRENT VULVOVAGINAL CANDIDIASIS

Definition

- Recurrent candida vulvovaginitis—more than 4 acute episodes per year

Predisposing factors

- Frequent vagina washing (reduces the normal vaginal flora)
- Antibiotic treatment
- Oestrogen-containing oral contraceptive pill or hormone replace therapy
- Diabetes
- Immunosuppression

Treatment

Induce symptom remission

- Option 1: fluconazole 50 mg PO daily
- Option 2: itraconazole 100 mg PO daily

If cannot tolerate azoles or for pregnant woman

- Nystatin* 100 000 units/5 g vaginal cream/pessary intravaginally nocte

Duration of induction

- Until remission of symptoms (2 weeks to 6 months)

Maintain remission

(For long term, may need to be continued until reach menopause)

- Option 1: fluconazole 150–300 mg PO weekly
- Option 2: itraconazole 100–200 mg PO weekly
- Option 3: clotrimazole 500 mg pessary intravaginally weekly
- Option 4: nystatin* 100 000 units/5 g vaginal cream/pessary intravaginally weekly

4. ANTIBIOTIC OR HRT-PREDISPOSED CANDIDIASIS

- **Antibiotic predisposed candidiasis**—patient may have to return to continuous antifungal therapy after the antibiotic course is completed
- **HRT-predisposed candidiasis**—HRT has to be suspended; when recovered, may restart HRT at a lower dose; if relapse, may need to cease HRT permanently or use intermittent antifungal therapy with low-dose HRT

5. MANAGEMENT OF MALE PARTNERS

- Male partner may develop postcoital itch with no rash (due to *Candida* secretions in vagina irritating the penile skin)—the itch usually resolves after the woman is treated

---

*Nystatin is less effective for *Candida albicans*, but better tolerated than clotrimazole

- To ease the man's itch
  - Option 1: clotrimazole 1% + hydrocortisone 1% cream (e.g. Hydrozole) top bid until itch goes
  - Option 2: miconazole 2% + hydrocortisone 1% cream (e.g. Resolve Plus 1.0) top bid until itch goes
- May cause male partner balanitis/balanoposthitis (itchy rash)—should be swabbed and treated (see Balanitis and balanoposthitis, p. 16)

CANDIDIASIS—ORAL

Other names: oral candidiasis, oral thrush, candidosis, moniliasis, pseudomembranous candidiasis, angular cheilitis

Pathogens

- *Candida albicans*
- *Candida glabrata*
- *Candida tropicalis*

Forms of oral candidiasis

- Pseudomembranous candidiasis (thrush)
- Erythematous candidiasis (denture-related)
- Hyperplastic candidiasis (white plaque cannot be wiped away)

Predisposing factors and risk groups

- Poor oral hygiene
- Wearing dentures
- Salivary gland hypofunction
- Poorly controlled diabetes
- Having taken antibiotics
- Inhaled corticosteroids for treatment of lung conditions (e.g. asthma or COPD)
- The immunocompromised (e.g. AIDS/HIV or chemotherapy)
- Newborn babies (mother may have received antibiotic before delivery)
- Pregnancy or on contraceptive pills

Clinical

- Creamy white plaques on mucosal membranes; once removed, leave an inflamed mucosa
- Hyperplastic candidiasis has a fixed white lesion that resembles oral cancer
- In babies the thrush is usually painless (breastfeeding mother can use miconazole gel on nipples before feeds)
- Adult candidosis may have discomfort or burning
- Angular cheilitis—cracking, peeling or ulceration on corners of mouth or lips

Laboratory

- Swab for microscopy and fungal culture
- Biopsy for the fixed white lesion (seen in hyperplastic candidiasis)

Treatment

- Allow the dentures to dry out at night when not worn
- Clean the dentures with a toothbrush and soap regularly (at least twice daily)
- Soak the dentures for 15–30 min in white vinegar (diluted 1 : 20) twice weekly

Mild case—use any of the following

- Amphotericin lozenges (e.g. Fungilin)* 10 mg sucked qid for 1–2 weeks
- Miconazole 2% oral gel (e.g. Daktarin) 2.5 mL (child 6 months–2 years: 1.25 mL) held in mouth as long as possible before swallowing, qid for 1–2 weeks
- Nystatin oral drops (e.g. Nilstat, Mycostatin) 1 mL retain in mouth as long as possible before swallowing, qid after food, for 1–2 weeks

Severe case, especially in the immunocompromised

- Option 1: fluconazole oral suspension (e.g. Diflucan) 6 mg/kg PO for day 1, then 3 mg/kg PO daily until symptoms disappear
- Option 2: fluconazole 100 mg PO for day 1, then 50 mg PO daily until symptoms disappear

CANDIDURIA AND *CANDIDA* CYSTITIS

Candiduria—asymptomatic presence of *Candida* spp in the urine
Candida cystitis—*Candida* infection of the bladder

Causes and risk factors

- Elderly women and pregnant women are at higher risk
- Contamination of the urine sample
- Vaginal *Candida* colonisation
- Urinary catheter and stenting
- Urinary tract procedures
- Antibiotic use
- Diabetes
- Urinary tract obstruction (may be related to fungal ball)
- Urinary tract tuberculosis
- Secondary to *Candida* vulvovaginitis (female) or *Candida* balanitis (male)
- As a part of disseminated candidiasis

---

*Do not use amphotericin lozenges in patients with severe dry mouth

Clinical

- Asymptomatic (urinary tract colonisation) in most patients with candiduria
- Candida cystitis—urinary symptoms are the same as bacteria cystitis
- Fever in patient with candiduria may be due to other bacterial infections or disseminated candidiasis

Laboratory

- MSU for microscopy and culture

Treatment

- Remove urinary catheter and stents if possible
- Treat the causes and risk factors
- Treat *Candida* vulvovaginitis and *Candida* balanitis (as the cause of urinary tract symptoms)
- Occasionally bladder irrigation with amphotericin B may be used

Indication for antifungal therapy

- Patients with urinary symptoms (need to exclude bacteria UTI)
- Patients with fever (need to exclude other infections)
- Patients with immunosuppression (e.g. neutropenia, HIV infection, post-chemotherapy)
- Patients undergoing urological procedures
- Patients with possible disseminated candidiasis

Antifungal therapy

- Fluconazole 200 mg (child: 3 mg/kg up to 200 mg) PO daily for 14 days

Patients undergoing urological procedures

- Fluconazole dose as above, take several days before and after the procedure

Patients with *Candida* pyelonephritis

- Fluconazole 400 mg (child: 6 mg/kg up to 400 mg) PO daily for 14 days

Bladder irrigation (if indicated)

- Amphotericin B 50 mg in 1 L sterile water, irrigate over 24 hours

For fluconazole-resistant or non-*albicans* candiduria

- Seek expert advice

CAT-SCRATCH DISEASE

Cat-scratch disease (CSD) is an infrequent self-limiting infectious disease characterised by painful regional lymphadenopathy following the scratch or bite of a cat (typically a kitten).

Pathogens

- *Bartonella henselae* and *B. clarridgeiae*—gram-negative bacteria

Transmission

- From the scratch, lick or bite of a cat

Incubation

- 1–2 weeks

Clinical

- **Skin disease (bacillary angiomatosis)**—inoculation lesion (a blister or bump at the site where the bacteria enter the body) with regional lymph node swelling, fever, fatigue, loss of appetite, headache, rash and sore throat
- **Internal organ disease (bacillary peliosis)**—infection involves liver, spleen, bones, joints, endocardium, eye, lungs, brain or spine; it may cause convulsions

Diagnosis

- History of cat scratch, lick or bite
- Regional lymphadenopathy (biopsy may show characteristic histology)
- *Bartonella* serology test—confirm the diagnosis

Treatment

- Generally self-limiting and most cases do not require antibiotic treatment
- Indication for antibiotic therapy:
    - Lymphadenopathy persists ≥1 month
    - Internal organ disease (see above)

Antifungal therapy

For extensive or persistent lymphadenopathy

- Azithromycin (PO) for 5 days

For *Bartonella* endocarditis

- Option 1: doxycycline (PO) for 6 weeks **plus** gentamicin (IV) for 2 weeks
- Option 2: doxycycline (PO) for 6 weeks **plus** rifampicin (PO) for 2 weeks

For infection in AIDS or other immunocompromised patients

- Seek expert advice

Dosage of above antibiotics

- Azithromycin 500 mg (child: 10 mg/kg up to 500 mg) PO on day 1, then 250 mg (child: 5 mg/kg up to 250 mg) PO daily on days 2–5
- Doxycycline 100 mg (child >8 years: 2 mg/kg up to 100 mg) PO q12h for 6 weeks
- Gentamicin (adult and child): 1 mg/kg IV q8h for 2 weeks (monitor blood levels, p. 459)
- Rifampicin 300 mg (child: 7.5 mg/kg up to 300 mg) PO q12h for 2 weeks

CELLULITIS

Cellulitis is infection of deep subcutaneous tissue of skin.

Pathogens

- *Streptococcus pyogenes*—often the cause of spontaneous cellulitis
- *Staphylococcus aureus*—important in wound-associated cellulitis
- *Aeromonas* or *Vibrio* spp—may cause cellulitis after a water-related injury
- Gram-negative bacteria, fungi and mycobacteria—may also be the cause of cellulitis in immunocompromised patients

Risk factors

- Insect bites, cuts, abrasions, blistering, animal bites, tattoos, pruritic skin rash, eczema, dry skin, fissured dermatitis, tinea pedis, injecting drugs, burns, boils, lymphoedema, previous DVT, vascular surgery and radiotherapy

Clinical

- Spreading erythema and swelling, with or without lymphangitis and lymphadenopathy, fever and systemic toxicity
- In adults, most often affects lower legs
- In children, often periorbital

Differential diagnosis

- Erysipelas (p. 110)
- Acute contact dermatitis
- Septic bursitis (p. 373)
- Reaction to insect bite
- Acute gout
- Acute lipoderatosclerosis

Treatment

- Search and treat underlying abnormalities:
  - Facial cellulitis—dental and sinuses examination
  - Lower leg cellulitis—foot fungal infection and circulation check
- Antibiotic therapy

Mild cellulitis

Empirical therapy (to cover *S. pyogenes* and *S. aureus*)

- Option 1: cefalexin (PO) for 5–10 days (preferred in children)
- Option 2: flucloxacillin (PO) for 5–10 days
- Option 3: clindamycin (PO) for 5–10 days (if immediate penicillin allergy)

If *S. pyogenes* is confirmed or for Indigenous patient in central and northern Australia

- Option 1: penicillin V (PO) for 5–10 days
- Option 2: procaine penicillin (IM) daily for 3–5 days

For water-related infections, see Wound infections—water-related (p. 448)

Dosage of above antibiotics

- Cefalexin 500 mg (child: 12.5 mg/kg up to 500 mg) PO q6h
- Flucloxacillin 500 mg (child: 12.5 mg/kg up to 500 mg) PO q6h
- Clindamycin 450 mg (child: 10 mg/kg up to 450 mg) PO q8h
- Penicillin V 500 mg (child: 10 mg/kg up to 500 mg) PO q6h
- Procaine penicillin 1.5 g (child: 50 mg/kg up to 1.5 g) IM daily

Severe cellulitis

- If patient has significant systemic symptoms or does not respond to oral therapy after 48 hours, commence IV therapy
- If there is significant systemic toxicity, consider underlying necrotising soft-tissue infections (see Gangrene, p. 123)
- Treat tinea pedis aggressively if it is the cause of cellulitis (see Tinea, p. 396)

Empirical therapy (to cover *S. aureus* and *S. pyogenes*)

- Option 1: cefazolin (IV)
- Option 2: flucloxacillin (IV)

If immediate penicillin allergy

- Option 1: vancomycin (IV)
- Option 2: clindamycin (IV)

If outpatient parenteral antimicrobial therapy is practical

- Cefazolin 2 g IV daily **plus** probenecid 1 g PO daily
or cefazolin 2 g IV twice daily

Once afebrile and the rash significantly improved, change to oral

- Option 1: cefalexin (PO) to complete a total 14-day course
- Option 2: flucloxacillin (PO) to complete a total 14-day course
- Option 3: clindamycin (PO) to complete a total 14-day course

Dosage of above antibiotics

- Cefazolin 2 g (child: 50 mg/kg up to 2 g) IV q8h
- Flucloxacillin 2 g (child: 50 mg/kg up to 2 g) IV q6h
- Vancomycin 25–30 mg/kg IV for the 1st dose (further dosing see p. 462)
- Clindamycin 600 mg (child: 10 mg/kg up to 600 mg) IV q8h
- Cefalexin 500 mg (child: 10 mg/kg up to 500 mg) PO q6h
- Flucloxacillin 500 mg (child: 12.5 mg/kg up to 500 mg) PO q6h
- Clindamycin 450 mg (child: 10 mg/kg up to 450 mg) PO q8h

Prevention of recurrent severe cellulitis

May use either:

Stand-by antibiotic for infrequent recurrence

- Have patient keep an oral antibiotic on hand for early use when cellulitis recurs

Long-term antibiotic prevention—for frequent recurrence

- Penicillin V 250 mg PO q12h for long term

CERVICAL LYMPHADENITIS

Causes

Viral

- Secondary to viral upper respiratory tract infections
- Epstein-Barr virus
- Parvovirus
- Rubella
- Cytomegalovirus

Bacterial

- Secondary to tonsillopharyngitis (*Streptococcus pyogenes*, *Mycoplasma pneumoniae*)
- Secondary to local skin infection (*Staphylococcus aureus*)
- Secondary to dental infection (anaerobic bacteria)
- *Yersinia* enteritis
- *Bartonella henselae*—cat-scratch disease (subacute)
- Tuberculosis and non-tuberculous mycobacteria (chronic)

Clinical

- Viral lymphadenitis—the lymph nodes are usually small and soft, more bilateral, no overlying skin changes and rarely suppurative
- Bacterial lymphadenitis—the lymph nodes are usually one-sided, rapidly developing, firm, tender and warm with erythema of the overlying skin; about 25% of these are fluctuant
- Cellulitis-adenitis syndrome—caused by group B streptococcus in neonates or infants <2 months old—sudden onset of fever, anorexia, irritability and submandibular swelling

Treatment

- Viral lymphadenitis resolves within 1–2 weeks; no specific treatment is required
- Fine-needle aspiration (FNA) or excision biopsy may be needed for diagnosis
- Abscess with fluctuation may require incision and drainage
- Antibiotic therapy is indicated for acute suppurative lymphadenitis
    - Option 1: flucloxacillin (PO) for 5–7 days
    - Option 2: cefalexin (PO) for 5–7 days
    - Option 3: clindamycin (PO) for 5–10 days (if immediate penicillin allergy)

Dosage of above antibiotics

- Flucloxacillin 500 mg (child: 12.5 mg/kg up to 500 mg) PO q6h
- Cefalexin 500 mg (child: 12.5 mg/kg up to 500 mg) PO q6h
- Clindamycin 300 mg (child: 7.5 mg/kg up to 300 mg) PO q8h

MYCOBACTERIAL LYMPHADENITIS

- Tuberculosis is the commonest cause in Indigenous children and migrants; atypical mycobacterial infections are more common in other Australian children
- Usually chronic or subacute and unilateral
- In early stages, nodes are well-demarcated, firm, mobile and non-tender; later, the nodes become soft, fluctuant and adhere to overlying skin, which may be erythematous; draining sinuses may develop
- Needle aspiration or excision of the infected nodes may be needed for diagnosis
- Mantoux test (tuberculin test) and interferon-gamma release assay (IGRA) can be helpful in diagnosis
- Treatment, see Extrapulmonary tuberculosis (p. 408) or Tuberculosis in children (p. 409)

CERVICITIS

Cervicitis is an inflammation of the uterine cervix. It is a sexually transmitted infection (STI).

Pathogens

- *Chlamydia trachomatis* (D-K serovars)—the commonest cause
- *Neisseria gonorrhoeae*—other important cause
- *Mycoplasma genitalium*—a significant minority of cases
- *Ureaplasma urealyticum*—a potential opportunistic pathogen
- Herpes simplex—potential cause
- *Trichomonas vaginalis*—potential cause
- Adenoviruses—potential cause

Transmission

- Usually via unprotected vaginal sex

Clinical

- Vaginal discharge, painful sexual intercourse; frequently coexists with urethritis
- Untreated cervicitis may cause pelvic inflammatory disease and infertility

Laboratory

- Urine or urethral/vaginal swab—for *C. trachomatis* and *N. gonorrhoeae* PCR testing
- Urine or urethral/vaginal swab—for *Mycoplasma genitalium* PCR testing
- Urethral or vaginal swab—Gram stain, microscopy and culture for *N. gonorrhoeae* (susceptibility testing is required on any isolated gonococci)

- Urethral or vaginal swab—microscopy for trichomonas
- APTIMA® assay for both *Chlamydia* and gonorrhoea—more sensitive and specific than PCR (requires green-topped urine container and APTIMA® swab collection kit)

Treatment

Empirical treatment—covers both *Chlamydia* and gonococci

- Ceftriaxone (IM **or** IV) **plus** azithromycin (**or** doxycycline) (PO) (doses see below)

Chlamydia infection

- Option 1: azithromycin 1 g PO st
- Option 2: doxycycline 100 mg PO q12h for 7 days

Gonococcal infection

- Ceftriaxone 500 mg in 2 mL 1% lidocaine (lignocaine) IM st **or** 500 mg IV st

If gonococci resistant to ceftriaxone*

- See expert advice

In remote Australia where penicillin-resistant *N. gonorrhoeae* is low

- Amoxicillin 3 g **plus** probenecid 1 g **plus** azithromycin 1 g PO st

Mycoplasma genitalium infection or no response to above treatment

- Option 1: doxycycline 100 mg PO q12h for 10 days
- Option 2: moxifloxacin 400 mg PO daily for 7–10 days

For disseminated gonococcal sepsis

- Ceftriaxone 1 g IV daily (**or** cefotaxime 1 g IV q8h)

Continue for 48 hours after defervescence and then switch to oral based on culture and susceptibility results

Total duration

- 7 days or 14 days (if symptoms persist)

Note

- If symptoms persist or recur—requires a second course of antibiotics and further investigation of aetiology (e.g. urine/urethral or vaginal swabs for *Mycoplasma/Ureaplasma* PCR)
- Sexual partners should be examined, investigated and treated empirically to prevent reinfection
- Post-treatment follow-up is recommended: a test of cure at 1 month; a test of reinfection at 3–6 months

---

*As cefalosporin-resistant gonorrhoea emerges, any suggestion of possible treatment failure in gonorrhoea should be reported to public health authorities and advice from a sexual health practitioner needs to be sought

CHANCROID

Other names: soft chancre

Chancroid is:

- A sexually transmitted infection (STI)
- A co-factor for HIV transmission
- Rare in Australia

Pathogens

- *Haemophilus ducreyi*—a fastidious gram-negative bacteria

Transmission

- Through sexual contact with the open sores/ulcers

Incubation

- 1 day to 2 weeks

Clinical

- Painful non-indurated genital/anogenital ulcers (sharp irregular borders, filled with pus), may persist for weeks or months
- Painful tender adenopathy (suppurative lymphadenitis)
- Chancroid is a risk factor for contracting HIV, due to their shared risk of exposure and biologically facilitated transmission of one infection by the other

Laboratory

- Wound (lesion) swab PCR for *Haemophilus ducreyi*

Compare to chancre

See Table 3.1

TABLE 3.1

COMPARE CHANCROID TO CHANCRE

	Chancroid	Chancre
Pathogen	*Haemophilus ducreyi*	*Treponema pallidum*
Pain	Painful	Painless
Exudate	Grey or yellow purulent	Non-exudative
Edge of ulcer	Soft (non-indurated)	Hard (indurated)
Progress	Persists for weeks or months	Heals within 3–6 weeks
Treatment	Usually required	Heals spontaneously

Treatment

- Option 1: azithromycin 1 g PO st
- Option 2: ceftriaxone 500 mg in 2 mL 1% lidocaine (lignocaine) IM st **or** 500 mg IV st
- Option 3: ciprofloxacin 500 mg PO q12h for 3 days

Prevention

- Limit the number of sexual partners
- Use a condom
- Carefully wash genitals after sexual intercourse
- If infected, avoid sexual contact and seek treatment
- Notify all sexual contacts immediately so they can obtain examination and treatment

CHICKENPOX

Other names: varicella

Pathogens

- Varicella zoster virus, a member of the herpes virus family

Incubation

- 10–21 days
- Shorter incubation in the immunocompromised
- Zoster immune globulin (ZIG) may prolong incubation to 28 days

Clinical

- Fever, irritability, malaise and headache
- More severe in adults
- Itchy papular red skin lesions (3–4 mm) with clear vesicles on the top, spreading from the trunk to the face and extremities; different stages of lesions can be seen at the same time

Complications

- Cerebellar ataxia, aseptic meningitis, transverse myelitis, thrombocytopenia, encephalitis and pneumonia

Treatment

Indications for antiviral therapy (not indicated for normal children)

1. All adults (≥16 years) with chickenpox
2. Children with chickenpox who have existing skin disease (e.g. dermatitis)
3. Patients with any complication of chickenpox (see above)
4. Immunocompromised patients with chickenpox

Antiviral therapy

Mild to moderate disease (above indications 1 and 2)—oral therapy

- Option 1: famciclovir 250 mg PO q8h for 7 days
- Option 2: valaciclovir 1 g PO q8h for 7 days
- Option 3: aciclovir 800 mg (child: 20 mg/kg) PO 5 times daily for 7 days (safe in pregnancy)

Severe disease (above indications 3 and 4)—IV therapy
- Aciclovir 10–12.5 mg/kg (child <5 years: 20 mg/kg; ≥5 years: 15 mg/kg) IV q8h

After improvement, switch to oral famciclovir for total (IV + PO) 7 days
- Famciclovir 500 mg PO q8h

Post-exposure prophylaxis

For non-immune household contacts (particularly children)
- Varicella vaccine 0.5 mL SC within 5 days of exposure, booster after 6 weeks

For pregnant women in contact with chickenpox or shingles (if seronegative)
- ZIG (zoster immunoglobulin)* 600 IU IM within 4 days of exposure

For neonate whose mother developed chickenpox (from 7 days before delivery to 28 days after delivery)
- ZIG (zoster immunoglobulin)* to neonate: 200 IU IM st

For immunocompromised household contacts (if seronegative)
- ZIG (zoster immunoglobulin)* 600 IU IM within 4–10 days of exposure

If ZIG is unavailable, may use normal human immunoglobulin (NHIG): 0.4–1.0 mL/kg IM

Immunisation (if no past history of chickenpox or negative varicella serology)

- MMRV (e.g. Prioris Tetra®) 0.5 mL SC/IM, 1 dose at 18 months

If missed 18-month immunisation
- Varicella vaccine (e.g. Varilrix®, Varivax®) 0.5 mL SC, 1 dose at 2–14 years of age

CHIKUNGUNYA FEVER

Chikungunya fever is an illness with symptoms similar to dengue fever. There is risk of importation of chikungunya fever into Australia by infected travellers. Australian mosquitoes are capable of spreading the virus.

Pathogen

- *Chikungunya* virus (CHIKV)

Transmission

- Naturally spread between mosquitoes and monkeys
- Spread to humans through the bites of infected mosquitoes: *Aedes aegypti* (the yellow fever mosquito) and *Aedes albopictus* (the Asian tiger mosquito)

---

*ZIG is available from the Australian Red Cross Blood Service

Distribution

- West, central and southern Africa and many areas of Asia (India, Sri Lanka, Thailand, Myanmar, Malaysia, Indonesia, Cambodia, Saudi Arabia and Papua New Guinea)
- No outbreak has been recorded in Australia, but given the current large CHIKV epidemics and worldwide distribution of *Aedes aegypti*, there is a risk of importation of CHIKV into Australia by infected travellers

Incubation

- 2–7 days (up to 12 days)

Clinical

- Fever, headache, photophobia, myalgia, arthralgia, fatigue, rash, nausea and vomiting, typically last a few days to a few weeks
- Some people experience fatigue or arthralgia for many weeks after the infection
- Some patients may have 'silent' CHIKV infection (infection without illness)
- CHIKV may occasionally cause severe infection, but it is rarely fatal

Laboratory

- *Chikungunya* virus isolation (takes 1–2 weeks)
- *Chikungunya* virus PCR testing
- *Chikungunya* serology (false positives can occur with infection via other related viruses)

Treatment

- Symptomatic treatment
- No vaccine or specific antiviral treatment is available
- CHIKV infection confers lifetime protection

Prevention

- Prevent from being infected—avoid mosquito bites
- Prevent infected persons from further mosquito exposure—staying indoors and/or under a mosquito net during the first few days of illness

CHLAMYDIA CONJUNCTIVITIS AND TRACHOMA

Other names: inclusion conjunctivitis
Chlamydia conjunctivitis and trachoma are common causes of blindness worldwide and they are still common in remote Indigenous communities.

Pathogens

- *Chlamydia trachomatis*

Transmission

- Direct contact
- Neonates acquire the infection from the mother

Clinical

- Typically affects sexually active teens and young adults
- Neonatal conjunctivitis (inclusion conjunctivitis)—the most common pathogen of neonata conjunctivitis; approximately 50% of neonates with chlamydia conjunctivitis develop *Chlamydia* pneumonia
- Eye signs: conjunctival injection, superficial punctate keratitis, superior corneal pannus, peripheral subepithelial infiltrates, iritis, follicle formation and mucopurulent or stringy discharge
- A palpable preauricular node is almost always present
- Trachoma is a form of chronic *C. trachomatis* conjunctivitis and it is the leading cause of preventable blindness in the world

Laboratory

- *Chlamydia* PCR—conjunctival swab or corneal scrapings

In trachoma, *Chlamydia* is not always detected by testing

Treatment

- Oral antibiotic only (eye drops/ointment provide no benefit)
- The mother of the infected neonate and her sexual contacts should also be treated
- In trachoma-prevalent areas, treat all household contacts of trachoma

For conjunctivitis

- Azithromycin 1 g (child: 20 mg/kg up to 1 g) PO as a single dose

For neonates

- Azithromycin 20 mg/kg PO daily for 3 days

For trachoma

- Azithromycin 1 g (child: 20 mg/kg up to 1 g) PO as a single dose

Prevention

- Regular face washing as a primary health measure
- Targeting young children who are at risk of trachoma
- If prevalence in children <10 years is ≥10%—consider **community-wide treatment**:
  - Azithromycin 1 g (child 1–10 years: 20 mg/kg up to 1 g) PO every 3 months

CHLAMYDIA STI

See also Lymphogranuloma venereum (p. 209)
Chlamydia remains the most common notifiable sexually transmitted infection (STI) in Australia.

Pathogen

- *Chlamydia trachomatis* (serovars B, D–K)

Transmission

- Sexually transmitted
- During vaginal delivery (neonatal infection)

Clinical

- In women, most cases of *Chlamydia* cervicitis are asymptomatic but may spread to cause pelvic inflammatory disease (p. 273); if untreated, infertility may result
- In men, *Chlamydia* urethritis is usually symptomatic (white discharge from penis with or without dysuria); it may spread to cause epididymo-orchitis (p. 106) and prostatitis (p. 338)

***Chlamydia* screening**

- All sexually active women and possibly men aged 16–25 should be screened annually for *Chlamydia* (especially after unprotected sex or partner change):
    - First-void urine for rapid *Chlamydia* antigen detection or for *Chlamydia* PCR
    - High vaginal swab for *Chlamydia* PCR—should be collected for women aged 16–30 when they present for a Pap smear

Laboratory

- PCR for *Chlamydia* and gonorrhoea—may use following specimens:
    - First-void urine (male and female)
    - Urethral (male), vagina swab (self-collected) or endocervix swab
    - Throat swab (if oral sex)
    - Anal swab (self-collected in men who engage in anal intercourse)
- APTIMA® assay for both *Chlamydia* and gonorrhoea—more sensitive and specific than PCR methods (requires green-topped urine container and APTIMA® swab collection kit)
- *Chlamydia* culture—remains useful in selected circumstances and is the test for non-genital specimens

Treatment

- Option 1: azithromycin 1 g PO st
- Option 2: doxycycline 100 mg PO q12h for 7 days
- Treat sexual partners simultaneously to prevent reinfection and complications:
    - Patient to ask partner to see doctor and get treatment
    - Patient-delivered partner therapy—treating doctor to prescribe azithromycin 1 g as a single dose for the partner
- Following treatment, no unprotected sex for 7 days and retest in 3 months (to check for reinfection)

CHOLANGITIS—ASCENDING

Pathogens

- Gram-negative bacilli—*Escherichia coli*, *Klebsiella* and *Enterobacter*
- Gram-positive cocci—enterococcus
- Anaerobes—*Clostridium*, *Bacteroides fragilis* and *Enterococcus faecalis*

Clinical

- A medical emergency
- Usually associated with biliary tract obstruction
- Abdominal pain, fever, rigors, malaise, jaundice, RUQ tenderness, septic shock and confusion

Laboratory

- Blood culture (aerobic and anaerobic)—before administering antibiotics
- Bile culture (aerobic and anaerobic)

Treatment

- Hospital admission, IV fluid
- Urgent biliary drainage—very important if there is biliary obstruction
- Prompt antibiotic treatment—prevent and treat sepsis

Antibiotic therapy

- Ampi(amoxi)cillin (IV) **plus** gentamicin (IV) **plus** metronidazole (IV)

If gentamicin is contraindicated or has been used for 3 days

- Piperacillin/tazobactam (IV) **or** ticarcillin/clavulanate (IV)

If non-immediate penicillin allergy

- Ceftriaxone (**or** cefotaxime)* (IV) **plus** metronidazole (IV)

If immediate penicillin allergy

- Gentamicin (IV) **plus** metronidazole (IV)

After improvement, change to oral

- Option 1: amoxicillin/clavulanate (PO)
- Option 2: cotrimoxazole **plus** metronidazole (PO) (if penicillin allergy)

Duration of therapy

- Total 7 days

Dosage of above antibiotics

- Ampi(amoxi)cillin 2 g (child: 50 mg/kg up to 2 g) IV q6h
- Gentamicin 4–7 mg/kg (child: 7.5 mg/kg up to 320 mg) IV for the 1st dose (further dosing see p. 459)
- Metronidazole 500 mg (child: 12.5 mg/kg up to 500 mg) IV q12h
- Piperacillin/tazobactam 4 g (child: 100 mg/kg up to 4 g) IV q8h
- Ticarcillin/clavulanate 3 g (child: 50 mg/kg up to 3 g) IV q6h
- Ceftriaxone 1 g (child >1 month: 50 mg/kg up to 1 g) IV daily

---

*Cefalosporins are not actively against enterococci

- Cefotaxime 1 g (child: 50 mg/kg up to 1 g) IV q8h
- Amoxicillin/clavulanate 875 mg (child: 22.5 mg/kg up to 875 mg) PO q12h
- Cotrimoxazole 160/800 mg (child >1 month: 4/20 mg/kg up to 160/800 mg) PO q12h
- Metronidazole 400 mg (child: 10 mg/kg up to 400 mg) PO q12h

Prevention of recurrent cholangitis

For patients with recurrent cholangitis associated with ongoing bile duct disease, long-term antibiotic suppressive therapy may reduce the recurrent infection

Antibiotic suppressive therapy (prophylaxis)
- Option 1: amoxicillin/clavulanate 875 mg (child: 22.5 mg/kg up to 875 mg) PO daily
- Option 2: cefalexin 500 mg (child: 10 mg/kg up to 500 mg) PO daily
- Option 3: norfloxacin 400 mg (child: 10 mg/kg up to 400 mg) PO daily
- Option 4: cotrimoxazole 160/800 mg (child: 4/20 mg/kg up to 160/800 mg) PO daily

Antibiotic rotation: the above antibiotics may be used in rotation to reduce the risk of developing bacterial antibiotic resistance (seek expert advice)

CHOLECYSTITIS

Cholecystitis is often associated with gallbladder stones, which may cause obstruction and result in secondary infection and serious complications.

Pathogens

- Aerobic bowel flora—*E. coli*, *Klebsiella* spp and *Enterococcus faecalis*
- Anaerobes (when obstructed)—Bacteroides spp

Clinical

- Epigastric or RUQ pain, vomiting, fever and positive Murphy's sign

Complications

- Perforation or rupture of the gall bladder
- Ascending cholangitis

Laboratory

- FBC, CRP, LFT, blood culture (if febrile) to assess whether patient is septic
- Ultrasound abdomen to see any gallstones or biliary obstruction

Treatment

- Most biliary colic with no septic signs—antibiotic treatment is not required
- If septic (rigor, fever, ↑WBC and CRP)—antibiotic treatment + urgent surgical referral
- Laparoscopic cholecystectomy should be considered early in acute presentation
  - Ampi(amoxi)cillin (IV) **plus** gentamicin (IV)

If gentamicin is contraindicated or has been used for 3 days
  - Piperacillin/tazobactam (IV) **or** ticarcillin/clavulanate (IV)

If non-immediate penicillin allergy
  - Ceftriaxone (**or** cefotaxime)* (IV)

If immediate penicillin allergy
  - Gentamicin (IV) as a single drug

If biliary obstruction is present, **add**
  - Metronidazole (IV or PO)

After improvement, change to oral
  - Option 1: amoxicillin/clavulanate (PO)
  - Option 2: cotrimoxazole (PO) (if penicillin allergy)

Duration of therapy

- Total 7 days

Dosage of above antibiotics

- Ampi(amoxi)cillin 2 g (child: 50 mg/kg up to 2 g) IV q6h
- Gentamicin 4–7 mg/kg (child: 7.5 mg/kg up to 320 mg) IV for the 1st dose (further dosing see p. 459)
- Amoxicillin/clavulanate 875 mg (child: 22.5 mg/kg up to 875 mg) PO q12h
- Ceftriaxone 1 g (child >1 month: 50 mg/kg up to 1 g) IV daily
- Cefotaxime 1 g (child: 50 mg/kg up to 1 g) IV q8h
- Metronidazole 500 mg (child: 12.5 mg/kg up to 500 mg) IV q12h **or** 400 mg (child: 10 mg/kg up to 400 mg) PO q12h
- Cotrimoxazole 160/800 mg (child >1 month: 4/20 mg/kg up to 160/800 mg) PO q12h

CHOLERA

Cholera is a disease characterised by severe diarrhoea and dehydration. There are occasional cases in international travellers and, very rarely, some cases have been acquired through ingestion of contaminated water in northern Australia.

Pathogens

- *Vibrio cholerae* serotypes O1 and O139, which produce enterotoxin

---

*Cefalosporins are not actively against enterococci

Transmission

- The bacteria are passed in faeces or vomit, and can survive up to 2 weeks in fresh water and 8 weeks in salty water
- Transmission is through food (especially shellfish) or water contaminated by faeces or vomit

Incubation

- Up to 5 days

Clinical

- Typically, sudden onset of severe painless diarrhoea ('rice-water' diarrhoea), results in intense dehydration and metabolic acidosis with muscular cramps; death from acute circulatory failure may occur within a few hours unless fluid and electrolytes are replaced
- However, the majority of infections cause only mild illness with slight diarrhoea

Laboratory

- Faeces cholera antigen detection
- Faeces microscopy, cultures (specific media)—for *Vibrio cholerae* O1 or O139

Treatment

- Rehydration—the mainstay of treatment
- Antibiotic treatment—reduces the volume and duration of diarrhoea
    - Option 1: azithromycin 1 g (child: 20 mg/kg up to 1 g) PO st
    - Option 2: ciprofloxacin 1 g (child: 20 mg/kg up to 1 g) PO st

If treatment failure (due to resistant strains)—choose antibiotics according to susceptibility testing

Vaccination

- Routine vaccination is not recommended, as the risk to travellers is very low
- **An oral cholera vaccine may be offered to the following people** who enter rural areas of highly endemic countries:
    - Reduced gastric acidity (e.g. on PPI)
    - Uncontrolled diabetes
    - Inflammatory bowel disease
    - HIV/AIDS and immunocompromised (lack of effect)
    - Significant cardiovascular disease
    - Aid workers going to work in disaster areas where cholera is endemic or epidemic
- Dukoral adult, child >6 years: 1 sachet PO, 2 doses 1–6 weeks apart, booster in 2 years (children 2–6 years: 3 doses 1–6 weeks apart, booster after 6 months)

If an interval is >6 weeks between the 2 doses, restart the vaccination course

The efficacy is between 60% and 80% and the protection occurs 2 weeks after completing the basic course and lasts 2–3 years

CIRRHOSIS AND HEPATIC ENCEPHALOPATHY

1. ANTIBIOTIC PROPHYLAXIS AND TREATMENT OF HEPATIC ENCEPHALOPATHY

- Ammonia and other toxic substances are generated and converted by intestinal bacteria
- Non-absorbable antibiotic can prevent or reverse hepatic encephalopathy by reducing intestinal bacteria

Prevention and treatment of hepatic encephalopathy

- Rifaximin (e.g. Xifaxan) 550 mg PO bid

2. ANTIBIOTIC PROPHYLAXIS IN CIRRHOTIC PATIENTS WITH GIT BLEEDING

Indication for prophylaxis

- Patient with cirrhosis who has active GIT bleeding

Aim of prophylaxis

- To reduce the risk of subsequent bacterial infections, such as bacteraemia, pneumonia, spontaneous bacterial peritonitis (SBP) and urinary tract infections

Short-term prophylaxis (to reduce quinolone resistance)

- Norfloxacin (PO) for 2 days

If oral therapy is not feasible
- Ceftriaxone (IV) for 2 days
- Ciprofloxacin (IV) for 2 days

Dosage of above antibiotics

- Norfloxacin 400 mg (child: 10 mg/kg up to 400 mg) PO q12h
- Ceftriaxone 1 g (child ≥1 month: 50 mg/kg up to 1 g) IV daily
- Ciprofloxacin 400 mg (child: 10 mg/kg up to 400 mg) IV q12h

CLOSTRIDIUM DIFFICILE

Other names: antibiotic-associated diarrhoea, pseudomembranous colitis

Pathogens

- *Clostridium difficile* and its toxins (hypervirulent strains: PCR ribotype 027 and 078)
- Hypervirulent community-acquired strains can be acquired zoonotically

Risk factors

- Antibiotic-associated *C. difficile* infection—associated with the use of broad-spectrum antibiotics such as cefalosporins, clindamycin, quinolones, amoxicillin/clavulanate or ticarcillin/clavulanate; however,

antibiotic use is not a prerequisite for development of *C. difficile* infection
- Community-acquired *C. difficile* infection—diarrhoea without prior exposure to antibiotics
- Proton-pump inhibitors (PPIs)—can increase susceptibility to *C. difficile*
- Cancer chemotherapy—can be associated with *C. difficile* infection

Clinical

- Diarrhoea can occur at any time during, or for some months after, a course of antibiotics
- Faeces may be watery or bloody and may progress to toxic bowel dilation

Laboratory

- Faeces *C. difficile* culture and CDT (*C. difficile* toxins)
    - Testing for CDT should be considered in patients with diarrhoea who have been on antibiotics or have had antibiotics over the last 6 weeks
    - Testing for CDT should also be considered in community patients with diarrhoea who have had no recent history of antibiotic exposure
    - In most cases no pathogen is isolated from faeces, but CDT are positive
- PCR for *C. difficile* toxin genes—the most sensitive and specific test
    - No need to test in young children (<2 years)—asymptomatic colonisation is common
    - No need to repeat the test for cure

Treatment

- Cease causative antibiotic(s)—up to 25% of patients will stop diarrhoea (if antibiotics cannot be stopped, seek expert advice)
- Antibiotic treatment—if *C. difficile* is confirmed and diarrhoea is persistent

For mild to moderate case
- Metronidazole (PO **or** via NGT) for 10 days

For severe case or if unresponsive or relapsing
- Option 1: vancomycin* (PO **or** via NGT) for 10 days
- Option 2: fidaxomicin (PO) for 10 days**

If patient has hypotension, ileus or megacolon
- Vancomycin (PO or via NGT +/– PR) **plus** metronidazole (IV) for 10 days

Early surgical referral for ? colectomy

---

*Injectable vancomycin can be used orally
**Fidaxomicin has lower rate of recurrence than vancomycin, but is expensive

For intractable recurrent colitis—seek specialist advice
- May try: bacitracin, rifaximin, sodium fusidate, tigecycline or nitazoxanide

Dosage of above antibiotics
- Metronidazole 400 mg (child: 10 mg/kg up to 400 mg) PO or via NGT q8h
- Vancomycin 125 mg (child: 3 mg/kg up to 125 mg) PO or via NGT q6h
- Fidaxomicin 200 mg PO q12h
- Vancomycin 500 mg in 100 mL normal saline PR q6h
- Metronidazole 500 mg (child: 12.5 mg/kg up to 500 mg) IV q8h
- Probiotics (e.g. *Lactobacillus* spp and *Bifidobacterium* spp) are reported effective at preventing and treating antibiotic-associated diarrhoea
- Faecal microbiota transplantation (FMT) ('stool transplant') (enema of bacterial flora from faeces of a healthy donor for 5–10 days) for recurrent or relapsing colitis when standard treatments have failed (near 95% success rate)

COMMON COLD

Other names: acute viral rhinitis

Pathogens
- Coronavirus
- Rhinovirus (>100 serotypes)
- Influenza virus
- Parainfluenza virus

Transmission
- By droplets

Incubation
- 1–4 days

Clinical
- Flu-like symptoms usually last 5–10 days (cough may persist for weeks)
- Purulent nasal discharge or sputum common after a few days of illness and does not necessarily require antibiotic treatment

Complications
- Otitis media
- Sinusitis
- Pneumonia
- Febrile convulsion

Treatment of common cold
- Good rest
- Analgesics (e.g. paracetamol)

- Keep drinking fluids
- Steam inhalation or nasal saline irrigation for nasal congestion and clearance of thick sticky secretion in nose
- Nasal decongestant (topical or oral) for nasal congestion and rhinorrhoea (short-term use only)
- Antihistamine in combination with a decongestant
- Ipratropium bromide nasal spray (e.g. Atrovent Nasal, Atrovent Nasal Forte)—for severe rhinorrhoea
- Vitamin C (high dose) may reduce the duration of symptoms

Antibiotics are not indicated for common cold

- Antibiotics have no effect on viruses, and may cause adverse effects and result in bacterial resistance

Antibiotics are indicated only for the following conditions

- Symptoms worsen after 5–7 days and develop focal symptoms and signs suggesting secondary bacterial infection (e.g. sinusitis, otitis media, bronchitis or pneumonia)
- Immunosuppressed patients, when bacterial infection is suspected

COMPOUND FRACTURE

Other names: open fractures

Pathogens

- Skin pathogens: *Staphylococcus aureus, Streptococcus pyogenes*
- Soil pathogens: *Clostridium* spp (e.g. *C. perfringens, C. septicum* and *C. novyi*)
- Water-related pathogens: *Vibrio* spp (e.g. *Vibrio vulnificus*) and *Aeromonas* spp

Treatment

- Urgent orthopaedic referral
- Irrigation and debridement—very important for preventing infection
- Tetanus prophylaxis (Table 2.1)

Empirical prophylaxis/early treatment

- All patients with open fractures require IV antibiotic prophylaxis or treatment

For 'clean' open fractures (prophylaxis)

- Cefazolin (IV) for 1–3 days

If immediate penicillin allergy

- Clindamycin (**or** lincomycin) (IV or PO) for 1–3 days

For severely soiled or damaged wounds or with soft-tissue infection

- Option 1: piperacillin/tazobactam (IV), **then** amoxicillin/clavulanate (PO) for 7 days

- Option 2: ticarcillin/clavulanate (IV), **then** amoxicillin/clavulanate (PO) for 7 days

If penicillin allergy

- Cefazolin (IV) **plus** metronidazole (IV), **then** cefalexin **plus** metronidazole (PO) for 7 days

If immediate penicillin allergy

- Ciprofloxacin (IV or PO) **plus** clindamycin (**or** lincomycin) (IV or PO) for 7 days

For water-contaminated wounds

- Ciprofloxacin (IV then PO) **plus** clindamycin (**or** lincomycin) (IV then PO) for 7 days

If bone infection established

- Treat as Osteomyelitis (p. 255)

Dosage of above antibiotics

- Cefazolin 2 g (child: 50 mg/kg up to 2 g) IV q8h
- Clindamycin 600 mg (child: 15 mg/kg up to 600 mg) IV q8h
- Clindamycin 450 mg (child: 10 mg/kg up to 450 mg) PO q8h
- Lincomycin 600 mg (child: 15 mg/kg up to 600 mg) IV q8h
- Piperacillin/tazobactam 4 g (child: 100 mg/kg up to 4 g) IV q8h
- Ticarcillin/clavulanate 3 g (child: 50 mg/kg up to 3 g) IV q6h
- Amoxicillin/clavulanate 875 mg (child: 22.5 mg/kg) PO q12h
- Cefazolin 2 g (child: 50 mg/kg up to 2 g) IV q8h
- Metronidazole 500 mg (child: 12.5 mg/kg up to 500 mg) IV q12h
- Cefalexin 1 g (child: 25 mg/kg up to 1 g) IV q6h
- Metronidazole 400 mg (child: 10 mg/kg up to 400 mg) IV q12h
- Ciprofloxacin 400 mg (child: 10 mg/kg up to 400 mg) IV q8h
- Ciprofloxacin 750 mg (child: 20 mg/kg up to 750 mg) PO q12h

CONJUNCTIVITIS

Conjunctivitis is inflammation of the conjunctiva.
If the patient presents with significant pain, photophobia or loss of vision—indicating acute keratitis or other serious disorders—prompt ophthalmologist referral is required.

1. VIRAL CONJUNCTIVITIS

Pathogens

- *Adenovirus*—the major cause, highly infectious

Clinical

- Begins as a unilateral red eye with a watery discharge and dense follicles; it may transfer with lesser intensity to the other eye after 2–3 days
- Often associated with viral upper respiratory tract infection and preauricular lymph node enlargement

Treatment

- Cold compresses (several times a day)
- Artificial tears
- Topic vasoconstrictor:
  - Phenylephrine 0.12% eye drops (e.g. Prefrin), 1–2 drops tds

2. BACTERIAL CONJUNCTIVITIS

Pathogens

- *Haemophilus influenzae* (especially in young children)
- *Streptococcus pneumoniae* or *Streptococcus pyogenes*
- *Staphylococcus aureus*
- *Neisseria gonorrhoeae* (particularly in central and northern Australia) (see Gonococcal conjunctivitis [p. 133] and Gonococcal neonate ophthalmia [p. 134])
- *Neisseria meningitidis* —may precede meningococcal invasive disease
- *Chlamydia trachomatis* (see *Chlamydia* conjunctivitis and trachoma [p. 52])

Laboratory

- Conjunctival swab/scraping—for bacteria culture, *Chlamydia* (PCR) and N. gonorrhoeae PCR and culture + sensitivity (specific medium)

Treatment

- Option 1: chloramphenicol eye drops +/– oint for 5–7 days
- Option 2: framycetin eye drops for 5–7 days

Gentamicin, tobramycin and quinolone eye drops are not recommended for empirical treatment

Dosage of above antibiotics

- Chloramphenicol 0.5% eye drops, 1–2 drops q2h initially, reduce to q6h as the infection improves +/– 1% chloramphenicol eye oint into conjunctival sac nocte
- Framycetin 0.5% eye drops, 1–2 drops q1–2h initially, reduce to q8h as the infection improves +/– 1% oint into conjunctival sac nocte

CREUTZFELDT-JAKOB DISEASE

Other names: prion disease, transmissible spongiform encephalopathy, Gerstmann-Sträussler-Scheinker syndrome (GSS), fatal familial insomnia (FFI), Alpers syndrome, kuru

Creutzfeldt-Jakob disease (CJD) is a rapidly progressive degenerative neurological disorder causing damage to the brain.

Pathogens

- Caused by prion—the infectious agent of CJD

Classification

1. **Sporadic CJD (sCJD)** (85–90% of cases)—affects one in every million people each year; in Australia, there are likely to be approximately 20 cases per year
2. **Hereditary or familial CJD (fCJD)** (13% of cases)—usually recognised from a family history of the illness; the disease is not always passed on
3. **Iatrogenic CJD (iCJD)**—occurs as a result of medical treatments, including:
   - Use of human pituitary extract growth hormone for infertility or short stature
   - Dura mater grafts used in brain surgery (5 cases in Australia)
   - Corneal grafts (3 cases worldwide)
   - Exposure to contaminated neurosurgical equipment (5 cases worldwide)
4. **Variant CJD (vCJD)**—the human form of bovine spongiform encephalopathy (BSE), (mad cow disease), from consumption of material from animals infected with BSE; it has not been found in Australia
5. **Kuru**—a human prion disease found only in the central highlands of New Guinea

Clinical

CJD is characterised by dementia and walking difficulties:

- Confusion or disorientation, which rapidly advances to a dementia
- Personality and behavioural changes
- Weakness, or loss of balance and muscle control, causing difficulty walking
- Muscle spasms
- Visual symptoms such as double vision or blindness
- Most patients die within 6 months

Laboratory (no firm diagnostic test has been found to confirm CJD)

- Extensive investigations are necessary to exclude other treatable diseases
- CSF analysis of 14-3-3 protein may help the diagnosis
- Brain biopsy after death is the only way to confirm CJD

Treatment

- There is currently no treatment or cure
- Quinacrine (a medicine originally created for malaria)—pilot studies showed quinacrine permanently cleared abnormal prion proteins from cell cultures

CHRONIC OBSTRUCTIVE PULMONARY DISEASE (COPD)—EXACERBATION

Other names: COAD (chronic obstructive airway disease), CAL (chronic airway limitation)

Pathogens

- Virus—common cause of exacerbations
- Bacteria:
  - *Haemophilus influenzae*, *Streptococcus pneumoniae* and *Moraxella catarrhalis*—frequently colonised in the lower airways of COPD patients and are most commonly involved in the exacerbation
  - *Mycoplasma pneumoniae* and *Chlamydia pneumoniae*—relatively frequently seen in the exacerbation
  - *Pseudomonas aeruginosa* and *Staphylococcus aureus*—often encountered in the later stages of COPD (when FEV_1 <35% predicted)
- Non-infectious causes—left ventricular failure, pulmonary embolus and air pollution

Laboratory

- Sputum culture is not recommended unless patient fails to respond to treatment (at least half of patients with COPD are persistently colonised with *H. influenzae*, *S. pneumoniae* or *M. catarrhalis*, hence a positive sputum culture is not necessarily indicative of acute infection)
- Serum procalcitonin assay may help distinguish bacterial infections from viral infections (elevated in bacterial infections and low in viral infections); it may serve as a guide for whether antibiotic treatment is appropriate
- Influenza testing (nasal/throat swabs for influenza antigen test) may be indicated in flu season
- Chest x-ray if suspect pneumonia

Management

- Quit smoking
- Bronchodilators
- Corticosteroids (oral or IV) for moderate to severe exacerbations
- Inhaled steroids may prevent exacerbations in more severe patients (there is concern regarding an increased risk of infection in patients who are on long-term inhaled steroids)
- Immunisation—reduces the risk of exacerbations, hospitalisation and death
  - influenza vaccination (yearly)
  - pneumococcal vaccination (5 yearly)
- Antibiotic therapy

Indication for antibiotic treatment

- Sputum turned to purulent
- Increase in coughing
- Increase in sputum volume
- Increase in dyspnoea
- Fever and leucocytosis

For mild exacerbation
  - Option 1: amoxicillin 500 mg PO q8h (or 1 g PO q12h) for 5 days
  - Option 2: doxycycline 200 mg PO for 1st dose, then 100 mg PO daily for 5 days

If does not respond in 3–5 days, or if resistant organisms are suspected (beta-lactamase-producing *H. influenzae* or penicillin-resistant *S. pneumoniae*)
  - Amoxicillin/clavulanate 875 mg PO q12h for 5–10 days

If penicillin allergy
  - Cefuroxime 500 mg PO q12h for 5–7 days

If immediate penicillin allergy
  - Option 1: doxycycline 100 mg PO q12h for 5–7 days
  - Option 2: moxifloxacin 400 mg PO daily for 5–7 days

For severe exacerbation (respiratory failure, confusion or pneumonia)
  - Hospital admission and IV antibiotic therapy

Prevention of recurrent exacerbations

- Long-acting bronchodilators
- Inhaled corticosteroids
- Long-term low-dose oral macrolides may reduce the frequency of exacerbations (expert advice is recommended before starting long-term antibiotic therapy)

CROUP

Other names: acute larygotracheobronchitis

Pathogens

- *Parainfluenza* virus (most)
- Other viruses
- Bacterial infections (rare)

Clinical

- Most common in children aged 1–3 years
- A coryzal prodrome
- Hoarseness or husky voice
- Biphasic stridor
- Harsh barking 'brassy' cough
- Generally self-limiting, with a course of 3–5 days
- Post-infective cough may last for weeks

Severity of croup

- **Mild croup**—croupy cough, mild chest wall retractions with no stridor at rest
- **Moderate croup**—mild stridor at rest, chest wall retractions, use of accessory muscles
- **Severe croup**—persisting stridor at rest, markedly decreased air entry, increasing fatigue and marked tachycardia
- **Life-threatening croup**—restlessness, decreased consciousness, cyanosis or pallor and hypotonia

Laboratory

- Investigation is not usually required
- Nasopharyngeal aspirate for viral detection may be considered for seriously ill children

Treatment

- Avoid throat examination or separating the child from the parent
- Oxygen therapy is rarely indicated
- Failure to respond to steroid treatment may be due to bacterial tracheitis (rare)
- Antibiotics are not indicated except for severe cases where failure to respond

Mild to moderate croup

- Option 1: budesonide (e.g. Pulmicort) 2 mg/kg neb as a single dose
- Option 2: prednisolone (e.g. Predmix, Redipred) 1 mg/kg PO as a single dose

If settles initially, but later develops stridor at rest with distress, send to the ED

Severe croup

- Adrenaline solution (neb) **plus** budesonide (neb) (**or** dexamethasone [PO or IM or IV] **or** prednisolone [PO])

Admission to intensive care if more than 1 dose of nebulised adrenaline is required

If good response to initial treatment, observe for 4 hours or overnight in the ED

Dosage of above agents

Severe croup

- Adrenaline 0.1% (1 : 1000, 1 mg/ mL) solution 5 mL neb, repeat after 30 min if no improvement
- Budesonide (e.g. Pulmicort) 2 mg/kg neb as a single dose
- Dexamethasone 0.15–0.3 mg/kg (max 12 mg) PO **or** IM **or** IV (if vomiting) as a single dose
- Prednisolone (e.g. Predmix, Redipred) 1 mg/kg PO as a single dose

CRYPTOSPORIDIOSIS

Other names: *Cryptosporidium parvum* gastroenteritis
Cryptosporidium parvum is one of the most common causes of water-borne diarrhoea in humans around the world. It is a leading cause of persistent diarrhoea in developing countries.

Pathogens

- *Cryptosporidium parvum*, an intracellular protozoon
- The sporocysts are resistant to most disinfectants but are susceptible to drying and sunlight

Transmission

- *Cryptosporidium* parasites live in bowels of humans and animals
- Contamination of hands after toileting, handling infected animals or changing nappies of infected infants
- Faecal–oral—infection is from ingesting contaminated foods, drinking contaminated water or unpasteurised milk, or swallowing contaminated swimming pool water
- Contamination of water supply—associated with large outbreaks

High-risk groups

- Young children (incidence is higher in childcare centres)
- Travellers
- People in close contact with animals
- Healthcare workers

Clinical

- **Intestinal cryptosporidiosis**—severe watery diarrhoea, vomiting, abdominal cramps and fever for 2–4 days, may come and go and may last for 1–4 weeks
- **Pulmonary and tracheal cryptosporidiosis** (in the immunocompromised)—coughing, low-grade fever, often accompanied by severe intestinal distress
- Immunocompetent patients—acute self-limiting gastroenteritis
- Immunocompromised patients (especially AIDS patients)—may have the disease for life, with the severe watery diarrhoea contributing to death

Laboratory

- Cryptosporidium antigen test (faeces)
- Faeces microscopy with acid fast staining—to identify cryptosporida oocysts
- Fluorescent antibody—to stain the oocysts isolated from faeces
- Intestinal biopsy for staining—for persistent diarrhoea
- Bronchoscopic biopsy for staining—for pulmonary and tracheal infection

Treatment

- Symptomatic treatment and rehydration, usually self-limiting within 14 days
- For immunocompromised patients, may use:
  - Nitazoxanide* 500 mg (child 1–3 years: 100 mg; 4–11 years: 200 mg) PO q12h for 3 days

Seek expert advice

CYCLOSPORIASIS

Other names: *Cyclospora cayetanensis* gastroenteritis

Pathogen

- *Cyclospora cayetanensis*, a coccidian intracellular protozoan parasite

Endemic regions

- Tropical/subtropical regions such as Peru, Brazil and Haiti

Transmission

- Faecal–oral—ingestion of oocysts in contaminated food or water
- No person-to-person transmission

Incubation

- 7 days

Clinical

- Traveller's diarrhoea—watery diarrhoea, abdominal bloating and cramping, nausea and vomiting, loss of appetite, increased flatulence, fatigue and low-grade fever; the diarrhoea may last from several days to several weeks and relapse if not treated
- More severe forms of disease can occur in immunocompromised patients such as those with AIDS

Diagnosis

- Suspect cyclosporiasis—persistent watery diarrhoea over several days, especially after travelling to an endemic region
- Faeces microscopy—for oocysts (tests may need to be repeated)
- After the oocysts are isolated—tests to identify *Cyclospora cayetanensis* (phase contrast microscopy, modified acid-fast staining or autofluorescence with UV)
- Faecal multiplex PCR testing—sensitivity 98–100%, result available in 24 hours

---

*Nitazoxanide is available via Special Access Scheme <www.tga.gov.au/hp/access-sas.htm> or from compounding chemist

Treatment

- Most diarrhoea caused by *C. cayetanensis* is self-limiting
- Antimicrobial treatment is indicated for:
  - Prolonged and relapsing diarrhoea
  - Immunocompromised patients

For prolonged and relapsing diarrhoea

- Cotrimoxazole (PO) for 7 days

If allergic to sulphonamide

- Option 1: ciprofloxacin (PO) for 7 days
- Option 2: nitazoxanide* (PO) for 3 days

For immunocompromised patients

- Cotrimoxazole (PO) for 10–14 days until symptoms resolve

To prevent relapse in HIV patients with CD4 cell count <200

- Continue with cotrimoxazole (PO) 3 times per week

Dosage of above antibiotics

- Cotrimoxazole 168/800 mg (child: 4/20 mg/kg up to 160/800 mg) PO q12h
- Ciprofloxacin 500 mg (child: 10 mg/kg up to 500 mg) PO q12h
- Nitazoxanide 500 mg (child 1–3 years: 100 mg; 4–11 years: 200 mg) PO q12h

CYSTIC FIBROSIS

Pathogens

- *Haemophilus influenzae*, *Staphylococcus aureus*—often the first organisms recovered in newly diagnosed cystic fibrosis (CF)
- *Pseudomonas aeruginosa*—after repetitive antibiotic exposure, *P. aeruginosa* is usually the predominant organism and may be present as several strains with different antibiotic sensitivities
- *Burkholderia* (formerly *Pseudomonas*) *cepacia*—also pathogenic
- Other gram-negative rods include *Xanthomonas xylosoxidans*, *B. gladioli* and occasionally *Proteus*, *Escherichia coli* and *Klebsiella*
- *Aspergillus fumigatus* (up to 50% and 10% of these patients have allergic bronchopulmonary aspergillosis) (see Aspergillosis, p. 11)

Laboratory

- Respiratory cultures (sputum or bronchoalveolar lavage)—at least annually and during respiratory exacerbations

---

*Nitazoxanide is available via Special Access Scheme <www.tga.gov.au/hp/access-sas.htm> or from compounding chemist

To limit transmission of *Pseudomonas* between patients

- Rigid segregation of both inpatients and outpatients
- Advise CF sufferers not to socialise together

Treatment of infection

For all antibiotic therapy, the choice, dose and duration must be decided in consultation with the specialist CF centre

Infection before *Pseudomonas aeruginosa* is established

- Option 1: flucloxacillin (PO or IV)
- Option 2: cefalexin (PO) (**or** cefazolin [IV])
- Option 3: clindamycin (PO or IV)
- Option 4: cotrimoxazole (PO)
- Option 5: amoxicillin/clavulanate (PO)

Duration of treatment

- 2–4 weeks

Early *Pseudomonas aeruginosa* infection (eradication)

- Option 1: piperacillin/tazobactam (IV) **plus** tobramycin (IV)
- Option 2: ticarcillin/clavulanate (IV) **plus** tobramycin (IV)
- Option 3: cefepime (IV) **plus** tobramycin (IV)
- Option 4: ceftazidime (IV) **plus** tobramycin (IV)
- Option 5: imipenem (IV) **plus** tobramycin (IV)

Duration of treatment

- IV therapy for 2 weeks
- Followed by 2–3 months of oral + inhaled antibiotics
  - Ciprofloxacin (PO) **plus** tobramycin (neb)

Chronic *Pseudomonas aeruginosa* infection (suppression)

Inhaled antibiotics continuously or alternating each drug monthly

- Option 1: tobramycin 300 mg add normal saline to 4 mL neb bid
- Option 2: colistin 150 mg add normal saline to 4 mL neb bid

Azithromycin long-term treatment is effective

- Azithromycin 500 mg (child: 20 mg/kg up to 500 mg) PO 3 times weekly

Burkholderia cepacia complex infection (eradication)

- Up to three IV antibiotics for 2 weeks, followed by oral ciprofloxacin **plus** inhaled tobramycin for up to 2 months

Dosage of above antibiotics

Infection before *Pseudomonas aeruginosa* is established

- Flucloxacillin 500 mg (child: 12.5 mg up to 500 mg) PO q6h
  or flucloxacillin 2 g (child: 50 mg/kg up to 2 g) IV q6h
- Cefalexin 500 mg (child: 25 mg/kg up to 500 mg) PO q6h

- Cefazolin 2 g (child: 50 mg/kg up to 2 g) IV q6h
- Clindamycin 450 mg (child: 10 mg/kg up to 450 mg) PO q8h
or clindamycin 600 mg (child: 15 mg/kg up to 600 mg) IV q8h
- Cotrimoxazole 160/800 mg (child <5 years: 0.4 mg/kg; 6–12 years: 80/400 mg) PO q12h
- Amoxicillin/clavulanate 875 mg (child: 50 mg/kg up to 875 mg) PO q12h

Early *Pseudomonas aeruginosa* infection

- Piperacillin 4 g (child: 100 mg/kg up to 4 g) IV q6–8h
- Tobramycin 4–7 mg/kg IV daily
- Piperacillin/tazobactam 4 g (child: 100 mg/kg up to 4 g) IV q8h
- Ticarcillin/clavulanate 100 mg/kg up to 6 g IV q8h
- Cefepime 1–2 g (child: 50 mg/kg up to 2 g) IV q8–12h
- Ceftazidime 2 g (child: 50 mg/kg up to 2 g) IV q8h
- Imipenem 500 mg–1 g (child: 15–25 mg/kg up to 500 mg–1 g) IV q6h
- Ciprofloxacin 750 mg (child: 15 mg/kg up to 750 mg) PO q12h
- Tobramycin 300 mg add normal saline to 4 mL neb bid

Aerosolised antibiotics play an important role in delaying exacerbations

- Option 1: tobramycin 300 mg add normal saline to 4 mL neb bid
- Option 2: gentamicin 80 mg add normal saline to 4 mL neb bid
- Option 3: ceftazidime 1 g add normal saline to 4 mL neb bid
- Option 4: colistin 150 mg add normal saline to 4 mL neb bid

CYTOMEGALOVIRUS

Pathogens

- Cytomegalovirus (CMV), commonly known as Human Herpesvirus 5 (HHV-5)
- All herpesviruses share a characteristic ability to remain latent in the body over long periods or lifelong

Transmission

- Person-to-person by repeated prolonged intimate exposure through saliva, urine, faeces, sexual contact, breastfeeding
- From transplanted organs
- From blood transfusions (rare)
- From mother to fetus

Clinical

- CMV is found all over the world and infects 50–80% of adults
- Healthy people—most are asymptomatic, some may have a glandular fever-like syndrome (CMV mononucleosis)
- Pregnant women—primary CMV infection occurs in about 1 in 300 pregnancies but the majority of women are asymptomatic

- Immunocompromised people (e.g. organ transplant, HIV infection, cancer, chemotherapy or haemodialysis)—CMV is much more aggressive in these patients and is a major cause of death

CMV infection may cause

- Immunocompromised people—CMV pneumonitis, CMV retinitis, CMV oesophagitis, CMV colitis and CMV hepatitis (may cause fulminant liver failure)
- Congenital CMV infection—CMV is the most common cause of congenital infection in humans and it is one of the TORCH infections (Toxoplasmosis, Rubella, CMV and Herpes simplex) that lead to fetal congenital abnormalities
- Infection is due to a primary infection or viral reactivation in pregnant woman
- Fetal infection occurs in 40% of pregnant women with primary CMV infection
- The infected fetus may have congenital abnormalities; including hearing loss; low birth weight; pneumonia; GIT, retinal and neurological abnormalities

Laboratory

- Microscopy: intranuclear inclusion bodies ('owl's eye')—urine, saliva, blood, tears, semen, or breast milk
- CMV serology
- PCR for CMV—blood, CSF or viral transport swab
- Biopsy—demonstration of CMV in tissue

Prophylaxis

CMV prophylaxis is indicated (either donor or recipient is CMV IgG positive):

- Solid organ transplant
- Allogeneic HSCT recipients
  - Valganciclovir 900 mg PO daily from day 10 to 3–6 months

In allogeneic HSCT recipients with graft-versus-host disease

  - Ganciclovir 5 mg/kg IV on 5–7 days per week from engraftment until day 100 (or until day 180 if significant ongoing immunosuppression at day 100)

Treatment

- Healthy individuals—no treatment is generally needed
- Immunocompromised patients—CMV antiviral drug therapy is indicated

Treatment of CMV retinitis, pneumonitis or colitis

  - Ganciclovir 5 mg/kg IV q12h for 2 weeks

Once a response to IV treatment has been established, may change to oral
- Valganciclovir 900 mg PO q12h to complete 2 weeks of treatment

If ganciclovir resistance is confirmed
- Option 1: foscarnet 90 mg/kg IV q12h for 2 weeks
- Option 2: cidofovir 5 mg/kg IV weekly with probenecid* for 2 weeks

For maintenance to prevent recurrence (if chronic severe immunosuppression)
- Option 1: valganciclovir 900 mg PO daily
- Option 2: ganciclovir 10 mg/kg IV 3 times weekly
- Option 3: foscarnet 90–120 mg/kg/day IV 5 times weekly

CMV immunoglobulin

- May be used with antiviral drugs in treatment of severe CMV infection
- Prevention of CMV infection in immunosuppressed patients at high risk of severe CMV infection (e.g. after bone marrow and renal transplants)—may be used with antiviral drugs to improve outcome
- May be used in high-risk pregnant women—treat primary infection and may protect fetus from congenital CMV infection
  - CMV immunoglobulin-VF 50 000 U/kg IV, repeat after 4–5 days, then every 10–14 days

CMV vaccine

- Still in research and development stage

Advice for pregnant women on prevention of CMV infection

- Good personal hygiene, handwashing with soap and water after contact with nappies or oral secretions (particularly in childcare settings)
- If develop a mononucleosis-like illness during pregnancy, check CMV serology and counsel about the possible risks to the unborn baby
- The benefits of breastfeeding outweigh the minimal risk of acquiring CMV from the breastfeeding mother

Newborn CMV testing

- Early (before 3 weeks of age) newborn CMV testing (saliva and blood samples) with antiviral treatment—could prevent hearing loss

---

*Probenecid 2 g PO 3 hours prior to cidofovir infusion, then 1 g PO at 2 hours and 8 hours after completion of cidofovir infusion (total of 4 g)

D

DACRYOCYSTITIS

Other name: tear sac infection

Dacryocystitis is an infection of the nasolacrimal sac (tear sac), usually associated with obstruction of the nasolacrimal duct.

Pathogens

- *Staphylococcus aureus*
- *Streptococcus pyogenes*
- *Pseudomonas* spp

Clinical

- **Acute dacryocystitis**—pain, swelling and redness over lacrimal sac at medial canthus with tearing, crusting and fever; digital pressure over lacrimal sac may extrude pus through punctum; delay of treatment may lead to local abscess
- **Chronic dacryocystitis**—blockage of nasolacrimal duct, swelling of lacrimal sac, usually painless, tearing may be the only symptom
- **Infantile dacryocystitis**—the nasolacrimal duct may not open at birth until the baby is 3 months old; the tear sac tends to be infected and produce sticky discharge

Treatment

1. Acute dacryocystitis

- Warm compresses, massage lacrimal sac and duct, decongestants
- Lacrimal discharge for culture (massage the tear sac)
- Early antibiotic therapy may prevent abscess formation

Mild cases

- Chloramphenicol (e.g. Chlorsig) eye drops, 1–2 drops qid for 5 days

More severe cases

- Flucloxacillin 500 mg (child: 12.5 mg up to 500 mg) PO q6h

If penicillin allergy

- Cefalexin 500 mg (child: 12.5 mg/kg up to 500 mg) PO q6h

If immediate penicillin allergy or MRSA is suspected

- Seek expert advice

If abscess has formed, refer to an ophthalmologist for external drainage

2. Chronic dacryocystitis

- Syringing the lacrimal system regularly
- If infection occurs, obtain cultures by aspiration
- Dacryocystorhinostomy (DCR) may be needed—refer to an ophthalmologist

3. Infantile dacryocystitis

- Teach the mother to massage the tear sac (to empty the contents) 4 times a day

- Antibiotic eye drops (e.g. gentamicin) to prevent/treat infection
- If the blockage persists after several months, probing of the duct under anaesthesia may be needed

DENGUE FEVER

Pathogens

- **Dengue fever**—dengue viruses (1–4), arbovirus
- **Dengue haemorrhagic fever**—dengue HF, a serotype of dengue virus different from dengue viruses 1–4

Distribution

- Australia (Queensland and Northern Territory), Southeast Asia, Africa and South America

Transmission

- Bite from day-biting mosquitoes (*Aedes aegypti* and *A. albopictus*)
- May also be transmitted via infected blood products and needle-stick injury

Incubation

- 2–7 days

Clinical

- **Dengue fever**—sudden onset of fever, headache, rash, nausea and vomiting, adenopathy, back pain along with severe myalgia ('break-bone fever') and arthralgia; red maculopapular rash that spares palms of hand and soles of feet
- **Dengue haemorrhagic fever (dengue HF)**—may cause thrombocytopenia, haemorrhagic complications
- **Dengue shock syndrome**—hypotension
- **Dengue meningoencephalitis**—severe headache with stiff neck and neurological signs

Infection with one serotype does not provide immunity to other serotypes

Laboratory

- FBC—may have leucopenia, thrombocytopenia (dengue HF)
- LFT—liver damage (serum aminotransferase elevation)
- Dengue virus PCR—early detection
- Dengue virus serology (blood or CSF)—positive IgM to dengue virus or dengue IgG seroconversion or ≥four-fold rise in titre (in the absence of IgM or IgG seroconversion to Murray Valley encephalitis virus, Kunjin virus and Japanese encephalitis virus)
- Dengue viral culture—from blood (in acute phase)

Differential diagnosis

For returned travellers with fever (Table 4.1)

TABLE 4.1

DIFFERENTIAL DIAGNOSIS FOR RETURNED TRAVELLERS WITH FEVER

	CRP	Leucocyte	Platelet
Dengue fever	Normal	Low ++	Low +
Malaria	High	Normal	Low ++
Enteric fever	High	Low +	Normal

Treatment

- Supportive treatment
- Avoid aspirin
- For dengue HF—hospital admission, fluid replacement, blood transfusion and corticosteroids

Prevention

- Mosquito control and avoidance
- Dengue vaccine against all 4 strains of the virus is in the stage of clinical trial

DENTAL INFECTION

Other names: tooth infection, toothache, tooth abscess

Dental infections

- **Gingivitis** (see Gingivitis, p. 129)
- **Dental caries** (see below)
- **Pulpitis and periapical abscess** (see below)
- **Periodontitis and periodontal abscess** (see below)
- **Deep dental infection** (see below)
- **Ludwig's angina** (see Ludwig's angina, p. 207)

1.   DENTAL CARIES

Dental caries damage the structures of teeth, cause tooth decay or cavities. They can lead to toothache, infection and tooth loss.

Pathogens

- Certain types of acid-producing bacteria (e.g. *Lactobacillus* spp, *Streptococcus mutans* and *Actinomyces* spp)

Prevention of caries

- Brushing, flossing, water picks and mouthwashes
- Chewing gum containing xylitol (wood sugar)
- Limiting sweet drinks and not giving bottles to infants during sleep

- Regular dental examinations and cleaning
- Water fluoridation, fluoride supplements, fluoride toothpaste or mouthwash
- Vaccines for dental caries are undergoing clinical trials

2. PULPITIS AND PERIAPICAL ABSCESS

Caries penetrate though tooth enamel and dentin into pulp cavity, leading to infection (pulpitis). The infection may find its way out and form periapical abscesses.

Treatment

- Antibiotic therapy—if facial swelling and systemic symptoms and signs are present (see Deep dental infection below)
- Root canal therapy
- Extraction of the tooth

3. PERIODONTITIS AND PERIODONTAL ABSCESS

Inflammation of the periodontium involving the gingiva, cementum, alveolar bone and periodontal ligaments. This causes progressive, irreversible bone loss around teeth, looseness of teeth and eventual loss of teeth. Sometimes pus is collected in the periodontal space (periodontal abscess).

Pathogens

- Anaerobes, Streptococcal spp, herpes virus

Clinical

- Gum bleeding while brushing teeth or biting into hard food (e.g. apple), recurrent gum swellings, halitosis and bad taste, gingival recession, deep pockets between teeth and gums and loose teeth
- Periodontitis is largely painless, but periodontal abscess (a localised gum swelling) may cause dull pain

Treatment

- Patient education on oral hygiene
- Smoking cessation
- Dental cleaning to remove calculus and plaque
- Periodontal surgery for advanced periodontal disease
- Antibiotic therapy if facial swelling and systemic symptoms and signs are present (see Deep dental infection below)

4. DEEP DENTAL INFECTION

Dental infection spreads from tooth to surrounding soft tissues or into upper neck, may cause trismus (difficulty in opening mouth due to spasm and pain) or airway obstruction.

Treatment

- Local surgical or dental treatment
- Antibiotic therapy is indicated if:
    - Facial swelling
    - Systemic symptoms and signs

Antibiotics should only be used as an adjunct to dental treatment

Mild dental infection

- Amoxicillin (**or** penicillin V) (PO) for 5 days

More severe dental infection

- Option 1: amoxicillin/clavulanate (PO) for 5 days
- Option 2: amoxicillin (PO) **plus** metronidazole (PO) for 5 days

If allergic to penicillin

- Clindamycin (PO) for 5 days

If fail to respond to antibiotic therapy

Prompt referral to a dentist or periodontist

Dosage of above antibiotics

- Amoxicillin 500 mg (child: 15 mg/kg up to 500 mg) PO q8h
- Penicillin V 500 mg (child: 10 mg/kg up to 500 mg) PO q6h
- Amoxicillin/clavulanate 875 mg (child: 22.5 mg/kg up to 875 mg) PO q12h
- Metronidazole 400 mg (child: 10 mg/kg up to 400 mg) PO q12h
- Clindamycin 300 mg (child: 10 mg/kg up to 300 mg) PO q8h

DIABETIC FOOT INFECTION

Pathogens

- Mixed gram-positive and gram-negative aerobes
- *Staphylococcus aureus*
- Anaerobes

Treatment

- Uninfected ulcers—cultures and antibiotic treatment are unnecessary
- Wound swab for culture if infected
- Surgical debridement and tissue sent for culture
- Good control of diabetes
- Antibiotic therapy—should cover both aerobes and anaerobes
- Hyperbaric oxygen therapy—may be used for severe or unresponsive infections

Mild to moderate infection

- Option 1: amoxicillin/clavulanate (PO) for at least 5 days
- Option 2: cefalexin (PO) **plus** metronidazole (PO) for at least 5 days

If immediate penicillin allergy
- Ciprofloxacin (PO) **plus** clindamycin (PO) for at least 5 days

Severe infection (systemic toxicity, deep ulceration, severe cellulitis, septic shock, necrosis or gangrene, or presence of osteomyelitis)

- Option 1: piperacillin/tazobactam (IV)
- Option 2: ticarcillin/clavulanate (IV)
- Option 3: ciprofloxacin (IV) **plus** clindamycin (IV) (If penicillin allergy)

If there is severe limb or life-threatening infection
- Vancomycin (IV) (added to any of above regimen)
- Adjust antibiotic—according to the susceptibility
- Outpatient parenteral antimicrobial therapy—if prolonged IV therapy is required
- Change to oral therapy—after substantial improvement
- Continue antibiotic therapy—until the infection has resolved
- After amputation—cease antibiotic therapy 2–5 days later

Dosage of above antibiotics

- Amoxicillin/clavulanate 875 mg PO q12h
- Cefalexin 500 mg PO q6h
- Metronidazole 400 mg PO q12h
- Ciprofloxacin 500 mg PO q12h
- Clindamycin 300–450 mg PO q8h
- Piperacillin/tazobactam 4 g IV q8h (q6h for *Pseudomonas aeruginosa*)
- Ticarcillin/clavulanate 3 g IV q6h
- Ciprofloxacin 400 mg IV q12h (q8h for *Pseudomonas aeruginosa*)
- Clindamycin 900 mg IV q8h (slow infusion)
- Vancomycin 25–30 mg/kg IV for the 1st dose (further dosing see p. 462)

DIARRHOEA—UNKNOWN CAUSE

Note

- Most diarrhoea is due to viral infection—does not require antibiotics
- Most cases of bacterial diarrhoea are self-limiting—do not usually require antibiotics
- Indications for antibiotic therapy in acute diarrhoea of unknown cause:
1. Severe diarrhoea that is likely to be bacterial in origin
2. Patient has serious underlying disease or is immunocompromised
3. Invasive bacterial diarrhoea (bloody diarrhoea [see Fig 4.1] and rigors/fevers)
4. Persistent diarrhoea (>1–2 weeks)—a trial of antibiotic therapy may be considered (see Fig. 4.2)

Antibiotic treatment should be started after collection of faecal samples for microscopic examination and culture

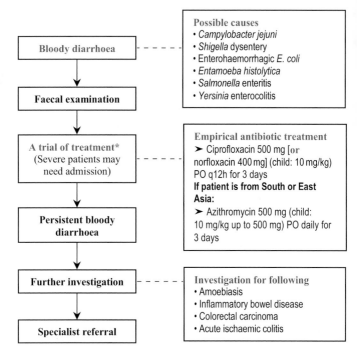

Possible causes
- *Campylobacter jejuni*
- *Shigella* dysentery
- Enterohaemorrhagic *E. coli*
- *Entamoeba histolytica*
- *Salmonella* enteritis
- *Yersinia* enterocolitis

Empirical antibiotic treatment
➤ Ciprofloxacin 500 mg [or norfloxacin 400 mg] (child: 10 mg/kg) PO q12h for 3 days
If patient is from South or East Asia:
➤ Azithromycin 500 mg (child: 10 mg/kg up to 500 mg) PO daily for 3 days

Investigation for following
- Amoebiasis
- Inflammatory bowel disease
- Colorectal carcinoma
- Acute ischaemic colitis

*Child with bloody diarrhoea without fever—do not use empirical antibiotic (potentially precipitating haemolytic uraemic syndrome if it is caused by enterohaemorrhagic *E. coli*).

FIGURE 4.1

Management of bloody diarrhoea

DIARRHOEA IN IMMUNOCOMPROMISED PATIENTS

Pathogens

- Bacteria
- Viruses (e.g. cytomegalovirus)
- Parasites (e.g. *Cryptosporidium* spp, Isospora *belli,* microsporidia spp)

Laboratory

- Cytomegalovirus testing
- Faecal parasites testing

Treatment

- Treat the pathogen(s) according to faecal test report
- If bacterial infection is suspected, even in mild disease, consider empirical antibiotic therapy

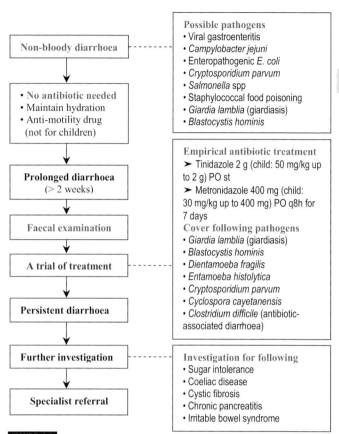

FIGURE 4.2

Management of non-bloody diarrhoea

DIENTAMOEBIASIS

Other names: *Dientamoeba fragilis* infection

Pathogen

- *Dientamoeba fragilis*—a non-flagellate trichomonad parasite

Prevalence

- In developed countries prevalence rate is 2–4%
- In developing countries (crowded and poor hygiene conditions) prevalence rate is 19–69%
- Higher infection rate in travellers to developing countries

Transmission

- Direct faecal–oral spread
- Possibly through coinfection of *Enterobius vermicularis* (pinworm)

Clinical

- The most common age group: children 5–10 years
- Many infected people do not have symptoms
- Symptoms—acute and relapsing diarrhoea with abdominal pain, bloating, fever, fatigue, loss of appetite and loss of weight
- Recurrent diarrhoea may be misdiagnosed as 'irritable bowel syndrome'

Laboratory

- Faeces OCP microscopy for *D. fragilis*—to find *D. fragilis* trophozoites
- Faecal multiplex PCR testing—sensitivity 98–100%, result available in 24 hours

Treatment

- Asymptomatic carrier—no treatment is required
- Symptomatic patient—antibiotic treatment
  - Option 1: doxycycline (PO) for 10 days
  - Option 2: metronidazole (PO) for 10 days

If no response, use either of following combination therapy

  - Doxycycline + secnidazole* (PO) for 10 days
  - Nitazoxanide* + furazolidone* + secnidazole* (PO) for 10 days

Dientamoeba fragilis + *Blastocystis hominis* infection coexisting

  - Option 1: doxycycline + cotrmoxazole + diloxanide furoate* + secnidazole* (PO) for 10 days
  - Option 2: doxycycline + nitazoxanide* + furazolidone* + secnidazole* (PO) for 10 days

Dosage of above antibiotics

  - Doxycycline 100 mg (child >8 years: 2 mg/kg up to 100 mg) PO bid
  - Metronidazole 400 mg (child: 10 mg/kg up to 400 mg) PO tds
  - Doxycycline 50 mg (child >8 years: 1 mg/kg up to 50 mg) PO bid
  - Secnidazole 400 mg PO tds
  - Nitazoxanide 500 mg PO bid
  - Furazolidone 100 mg PO tds
  - Cotrmoxazole 160/800 mg PO bid
  - Diloxanide furoate 500 mg PO tds

---

*Available via Special Access Scheme <www.tga.gov.au/hp/access-sas.htm> or from compounding chemist

Note

- Repeat stool test 4–6 weeks after treatment to determine the eradication
- All family members (particularly siblings) should have stool test for *D. fragilis* and other infestations such as *E. vermicularis* (pinworm)

DIPHTHERIA

Diphtheria may occur in returned travellers from overseas.

Pathogens

- *Corynebacterium diphtheriae*, an aerobic gram-positive bacillus
- Its exotoxin causes an adherent pseudomembrane on the respiratory tract
- The toxin also acts on cells of the myocardium, nervous system and adrenals

Transmission

- By droplets or direct contact with skin sores or articles soiled by infected persons
- It is infectious for up to 4 weeks; carrier may shed bacteria for longer

Incubation

- 2–5 days

Clinical

- Pharyngeal diphtheria—fever, sore throat, tonsillitis, white nasal/throat membrane, hoarseness, dysphagia; may have airway obstruction

Complications

- Cardiomyopathy
- Neuropathy
- Shock (may be fatal)

Laboratory

- Nasal/throat swab—culture for *C. diphtheriae* (specific transport and culture media)
- Histopathological diagnosis of diphtheria

Treatment

- Isolate patient and treat urgently—do not wait for bacteriological confirmation
- Intubation or a tracheotomy—if airway obstruction occurs; ECG monitoring
- Diphtheria antitoxin—should be given immediately
- Antibiotic—hastens recovery and prevents spread of disease to others

Diphtheria antitoxin

- Diphtheria antitoxin* (first give a test dose to exclude hypersensitivity) IM or IV

If hypersensitive to diphtheria antitoxin

- Administer diphtheria antitoxin under corticosteroid, adrenaline and antihistamine

Antibiotic treatment

- Benzylpenicillin 1.2 g (child: 30 mg/kg up to 1.2 g) IV q6h for 10 days

Prophylaxis for close contacts (take throat swabs for culture)

- Diphtheria vaccine booster (e.g. ADT or dTpa) 0.5 mL IM st
- Erythromycin 250 mg PO q6h for 10 days

Therapeutic dose of antitoxin will depend on patient's clinical condition

Diphtheria vaccination

- Primary course: DTPa 0.5 mL IM, 3 doses at (6 weeks or) 2, 4 and 6 months of age
- 1st booster: DTPa 0.5 mL IM, at 3.5–4 years of age
- 2nd booster: dTpa 0.5 mL IM, at 10–17 years of age
- Further booster: dTpa 0.5 mL IM, at 50 years of age (if no dT in previous 10 years)

DIVERTICULITIS

Other names: diverticular disease, diverticulosis

Pathogens

- Overgrowth of normal colonic bacteria

Clinical

- More common in elderly and obese people; 20% of cases <50 years of age
- Left-sided (95%) abdominal pain, nausea, fever and left lower quadrant tenderness
- May have constipation/alteration in bowel habits
- WBC and CRP elevation; CT abdomen confirms the diagnosis

Treatment

Mild diverticulitis

- If no improvement in 2–3 days—CT abdomen to exclude intra-abdominal abscess
  - Option 1: amoxicillin/clavulanate (PO) for 5 days
  - Option 2: cefalexin **plus** metronidazole (PO) for 5 days

---

*Available via Special Access Scheme <www.tga.gov.au/hp/access-sas.htm>

- Option 3: cotrimoxazole **plus** metronidazole (PO) for 5 days (if penicillin allergy)

Dosage of above antibiotics

- Amoxicillin/clavulanate 875 mg PO q12h
- Cefalexin 500 mg PO q6h
- Metronidazole 400 mg PO q12h
- Cotrimoxazole 160/800 mg PO q12h

Severe diverticulitis with or without bowel perforation

- Significant systemic signs, fever or with peritonism
- Hospital admission
- Nil-by-mouth, IV fluids, analgesia, IV antibiotics
- CT abdomen; if bowel perforation, abscess or rectal bleeding—surgical referral
  - Ampi(amoxi)cillin **plus** gentamicin **plus** metronidazole (IV)
- If gentamicin treatment >72 hours or is contraindicated
  - Piperacillin/tazobactam (**or** ticarcillin/clavulanate) (IV)
- If non-immediate penicillin allergy
  - Ceftriaxone (**or** cefotaxime) (IV) **plus** metronidazole (IV) **plus** metronidazole (IV)
- If immediate penicillin allergy
  - Gentamicin **plus** clindamycin (IV)

Switch to oral therapy once afebrile for 1–2 days (see mild diverticulitis above)

Dosage of above antibiotics

- Ampi(amoxy)cillin 2 g IV q6h
- Gentamicin 4–7 mg/kg IV for the 1st dose (further dosing see p. 459)
- Metronidazole 500 mg IV q12h
- Piperacillin/tazobactam 4 g IV q8h
- Ticarcillin/clavulanate 3 g IV q6h
- Ceftriaxone 1 g IV daily
- Cefotaxime 1 g IV q8h
- Clindamycin 600 mg (child: 15 mg/kg up to 600 mg) IV q8h

DONOVANOSIS

Other names: *Granuloma inguinale, Granuloma venereum*
Donovanosis is a chronic destructive bacterial infection of the genital region with ulceration and epitheliomatous hyperplasia.

Distribution

- It is found in central and northern Australia and overseas (Papua New Guinea, India and southern Africa)

Pathogen

- *Klebsiella granulomatis* (formerly known as *Calymmatobacterium granulomatis*)—a gram-negative rod

Transmission

- Sexually transmitted through contact with open sores

Incubation

- 1–12 weeks

Clinical

- Initially a painless, red nodule that slowly grows into one or more round and raised lumps
- Later the lumps burst and create open, fleshy, oozing ulcers
- The infection continues to destroy tissue until treated
- Sites of infection include penis, scrotum, groin and thighs in men; and vulva, vagina, groin and perineum in women
- Extragenital lesions may occur in mouth, lips, throat and face

Laboratory

- Microscopy of scrapings, aspirates, snip or punch biopsy—intracellular Donovan bodies (cytoplasmic inclusions)
- PCR for *Klebsiella granulomatis* (from a specimen of a lesion)

Treatment

- Directly observed therapy or hospital admission for supervised therapy may be necessary
- Normally, the infection will begin to subside within a week of treatment
- Follow-up is important as resolution may be slow and recurrence can occur
- If lesions have not healed after 6 weeks, biopsy to exclude other diagnosis
  - Option 1: azithromycin 1 g PO weekly for at least 4 weeks and until resolution
  - Option 2: azithromycin 500 mg PO daily for 7 days
  - Option 3: doxycycline 100 mg PO q12h for at least 4 weeks and until resolution

Prevention

- Avoid sexual contact with individuals in endemic regions
- STI testing before beginning a sexual relationship
- Children born via vaginal delivery to women with active donovanosis should receive prophylactic azithromycin (seek expert advice)

ENCEPHALITIS—VIRAL

Other names: aseptic encephalitis

Pathogens

1. Herpesviruses

- Herpes simplex virus (HSV-1 and HSV-2)—the most common cause of sporadic viral encephalitis worldwide (see Herpes simplex encephalitis, p. 160)
- Varicella zoster virus (HHV-3) (VZV) (see Herpes zoster, p. 162)
- Epstein-Barr virus (HHV-4) (see Glandular fever, p. 132)
- Cytomegalovirus (HHV-5) (see Cytomegalovirus, p. 73)
- Human herpes virus 6 (HHV-6) and 7 (HHV-7)

2. Enteroviruses

- Enterovirus (serotypes 68–71)—the major cause of viral encephalitis in children (see *Enterovirus 71*, p. 105)
- Polioviruses (3 serotypes) (see Poliomyelitis, p. 312)
- Coxsackievirus A (23 serotypes)
- Coxsackievirus B (6 serotypes)
- Echovirus (31 serotypes)
- Parechovirus

3. Arboviruses

- West Nile virus (WNV)—the most common seasonal viral encephalitis in Australia (see West Nile virus, p. 439)
- Murray Valley encephalitis (MVE) virus—the most common flavivirus encephalitis in Australia (see Murray Valley encephalitis, p. 239)
- Dengue virus (see Dengue fever, p. 77)
- Kunjin virus (see Kunjin virus, p. 195)
- Eastern and Western equine encephalitis virus
- Japanese encephalitis virus (see Japanese encephalitis, p. 188)
- Yellow fever virus (see Yellow fever, p. 454)
- Tick-borne encephalitis
- St Louis encephalitis virus
- California encephalitis virus (*Bunyavirus* group, including La Crosse encephalitis virus)

4. Other viruses

- Measles virus (a paramyxovirus) and measles vaccine (see Measles, p. 216)
- Lymphocytic choriomeningitis (LCM) virus
- Human immunodeficiency virus (HIV)
- Mumps virus (a paramyxovirus) (see Mumps, p. 238)
- Adenovirus (serotypes 1, 6, 7, 12 and 32) (see Adenovirus, p. 4)
- Influenza virus and parainfluenza virus (see Influenza, p. 184)

- Hendra virus (HeV) and Nipah virus (see Hendra and Nipah viruses, p. 144)
- Australian bat lyssavirus (ABL) (see Rabies and Australian bat lyssavirus, p. 345)
- Rabies virus (see Rabies and Australian bat lyssavirus, p. 345)
- Rotavirus (see Rotavirus, p. 352)

Clinical

- Viral illness—flu-like symptoms, headache, fever, malaise
- Rapid decline in mental status—confusion
- Focal neurological signs—ataxia, hemiparesis, aphasia, cranial nerve signs
- Seizures—in 50% patients

Some clues suggest specific viral encephalitis

- Aphasia, hallucinations and acute personality changes—HSV encephalitis
- Child with high fever + skin blisters/mouth ulcers + flaccid paralysis—enterovirus encephalitis (EV71)
- Recent travel, outdoor exposure and tick bites—an arbovirus infection
- Parotitis, orchitis and pancreatitis—mumps encephalitis
- Skin vesicular outbreak—VZV or HSV encephalitis

Diagnosis

- Diagnosis of viral encephalitis—viral illness + mental status change/focal neurological signs + exclude other causes of brain damage
- Identify causative virus—history of travel/animal exposure/vaccination (to narrow possible causative viruses) + viral testing

Travel

- Northern Australia—MVE (at times of high regional rainfall), Kunjin, scrub typhus, Japanese encephalitis, Hendra, dengue, Australian bat lyssavirus
- Southeast Asia—Japanese encephalitis, rabies, tick-borne encephalitis, scrub typhus, dengue, Nipah
- America—rabies, Eastern and Western equine encephalitis, Venezuelan equine encephalitis, St Louis encephalitis
- Europe—West Nile, tick-borne encephalitis

Animal exposure

- Bats (Australia)—Australian bat lyssavirus
- Canid spp (endemic countries)—rabies
- Arthropods (Australia and overseas)—MVE/Kunjin, scrub typhus, Q fever, Japanese encephalitis
- Horses (Australia)—Hendra virus
- Rodents (Australia and overseas)—murine typhus, Hantavirus
- Monkeys (overseas, research facilities)—herpes simian B virus

Laboratory

Contact laboratory for available tests

- Rapid serum procalcitonin test—may help distinguish viral meningitis from bacterial meningitis (high in bacterial infections and low in viral infections)
- Throat and faecal viral culture—for enterovirus
- Viral serology—for enterovirus, CMV, EBV, VZV, WNV and HIV
- Convalescent serological tests at week 4—for HSV, flaviviruses and VZV (antibody titres four-fold rise is diagnostic)
- Blood viral isolation—for WNV, lymphocytic choriomeningitis (early in disease)
- Urine viral isolation—for lymphocytic choriomeningitis (later in disease)
- CSF microscopy—non-traumatic elevation of RBC suggests HSV encephalitis or other haemorrhagic encephalitis
- CSF PCR—for HSV, enteroviruses, CMV, EBV, VZV, WNV, HIV
- CSF viral antibodies—HSV, WNV, MVE/Kunjin, Japanese encephalitis
- CSF viral culture—for enteroviruses, lymphocytic choriomeningitis virus, mumps virus and some arboviruses (contact laboratory)
- CT, MRI—identify the region of involvement and exclude other processes; HSV encephalitis, Japanese encephalitis and enterovirus 71 encephalitis have characteristic findings on MRI
- EEG—temporal lobe involvement—suggests HSV encephalitis
- Brain biopsy and viral culture—reserved for patients who demonstrate clinical decline despite empirical therapy

Treatment

- Most viral encephalitis—mild; recover spontaneously
- Small number of cases can be very serious, leading to brain damage, coma and death
- Supportive treatment and seizure control
- Antiviral treatment only available for following viral encephalitis

1. HSV encephalitis

Start empirical aciclovir therapy if HSV is suspected:

- Fever + confusion and acute personality changes +/- seizure
- EEG—abnormalities in the temporal lobe(s)
- MRI brain—characteristic changes in the temporal lobes
- CSF HSV PCR—positive (treatment should start early without waiting for the result)

Early treatment (within 48 hours) reduces mortality

- Aciclovir 10 mg/kg (child <5 years: 20 mg/kg; >5 years: 15 mg/kg) IV q8h for 2–3 weeks

If CSF PCR for HSV is positive, repeat CSF PCR in 2 weeks
If the 2nd CSF PCR becomes negative, aciclovir can be stopped

2. VZV

Aciclovir or ganciclovir
- Option 1: aciclovir 10 mg/kg IV q8h for 1–2 weeks
- Option 2: ganciclovir 5 mg/kg IV q12h for 1–2 weeks

3. CMV

Ganciclovir + foscarnet

- Ganciclovir 5 mg/kg IV q12h **plus** foscarnet 60 mg/kg IV q8h for 2–3 weeks

4. EBV

Aciclovir (limited effect) or cidofovir

- Empirical: aciclovir 10 mg/kg IV q8h for 1–2 weeks
- Confirmed: cidofovir 5 mg/kg IV weekly for 2 weeks + probenecid

5. HHV-6

Ganciclovir or foscarnet
- Option 1: ganciclovir 5 mg/kg IV q12h for 2–3 weeks
- Option 2: foscarnet 60 mg/kg IV q8h for 2–3 weeks

6. Enteroviruses (including EV71)

May use pleconaril (binds to a cleft in enteroviruses and prevents host cell–receptor interaction with the virus)

ENDOCARDITIS—EMPIRICAL THERAPY

Management

- Blood cultures with minimum inhibitory concentration (MIC) for penicillin:
    - 3 sets of blood from different sites prior to antibiotic therapy
    - may withhold empirical therapy in stable patients until the causative pathogen is isolated
    - if cultures remain negative after 2–3 days, send additional 2–3 blood cultures
- Patients with acute endocarditis or with deteriorating haemodynamics who may require urgent surgery should be treated empirically immediately after initial blood cultures are obtained
- Serology tests may be used for some uncommon pathogens, such as *Brucella*, *Bartonella*, *Legionella* (urinary antigen test), *Chlamydia*, *Mycoplasma* and *Coxiella burnetii* (Q fever pathogen) (see Endocarditis—culture-negative, p. 101)
- PCR for unique microbial DNA or 16S rRNA—to identify pathogens
- Consult with a cardiologist, an infectious disease practitioner or a clinical microbiologist

- Consult with a cardiovascular surgeon if the infection is fulminant or complicated, or if it involves aneurysms or intravascular prostheses

1. NATIVE VALVE ENDOCARDITIS

Empirical therapy

- Benzylpenicillin (IV) **plus** flucloxacillin (IV) **plus** gentamicin (IV)

If MRSA is suspected* or for fulminant endocarditis

- Vancomycin (IV) **plus** flucloxacillin (IV) **plus** gentamicin (IV)

If penicillin allergy

- Vancomycin (IV) **plus** cefalotin (**or** cefazolin) (IV) **plus** gentamicin (IV)

If immediate penicillin allergy

- Vancomycin (IV) **plus** gentamicin (IV)

Modify regimens once causative organism and susceptibility are available
Gentamicin may be continued only for streptococcal and enterococcal endocarditis

Dosage of above antibiotics

- Benzylpenicillin 1.8 g (child: 50 mg/kg up to 1.8 g) IV q4h
- Flucloxacillin 2 g (child: 50 mg/kg up to 2 g) IV q4h
- Gentamicin IV once daily (dosing see p. 459)
- Vancomycin IV (dosing see p. 462)
- Cefalotin 2 g (child: 50 mg/kg up to 2 g) IV q4h
- Cefazolin 2 g (child: 50 mg/kg up to 2 g) IV q8h

2. PROSTHETIC VALVE AND PACEMAKER lEAD ENDOCARDITIS

Pathogens

- *Staphylococcus aureus*
- Coagulase-negative staphylococci
- *Corynebacterium* spp
- *Streptococcus* spp
- Enterococci
- Enteric gram-negative rods
- *Pseudomonas aeruginosa*
- *Candida albicans* and other fungi

Management

- Transoesophageal echocardiography for diagnosis
- Scrupulous surgical technique and antibiotic prophylaxis—reduce the risk of infection
- Removal of pacing device and leads transvenously or at open-heart surgery
- Removal of all infected material in pocket infection

---

*MRSA is suspected if the infection is healthcare-associated or in IV drug users

- May need insertion of a temporary pacing wire at the same procedure
- Early consultation with a cardiologist, cardiac surgeon and infectious disease practitioner

Empirical therapy

- Vancomycin (IV) **plus** flucloxacillin (IV) **plus** gentamicin (IV)

If penicillin allergy

- Vancomycin (IV) **plus** cefalotin (**or** cefazolin) (IV) **plus** gentamicin (IV)

If immediate penicillin allergy

- Vancomycin (IV) **plus** gentamicin (IV)

Modify regimen once causative organism and susceptibility are available

Gentamicin may be continued only for streptococcal and enterococcal endocarditis

Duration of therapy after valve surgery

At the time of valve surgery take valve tissues for culture:

- if valve culture is negative, complete the recommended duration or for at least a further 2 weeks, whichever is longer
- if valve culture is positive, 4–6 weeks postoperative treatment

Dosage of above antibiotics

- Vancomycin IV (dosing see p. 462)
- Flucloxacillin 2 g (child: 50 mg/kg up to 2 g) IV q4h
- Gentamicin IV once daily (dosing see p. 459)
- Cefalotin 2 g (child: 50 mg/kg up to 2 g) IV q4h
- Cefazolin 2 g (child: 50 mg/kg up to 2 g) IV q8h

3. INFECTED ANEURYSMS AND INTRAVASCULAR PROSTHESES

Pathogens

- Staphylococci
- Gram-negative bacteria (including *Salmonella*)

Management

- Consult with a cardiac surgeon and infectious disease practitioner or clinic microbiologist
- While waiting for results of blood cultures, give empirical therapy

Empirical therapy

- Vancomycin (IV) **plus** ceftriaxone (**or** cefotaxime) (IV)

For early or fulminant infection

- Vancomycin (IV) **plus** ceftriaxone (**or** cefotaxime) (IV) **plus** flucloxacillin (IV)

Modify regimen once causative organism and susceptibility are available

Dosage of above antibiotics

- Vancomycin IV (dosing see p. 462)
- Ceftriaxone 2 g (child ≥1 month: 50 mg/kg up to 2 g) IV daily

- Cefotaxime 2 g (child: 50 mg/kg up to 2 g) IV q8h
- Flucloxacillin 2 g (child: 50 mg/kg up to 2 g) IV q4h

ENDOCARDITIS—DIRECT THERAPY

1. STREPTOCOCCAL ENDOCARDITIS

Pathogens

- **Viridans streptococci**—*S. sanguis, S. mitior, S. milleri, S. mutans, S. mitis, S. salivarius*
- **Nutritional variant streptococci**—*Granulicatella* and *Abiotrophia* spp
- ***Streptococcus bovis* group**—*S. gallolyticus* or *S. infantarius*; treatment should be based on the minimum inhibitory concentration (MIC) for penicillin

Antibiotic therapy

If sensitive to penicillin (MIC ≤0.12 mg/L)

1. For uncomplicated case

- Option 1: benzylpenicillin (IV) **plus** gentamicin (IV) for 2 weeks
- Option 2: benzylpenicillin (IV or IV infusion) for 4 weeks (may use home-based IV therapy)

If penicillin allergy
- Ceftriaxone (IV) **plus** gentamicin (IV) for 2 weeks

If immediate penicillin allergy
- Vancomycin (IV) for 2 weeks

2. For complicated case (prolonged illness >3 months, large vegetation, multiple emboli or septic foci)

- Benzylpenicillin (IV) for 4 weeks **plus** gentamicin (IV) for first 2 weeks

If penicillin allergy
- Ceftriaxone (IV) for 4 weeks **plus** gentamicin (IV) for first 2 weeks

If immediate penicillin allergy
- Vancomycin (IV) **plus** gentamicin (IV) for 2 weeks

If mildly resistant to penicillin (MIC 0.13–0.5 mg/L)
- Benzylpenicillin (IV) for 4 weeks **plus** gentamicin (IV) for first 2 weeks

If penicillin allergy
- Ceftriaxone (IV) for 4 weeks **plus** gentamicin (IV) for first 2 weeks

If immediate penicillin allergy
- Vancomycin (IV) **plus** gentamicin (IV) for 2 weeks

If moderately resistant to penicillin (MIC 0.6–2 mg/L)
- Benzylpenicillin (IV) **plus** gentamicin (IV) for 4–6 weeks

If penicillin allergy
- Ceftriaxone (IV) **plus** gentamicin (IV) for 4–6 weeks

If immediate penicillin allergy
- Vancomycin (IV) **plus** gentamicin (IV) for 4 weeks

If resistant to penicillin (MIC >2 mg/L)
- Vancomycin (IV) **plus** gentamicin (IV) for 4–6 weeks

Dosage of above antibiotics

- Benzylpenicillin 1.8 g (child: 50 mg/kg up to 1.8 g) IV q4h
- Gentamicin (adult and child) 1 mg/kg IV q8h (monitor blood levels and adjust dose, see p. 459)
- Benzylpenicillin 10.8 g/24 hours by continuous IV infusion (home-based IV therapy)
- Ceftriaxone 2 g (child: 50 mg/kg up to 2 g) IV daily
- Vancomycin IV daily (monitor blood levels and adjust dose, see p. 462)

2. ENTEROCOCCAL ENDOCARDITIS

Pathogens

- *Enterococcus faecalis*
- *Enterococcus faecium*

All isolates must be tested for

- MIC of penicillin
- High-level aminoglycoside resistance
- Beta-lactamase enzyme production

Antibiotic therapy

Patients often need cardiac surgery

If penicillin sensitive (MIC <8 mg/L)
- Option 1: benzylpenicillin (IV) **plus** gentamicin (IV) for 4–6 weeks
- Option 2: ampi(amoxi)cillan (IV) **plus** gentamicin (IV) for 4–6 weeks

If allergic to penicillin
- Vancomycin (IV) **plus** gentamicin (IV) for 4–6 weeks
- Consider rapid penicillin desensitisation

If penicillin resistant (MIC >8 mg/L)
- Vancomycin (IV) **plus** gentamicin (IV) for 4–6 weeks

If high-level aminoglycoside resistance (surgery may be required)
- Option 1: benzylpenicillin (IV) **or** ampicillin (IV) monotherapy for 4–6 weeks
- Option 2: benzylpenicillin (IV) **plus** ceftriaxone (IV) for 6 weeks (for *E. faecalis* only)
- Option 3: vancomycin (IV) **plus** streptomycin* (IM) for 4–6 weeks

If highly resistant to vancomycin (seek expert advice)
- Option 1: linezolid (IV) for 4–6 weeks
- Option 2: teicoplanin (IV) for 4–6 weeks
- Option 3: daptomycin (IV) for 4–6 weeks (often with surgery)

---

*Available via Special Access Scheme <www.tga.gov.au/hp/access-sas.htm>

Dosage of above antibiotics

- Benzylpenicillin 2.4 g (child: 50 mg/kg up to 2.4 g) IV q4h
- Ampicillin or amoxicillin 2 g (child: 50 mg/kg up to 2 g) IV q4h
- Gentamicin (adult and child) 1 mg/kg IV q8h (monitor blood levels and adjust dose, see p. 459)
- Vancomycin IV daily (monitor blood levels and adjust dose, see p. 462)
- Ceftriaxone 2 g (child: 50 mg/kg up to 2 g) IV q12h
- Linezolid 600 mg (child: 10 mg/kg up to 600 mg) IV or PO q12h enterococci resistant to linezolid have been isolated
- Teicoplanin 800 mg (child: 10 mg/kg up to 800 mg) IV q12h for 3 doses, then 400 mg (child: 6–10 mg/kg up to 400 mg) IV once daily
- Daptomycin 6 mg/kg (child: 6–8 mg/kg) IV daily

3. STAPHYLOCOCCAL ENDOCARDITIS

Pathogens

- *Staphylococcus aureus*
- *Staphylococcus epidermidis*
- *Staphylococcus lugdenensis* (coagulase-negative)

1. Staphylococcal left-sided valve endocarditis

Treatment

- Early consultation with a cardiac surgeon for all cases
- Repeat blood culture after 72 hours of therapy

Methicillin-susceptible staphylococci (MSSA)

- Flucloxacillin (IV) for 4–6 weeks

Once stable after 2 weeks, may switch to home-based IV therapy

- Flucloxacillin (IV via infusion pump) to complete the course

Methicillin-resistant staphylococci (MRSA)

- Vancomycin (IV) for 6 weeks

Once stable, may switch to home-based IV therapy

- Vancomycin (IV) at home to complete the course

If the above therapy fails and unable to have surgery

- Vancomycin **plus** two other active drugs (seek expert advice)

Vancomycin-intermediate *S. aureus* (VISA) Vancomycin-resistant *S. aureus* (VRSA)

- Option 1: daptomycin (IV) for 4–6 weeks
- Option 2: linezolid (IV) for 4–6 weeks
- Option 3: quinupristin/dalfopristin (IV) for 4–6 weeks

Seek expert advice

Dosage of above antibiotics

- Flucloxacillin 2 g (child: 50 mg/kg up to 2 g) IV q4h
- Flucloxacillin 12 g/day IV daily continuous infusion or divided doses via an infusion pump
- Vancomycin IV daily (monitor blood levels and adjust dose, see p. 462)
- Daptomycin 6 mg/kg (child: 6–8 mg/kg) IV daily
- Linezolid 600 mg (child: 10 mg/kg up to 600 mg) IV or PO q12h

2. Staphylococcal right-sided (tricuspid) valve endocarditis

- Almost exclusively occurs in injecting drug users
- Prognosis is generally better than for left-sided endocarditis

Treatment
Methicillin-susceptible *S. aureus* (MSSA) infection

- Flucloxacillin (IV) for 2–4 weeks*

If non-immediate penicillin allergy

- Option 1: cefazolin (IV) for 2–4 weeks
- Option 2: consider rapid penicillin desensitisation

If immediate penicillin allergy

- Vancomycin (IV) for 2–4 weeks

Methicillin-resistant *S. aureus* (MRSA) infection

- Option 1: vancomycin (IV) for 2–4 weeks
- Option 2: quinupristin/dalfopristin (IV) for 2–4 weeks
- Option 3: daptomycin (IV) for 2–4 weeks

Seek expert advice

Dosage of above antibiotics

- Flucloxacillin 2 g (child: 50 mg/kg up to 2 g) IV q4h
- Cefazolin 2 g (child: 50 mg/kg up to 2 g) IV q8h
- Vancomycin IV daily (monitor blood levels and adjust dose, see p. 462)
- Linezolid 600 mg (child: 10 mg/kg up to 600 mg) IV or PO q12h
- Quinupristin/dalfopristin adult and child: 7.5 mg/kg IV q8h
- Daptomycin 6 mg/kg IV daily

---

*Give ≥4 weeks treatment if:

- Presence of metastatic foci of infection (e.g. osteomyelitis, lung abscess and empyema) or left-sided valve is involved
- Presence of right heart failure or acute respiratory failure
- Vegetation ≥2 cm
- No improvement after 3–4 days of initial treatment
- HIV-infected patient, CD4 cell count <200/mL

4. ENDOCARDITIS CAUSED BY HACEK GROUP

Pathogens

- *H*aemophilus aphrophilus, H. parainfluenzae
- *A*ggregatibacter (Actinobacillus) actinomycetemcomitans
- *C*ardiobacterium hominis
- *E*ikenella corrodens
- *K*ingella kingae (fastidious gram-negative bacteria)

Incubation

- 7–14 days

Clinical

- HACEK accounts for 5% of endocarditis cases; prosthetic valves in 30% of cases
- Usually slow onset and progress
- Often difficult to diagnose because of their slow growth in traditional media
- May require special microbiological techniques for isolation

Treatment

Treat as if they are penicillin-resistant

- Option 1: ceftriaxone (IV) for 4–6 weeks
- Option 2: cefotaxime (IV) for 4–6 weeks

Gentamicin may be used for synergy in the first 2 weeks
Modify antibiotic once bacterial sensitivity is known
Seek expert advice

Dosage of above antibiotics

- Ceftriaxone 2 g (child >1 month: 50 mg/kg up to 2 g) IV daily
- Cefotaxime 2 g (child: 50 mg/kg up to 2 g) IV q8h

5. CANDIDA ENDOCARDITIS

Pathogen

- *Candida* spp

Risk factors

- IV drug users (predominant)
- Immunosuppressed
- Intravenous catheter
- Prosthetic heart valve

Treatment

Early surgery is usually required

- Option 1: amphotericin B (IV) **plus** flucytosine (IV)
- Option 2: caspofungin (IV)

Long-term suppression with an oral azole may be needed

Dosage of above antibiotics

- Amphotericin B 0.5–1 mg/kg IV daily
- Flucytosine 37.5–50 mg/kg IV q6h
- Caspofungin 50 mg IV daily

6.   PNEUMOCOCCAL ENDOCARDITIS

Treatment

Penicillin sensitive

- Benzylpenicillin (IV) for 4 weeks

Penicillin resistant or if concurrent meningitis is suspected

- Ceftriaxone (IV) **plus** vancomycin (IV) for 4–6 weeks

Dosage of above antibiotics

- Benzylpenicillin 1.8 g (child: 50 mg/kg up to 1.8 g) IV q4h
- Ceftriaxone 2 g (child: 50 mg/kg up to 2 g) IV daily
- Vancomycin IV daily (monitor blood levels and adjust dose, see p. 462)

7.   NEISSERIA GONORRHOEAE ENDOCARDITIS

Treatment

Choose regimen according to susceptibility testing results

- Option 1: ceftriaxone 1 g (child: 25 mg/kg up to 1 g) IV daily for 4 weeks
- Option 2: cefotaxime 1 g (child: 25 mg/kg up to 1 g) IV q8h for 4 weeks

Seek expert advice
Note: As cefalosporin-resistant gonorrhoea emerges, any suggestion of possible treatment failure in gonorrhoea should be reported to public health authorities

8.   ENTEROBACTERIACEAE ENDOCARDITIS

Treatment

- Ceftriaxone (**or** cefotaxime) (IV) **plus** gentamicin (IV) for 4–6 weeks

Dosage of above antibiotics

- Ceftriaxone 1 g (child: 25 mg/kg up to 1 g) IV daily
- Cefotaxime 1 g (child: 25 mg/kg up to 1 g) IV q8h

- Gentamicin (adult and child) 1 mg/kg IV q8h (monitor blood levels and adjust dose, see p. 459)

9. *PSEUDOMONAS AERUGINOSA* ENDOCARDITIS

Treatment

Frequently require cardiac surgery

- Ticarcillin/claviculate (**or** piperacillin) (IV) **plus** tobramycin (IV)

Consult a cardiac surgeon

Dosage of above antibiotics

- Ticarcillin/claviculate 3 g (child: 50 mg/kg up to 3 g) IV q4–6h
- Piperacillin 3–4 g (child: 50–75 mg/kg up to 4 g) IV q6h
- Tobramycin (adult and child) 2.5 mg/kg IV q8h (monitor blood levels and adjust dose, see p. 459)

10. *CORYNEBACTERIUM DIPHTHERIAE* ENDOCARDITIS

Treatment

- Benzylpenicillin (IV) **plus** gentamicin (IV) for 4–6 weeks

If resistant or allergic to penicillin

- Vancomycin (IV) for 4–6 weeks

Dosage of above antibiotics

- Benzylpenicillin 1.8 g (child: 50 mg/kg up to 1.8 g) IV q4h
- Gentamicin (adult and child) 1 mg/kg IV q8h (monitor blood levels and adjust dose, see p. 459)
- Vancomycin IV (monitor blood levels and adjust dose, see p. 462)

ENDOCARDITIS—CULTURE-NEGATIVE

- Up to 5–10% of endocarditis cases are culture-negative
- May be due to prior antibiotic treatment
- May be due to unusual organisms—fastidious gram-positive cocci, HACEK bacteria, anaerobic, *Brucella* spp (cat-scratch disease), *Bartonella* spp, *Legionella* spp, *Coxiella burnetii* (Q fever), *Tropheryma whipplei* (Whipple disease) or fungi
- Marantic endocarditis must be excluded

Special tests can be used to screen for some uncommon pathogens

Brucella spp (undulant fever)

- *Brucella* agglutination test (a single titre >1 : 160 or four-fold rise over 4-week period)
- *Brucella* PCR test (very sensitive and specific)
- *Brucella* cultures (blood, bone marrow or CSF)

Bartonella spp (cat-scratch disease)

- *Bartonella* serology test

Coxiella burnetii (Q fever)

- Q fever serology (four-fold rise in antibody titre over 10–14 days)
- *Coxiella burnetii* 16 rRNA sequencing of heart valve specimens after valve surgery

Legionella spp

- *Legionella* urinary antigen test

Mycoplasma hominis

- Blood culture for mycoplasma (special media—consult pathologist)

Empirical antibiotic therapy

Seek expert advice

- Benzylpenicillin (IV) **plus** gentamicin (IV) for 4–6 weeks
- Ceftriaxone (IV) **plus** gentamicin (IV) for 4–6 weeks (if non-immediate penicillin allergy)

If prosthetic valves are involved

- Ceftriaxone (IV) **plus** gentamicin (IV) **plus** vancomycin (IV) for 4–6 weeks

Dosage of above antibiotics

- Benzylpenicillin 2.4 g (child: 50 mg/kg up to 2.4 g) IV q4h
- Ceftriaxone 2 g (child: 50 mg/kg up to 2 g) IV daily
- Gentamicin (adult and child) 1 mg/kg IV q8h (monitor blood levels and adjust dose, see p. 459)
- Vancomycin IV daily (monitor blood levels and adjust dose, see p. 462)

1.   Q FEVER ENDOCARDITIS

Pathogen

- *Coxiella burnetii*

Laboratory

Pre-existing valve disease + fever + negative blood culture should send blood for:

- *Coxiella burnetii* PCR
- Q fever serology (four-fold rise in antibody titre over 10–14 days)

Treatment

- Cardiac surgery may be required
- Serological monitoring for at least 5 years
  - Doxycycline (PO) **plus** rifampicin (**or** hydroxychloroquine) (PO) for 18 months (for 24 months if having prosthetic valves) (seek expert advice)

Dosage of above antibiotics

- Doxycycline 100 mg (child >8 years: 2 mg/kg up to 100 mg) PO q12h
- Rifampicin 600 mg (child: 20 mg/kg up to 600 mg) PO daily
- Hydroxychloroquine (seek expert advice for dosage)

2. BARTONELLA ENDOCARDITIS

Pathogen

- *Bartonella henselae* (cat-scratch disease)

Laboratory

- *Bartonella* serology test

Treatment

- Option 1: doxycycline (PO) for 6 weeks **plus** gentamicin (IV) for first 2 weeks
- Option 2: doxycycline (PO) for 6 weeks **plus** rifampicin (PO) for first 2 weeks

Dosage of above antibiotics

- Doxycycline 100 mg (child >8 years: 2 mg/kg up to 100 mg) PO q12h
- Gentamicin (adult and child) 1 mg/kg iv q8h (monitor blood levels, see p. 459)
- Rifampicin 300 mg (child: 7.5 mg/kg up to 300 mg) PO q12h

3. BRUCELLA ENDOCARDITIS

Pathogen

- *Brucella* spp

Laboratory

- *Brucella* agglutination test (a single titre >1 : 160 or four-fold rise over 4-week period)
- *Brucella* PCR test (very sensitive and specific)
- *Brucella* cultures (blood, bone marrow or CSF)

Treatment

- *Brucella* endocarditis requires a longer duration of treatment and may require alternative combination regimens—seek expert advice

ENTEROCOCCI—VANCOMYCIN-RESISTANT

Enterococci are part of the normal flora in the bowel and female genital tract and are often found in the environment. When exposed to antibiotics (e.g. vancomycin), drug-resistant strains (e.g. vancomycin-resistant enterococci, VRE) may survive and overgrow in the bowel. The colonised VRE may cause infections.

Pathogens

- *Enterococcus faecium*
- *Enterococcus faecalis*

Transmission

- Most infections are from the patient's own VRE flora
- Healthcare workers may carry VRE on their hands and transmit to patients
- Indirect transmission by contaminated environmental surfaces and equipment
- VRE has the potential to be transmitted to other gram-positive bacteria, such as *Staphylococcus aureus*

Risk factors

- Broad-spectrum antibiotics (particularly third-generation cefalosporins)—risk factor for VRE colonisation and also MRSA amplification
- Vancomycin therapy (oral or IV)
- Prolonged hospital stay and critically ill patients (e.g. ICU patients)
- Immunosuppressed
- Intra-abdominal or cardio-thoracic surgery
- Central venous catheter

Laboratory

- Culture of clinical samples (urine, faeces, swabs or blood)
- VRE PCR test

Infection control

- Control antibiotic use—reduce the use of vancomycin and broad-spectrum antibiotics whenever possible
- A patient with VRE should be isolated in a single room with own toilet
- Wear gloves and long-sleeved gown prior to contact with the patient
- Handwashing with soap and water or use alcohol-based hand gel
- Yoghurt containing *Lactobacillus rbamnosus* GG (LGG) has been reported to be effective against VRE
- Patient care equipment should be left in the room during the patient's stay and decontaminated after use
- The patient's charts and notes should be kept outside the patient's room
- Visitors must wear protective gown and wash hands before leaving the room
- Regular auditing of antibiotic use can assist hospital drug committees in defining areas for targeted intervention

ENTEROVIRUS 71

Enterovirus 71 (EV71) is one of the viruses that cause hand, foot and mouth disease (HFMD). It can also cause fatal neurological disease in young children. Outbreaks of HFMD and EV71 neurological disease have been reported in Australia.

Pathogen

- *Enterovirus* 71

Transmission

- Direct contact—fluid from blisters, mucus, saliva or faeces of an infected person
- Virus continues to be excreted in faeces for many weeks after symptoms develop
- Typically occurs in small epidemics in nursery schools or kindergartens, usually during summer and autumn months

Incubation

- 3–7 days

Clinical

Highly infectious, commonly affects children and may also affect immunosuppressed adults

- **HFMD**—slight fever, sore throat, followed by blisters on hands and feet and ulcers in mouth; rash and blisters may also occur on other parts of the body; the child usually recovers within a week
- **EV71 neurological disease**—occasionally, EV71 can cause high fever with acute flaccid paralysis, aseptic meningitis, encephalitis or pulmonary oedema/pulmonary haemorrhage; death may follow

Diagnosis

Consider EV71 neurological disease in any child who has high fever + neurological signs (sleep myoclonus, paralysis, stiff neck or mental status change), particularly if skin blisters and mouth ulcers are present

- EV71 virus isolation—from viral swabs (throat, mouth ulcers or skin lesions), faeces samples or CSF
- Enterovirus serology (IgM)—later diagnosis

Treatment

- HFMD—symptomatic treatment
- EV71 neurological disease:
  - admission, supportive treatment including ventilation
  - *pleconaril* (binds to a cleft in enteroviruses and prevents host cell–receptor interaction with the virus) (the drug is not available in Australia)

Prevention

- Wash hands with soap and water after toileting, before eating and after touching skin lesions
- School exclusion until blisters and ulcers have healed
- EV71 vaccines and antiviral agents are being worked on

EPIDIDYMO-ORCHITIS

Pathogens

- Secondary to sexually transmitted infection—*Chlamydia trachomatis*, *Neisseria gonorrhoea*, *Ureaplasma urealyticum* and *Mycoplasma genitalium* (from a urethral infection); enteric gram-negative bacteria (from anal intercourse)
- Secondary to urine infection—*E. coli* and other enteric gram-negative bacteria
- Secondary to recent urinary tract instrumentation—enteric gram-negative bacteria
- Haematogenous spread—as a complication of other systemic infections
- Mumps virus—now uncommon since MMR immunisation
- Other causes—tuberculosis, syphilis, brucellosis, melioidosis and schistosomiasis

Clinical

- Onset may be insidious; fever, vomiting, urinary symptoms with red, tender and swollen hemiscrotum; pyuria may be present

Laboratory

- MSU—for microscopy, culture and susceptibility
- First-void urine—for *Chlamydia* and gonorrhoea PCR. If negative, consider urine PCR testing for *Ureaplasma urealyticum* and *Mycoplasma genitalium*
- Urethral swab—for Gram stain, culture and gonorrhoea culture

Treatment

- Vasectomy may be indicated for prevention of recurrent infection

1. Sexually acquired infection
- Contact tracing is important to prevent the recurrence of infection
  - Option 1: ceftriaxone (IM **or** IV) **plus** azithromycin (PO) **plus** doxycycline (PO)
  - Option 2: ceftriaxone (IM **or** IV) **plus** azithromycin (PO) weekly for 2 weeks

Severe infection—oral treatment may need to be continued for 3 weeks
If immediate penicillin allergy, seek expert advice

Dosage of above antibiotics

- Ceftriaxone 500 mg in 2 mL 1% lidocaine (lignocaine) IM **or** 500 mg IV as a single dose
- Azithromycin 1 g PO as a single dose **or** 1 g PO weekly for 2 weeks (if unable to take doxycycline) **or** 1 g PO weekly for 3 weeks (if severe infection)
- Doxycycline 100 mg PO q12h for 2 weeks **or** 3 weeks (if severe infection)

2. **Non-sexually acquired infection**

Mild to moderate infection
- Option 1: cefalexin (PO) for 2 weeks
- Option 2: amoxicillin/clavulanate (PO) for 2 weeks
- Option 3: trimethoprim (PO) for 2 weeks

If pathogen is resistant to above antibiotics and is susceptible to quinolones
- Norfloxacin (PO) for 2 weeks

Severe infection
- Ampicillin (IV) **plus** gentamicin (IV)

If penicillin allergy
- Gentamicin (IV)

If gentamicin is contraindicated
- Ceftriaxone (**or** cefotaxime) (IV)

Switch to oral therapy when significantly improved
- Option 1: cefalexin 12.5 mg/kg up to 500 mg PO q6h
- Option 2: amoxicillin/clavulanate 22.5 mg/kg up to 875 mg PO q12h
- Option 3: cotrimoxazole 4/20 mg/kg up to 160/800 mg PO q12h

After improvement change to above oral therapy to complete a 2-week course

Dosage of above antibiotics

Mild to moderate infection
- Cefalexin 500 mg (child: 12.5 mg/kg up to 500 mg) PO q12h
- Amoxicillin/clavulanate 500 mg (child: 12.5 mg/kg up to 500 mg) PO q12h
- Trimethoprim 300 mg (child: 6 mg/kg up to 300 mg) PO q12h
- Norfloxacin 400 mg PO q12h (avoid in children)

Severe infection
- Ampicillin 2 g (child: 50 mg/kg up to 2 g) IV q6h
- Gentamicin 4–7 mg/kg IV for the 1st dose (further dosing see p. 459)
- Ceftriaxone 1 g (child>1 month: 50 mg/kg up to 1 g) IV daily
- Cefotaxime 1 g (child: 50 mg/kg up to 1 g) IV q8h

EPIDURAL ABSCESS

Pathogens

- *Staphylococcus aureus*
- *Escherichia coli*

- Mixed anaerobes
- Rarely, a tuberculous abscess develops with Pott's disease of the thoracic spine

Causes

- An adjacent infection spreads to the spinal area
- About a third of cases develop without any known cause

Diagnosis

- MRI to find the location of the abscess and assess the pressure on the spinal cord (CT may miss the abscess)
- Blood culture if septic

Treatment

- Start empirical antibiotic therapy as soon as clinical suspicion arises
- Urgent surgical assessment and operation to drain the abscess and relieve the pressure on the spinal cord
- Operative materials should be sent for Gram stain and culture

Empirical therapy or if MSSA is isolated

- Flucloxacillin (IV) **plus** gentamicin (IV)

If non-immediate penicillin allergy or gentamicin is contraindicated

- Ceftriaxone (**or** cefotaxime) (IV)

For post-neurosurgical infection or if MRSA is suspected

- **Add** vancomycin (IV)

If immediate penicillin allergy

- Vancomycin (IV) **plus** gentamicin (IV)

If susceptibility is unavailable in 3 days

Cease gentamicin-containing regimen

- Ceftriaxone (**or** cefotaxime) (IV)

Further treatment

Direct therapy—as for Osteomylitis (see p. 256)

Duration of therapy

- For at least 6 weeks

Dosage of above antibiotics

- Flucloxacillin 2 g (child: 50 mg/kg up to 2 g) IV q4–6h
- Gentamicin 4–7 mg/kg (child: 7.5 mg/kg up to 320 mg) IV for the 1st dose (further dosing see p. 459)
- Ceftriaxone 4 g (child >1 month: 100 mg/kg up to 4 g) IV daily **or** 2 g (child >1 month: 50 mg/kg up to 2 g) IV q12h
- Cefotaxime 2 g (child: 50 mg/kg up to 2 g) IV q6h
- Vancomycin 25–30 mg/kg IV for the 1st dose (further dosing see p. 462)

EPIGLOTTITIS

Other names: Supraglottitis
Do not examine the throat without skilled intubation and general anaesthesia being available

Pathogens

- *Haemophilus influenzae* type b (Hib)
- *Streptococcus pneumoniae*
- *Streptococcus pyogenes*

Clinical

- Typically affects children; child often appears acutely ill, anxious, fever, dysphagia, drooling, stridor and cyanosis
- Adult cases are commonly seen in crack cocaine abusers and have a more subacute presentation

Diagnosis

- Direct inspection using laryngoscopy (do not use tongue presser—may provoke airway spasm!)—the epiglottis and arytenoids are cherry-red and swollen
- Lateral neck x-ray—dilation of the hypopharynx and a swollen epiglottis (the thumbprint sign) suggests epiglottitis
- Blood culture (do not swab the throat unless patient has been intubated!)

Treatment

- Maintain the airway—may need urgent endotracheal intubation by an experienced anaesthetist; if intubation fails, tracheotomy is required
- Humidified oxygen by mask
- All patients require intensive monitoring—seek expert advice
  - Ceftriaxone (**or** cefotaxime) (IV) for 5 days

If immediate penicillin allergy
  - Chloramphenicol (IV) for 5 days

Adjunctive use of corticosteroid to reduce airway inflammation

  - Dexamethasone (IV) st, repeat at 24 hours if required

To eliminate carriage of Hib in contacts

  - Option 1: rifampicin (PO) for 4 days
  - Option 2: ceftriaxone (IM) for 2 days

Dosage of above agents

  - Ceftriaxone 1 g (child >1 month: 50 mg/kg up to 1 g) IV daily
  - Cefotaxime 1 g (child: 50 mg/kg up to 1 g) IV q8h
  - Chloramphenicol adult and child: 12.5–25 mg/kg up to 1 g IV q6h
  - Dexamethasone 10 mg (child 0.15 mg/kg up to 10 mg) IV st, repeat at 24 hours if required

- Rifampicin 600 mg (neonate: 10 mg/kg; child: 20 mg/kg up to 600 mg) PO daily
- Ceftriaxone 1 g in 3.5 mL 1% lignocaine (child: 50 mg/kg up to 1) IM daily

Vaccination

- If index case is <2 years—commence a full course of Hib vaccination after recovery regardless of any previous Hib immunisation
- For unvaccinated contacts <5 years—start Hib immunisation ASAP

ERYSIPELAS

Erysipelas is a superficial infection of the dermis and upper subcutaneous layer that presents with a well-defined edge. Erysipelas and cellulitis often coexist.

Pathogens and risk factors

- *Streptococcus pyogenes*—almost always the cause of infection
- May be associated with underling facial or dental infection

Clinical

- A small red patch that progresses to an indurate plaque; often affects face or legs with fever and rigors; may rapidly progress to cellulitis

Treatment

- Search and treat underlying abnormalities (e.g. dental and sinus examination, feet for fungal infection and circulation check)
- Antibiotic therapy
  - Option 1: cefalexin (PO) for 5–10 days
  - Option 2: flucloxacillin (PO) for 5–10 days
  - Option 3: clindamycin (PO) for 5–10 days (if immediate penicillin allergy)
- If *S. pyogenes* is isolated or patient is in Indigenous community
  - Option 1: penicillin V (PO) for 5–10 days
  - Option 2: procaine penicillin (IM) for 3–5 days
- If severe with systemic toxicity
  - Option 1: benzylpenicillin (IV)
  - Option 2: cefazolin (IV)
  - Option 3: clindamycin (IV)

Prophylaxis

- Penicillin V (PO) for 6 months or longer
- If frequently recurs, consider continuous antibiotic prevention

Dosage of above antibiotics

- Cefalexin 500 mg (child: 12.5 mg/kg up to 500 mg) PO q6h
- Flucloxacillin 500 mg (child: 25 mg/kg up to 500 mg) PO q6h
- Clindamycin 450 mg (child: 10 mg/kg up to 300 mg) PO q8h

- Penicillin V 500 mg (child: 10 mg/kg up to 500 mg) PO q6h
- Procaine penicillin 1.5 g (child: 50 mg/kg up to 1.5 g) IM daily
- Benzylpenicillin 1.2 g (child: 30 mg/kg up to 1.2 g) IV q6h
- Cefazolin 1 g (child: 25 mg/kg up to 1 g) IV q6h
- Clindamycin 600 mg (child: 15 mg/kg up to 600 mg) IV q8h
- Penicillin V 250 mg (Child <5 years: 125 mg) PO q12h

ERYSIPELOID

Erysipeloid is an acute bacterial infection of the skin and other organs. It is an occupational disease.

Pathogen

- *Erysipelothrix rhusiopathiae* (*insidiosa*)

Transmission

- Human infection is acquired through direct contact with the meat of infected animals, poultry, fish and shellfish
- The organism enters the skin through abrasions, scratches, cut or pricks

Risk groups

- Fishermen, farmers, butchers, abattoir workers, veterinary surgeons and cooks

Clinical

- **Skin form**—well-demarcated, purplish-red plaques with a smooth, shiny surface, often on fingers, hands or forearms, usually with no systemic symptoms
- **Systemic form**—organism may spread to joints, heart, CNS and lungs; patient may die of sepsis if diagnosis is not made and treatment is not initiated early

Laboratory

- Blood culture—aids in diagnosis of systemic erysipeloid
- Skin biopsy and culture—confirms the diagnosis

Complications

- Permanent neurological damage (e.g. cerebrovascular accident)
- Endocarditis with long-term valvular heart disease
- Septic arthritis with long-term joint diseases

Treatment

- Skin forms of erysipeloid—self-limited and may remit spontaneously within 2–4 weeks; however, antibiotic treatment may hasten recovery and limit further progression of disease
- Systemic form—needs IV antibiotic treatment

Skin form

- Option 1: penicillin V (PO) for 7–10 days
- Option 2: doxycycline (PO) for 7–10 days

Systemic form

- Benzylpenicillin (IV) for 4 weeks

Dosage of above antibiotics

- Penicillin V 500 mg (child: 12.5 mg/kg up to 500 mg) PO q6h
- Doxycycline 200 mg (child >8 years: 4 mg/kg up to 200 mg) PO on day 1, then 100 mg (child >8 years: 2 mg/kg up to 100 mg) PO daily
- Benzylpenicillin 1.8 g (child: 50 mg/kg up to 1.8 g) IV q4–6h

ERYTHEMA INFECTIOSUM

Other names: fifth disease, slapped cheek disease, B19 infection
Erythema infectiosum is a common viral infection of childhood.

Pathogen

- *Parvovirus* B19

Transmission

- Mainly via droplets
- Can be transmitted through blood transfusion
- Intrauterine transmission from mother to baby

Incubation

- 4–14 days, may take 3 weeks

Clinical

- Most common in young school-aged children
- Flu-like illness, malaise, fever, sore throat and cervical lymphadenopathy
- A few days later may develop bright macular red rash on the face ('slapped cheek' rash) with a pale ring around the mouth ('circumoral pallor'); a fainter 'lace-like' rash may also be seen on the trunk and extremities; the rash usually lasts for 2–3 days, but may reappear
- Severe joint pain may occur, more common in adult patients, lasts 1–2 weeks
- Immunosuppressed people are at risk of chronic parvovirus B19 infection

Complications

- In pregnant women (mainly before 20 weeks of gestation)—may cause fetal death or fetal hydrops
- In people with sickle cell disease—can cause aplastic crisis

Laboratory

Laboratory test only for post-exposure or symptomatic pregnant women or immunosuppressed people:

- Parvovirus B19 serology—IgM confirms current infection, IgG indicates past infection
- Parvovirus B19 PCR (blood or amniotic fluid)—for diagnosis of seronegative B19 infection or fetal B19 infection

Treatment

- Symptomatic treatment
- Pregnant women who are exposed to parvovirus infection or have symptoms should have parvovirus B19 serological testing—if B19 IgM positive, should have serial obstetric ultrasounds (look for signs of fetal hydrops/death)
- Immune globulin (IV)—may help severe cases, such as aplastic crises, or may be used in immunosuppressed people and HIV-infected children
- School exclusion is not necessary (by the time the rash appears the child is no longer contagious)
- Infection probably confers lifelong immunity

ERYTHRASMA

Erythrasma is a skin disease with pink patches and brown scales. It is found worldwide, more frequently in subtropical and tropical areas.

Pathogens

- *Corynebacterium minutissimum*, a gram-positive filamentous rod
- It is a normal skin flora, most commonly found in folds of skin

Predisposing factors

- Excessive sweating/hyperhidrosis
- Delicate skin barrier
- Obesity
- Diabetes
- Warm climate
- Poor hygiene

Clinical

- The incidence is around 4%, higher in black people
- Typical appearance—well-demarcated, brown-red macular patches; the skin has a wrinkled appearance with fine scales; toe web lesions appear as maceration; dark discolouration on body folds
- Usually asymptomatic, but can be pruritic
- Infection is commonly seen over inner thighs, scrotum, foot region and toe webs; less common in axillae, submammary area, periumbilical

region and intergluteal fold; widespread involvement of trunk and limbs is possible
- Duration of the infection ranges from months to years

Complications

- In immunocompromised patients—may become widespread and invasive (abscess formation, bacteraemia, intravascular catheter–related infections, peritoneal catheter–related infections, endocarditis and pyelonephritis)

Laboratory

- Wood light examination—reveals coral-red fluorescence of lesions (results may be negative if the patient is bathed prior to examination)
- Gram stain and culture

Treatment

Antibacterial and/or antifungal agents are used to eradicate *C. minutissimum* and possible concomitant infections
- Option 1: azithromycin 1 g (child 15 mg/kg up to 1 g) PO st
- Option 2: erythromycin 500 mg (child: 15–25 mg/kg up to 250 mg) PO q12h for 7–14 days

Topical treatment

- Option 1: clindamycin 1% lotion (e.g. Dalacin) top bid for 2 weeks
- Option 2: miconazole 2% lotion/cream (e.g. Daktarin) top bid for 2 weeks

ESCHERICHIA COLI INFECTION

Pathogens

- *Escherichia coli* (*E. coli*)—aerobic gram-negative non-sporing rods
- Most *E. coli* strains are harmless, but some virulent strains can cause gastroenteritis, urinary tract infections, neonatal meningitis, haemolytic uraemic syndrome (HUS), peritonitis, septicaemia and pneumonia

1. ENTEROHAEMORRHAGIC *E. COLI* (EHEC), SHIGATOXIGENIC *E. COLI* (STEC) AND VEROTOXIGENIC *E. COLI* (VTEC)

Pathogenicity

- The most important strains are O157:H7, O111:H8 and O26:H11
- EHEC can cause HUS and sudden renal failure
- Shigatoxigenic *E. coli* produce Shiga toxins
- Verotoxigenic *E. coli* produce Vero toxins

Transmission

- Faecal–oral (the infective dose is very low)

Incubation

- 2–8 days

Clinical

- **Haemorrhagic colitis**—bloody diarrhoea, abdominal pain, fever and vomiting
- **HUS**—10% of patients may develop HUS with acute renal failure, haemolytic anaemia and thrombocytopenia (HUS is the most common cause of acute renal failure in young children)
- Neurological complications (seizure, stroke and coma)—25% of HUS patients
- Chronic renal sequelae (usually mild)—50% of survivors

HUS should be considered in the presence of the following:

- Acute microangiopathic anaemia on peripheral blood smears
- Acute renal impairment
- Thrombocytopenia, particularly during the first 7 days of illness
- Duration of symptoms: 2–9 days

Laboratory

- Faecal cultures, bloody cultures—for EHEC and STEC/VTEC (must be specifically requested); one negative faeces culture is not exclusionary
- Food samples culture—for EHEC and STEC/VTEC
- Identification of Shiga toxin or Vero toxin—from a clinical isolate of *E. coli*
- PCR for EHEC
- PCR for toxin-associated gene on isolate or bloody diarrhoea

Treatment

- HUS must be notified immediately by telephone and then by written notification within 5 days (see Appendix 7)
- Symptomatic treatment—most patients recover within 10 days
- **Antibiotics should be avoided**—no evidence that antibiotics improve the course of disease and some antibiotics may increase toxin release from the bacteria and precipitate kidney complications
- Anti-diarrhoeal agents should be avoided
- HUS is usually treated in an intensive care unit; blood transfusions and kidney dialysis are often required

Prevention

- Education in hygienic handling of foods for abattoir workers and those involved in the production of raw meat
- Education of farm workers in good hygienic practice
- Eliminating EHEC from foods through heat or radiation
- Good food hygiene practice can prevent the transmission of pathogens

2. ENTEROTOXIGENIC *E. COLI* (ETEC)

Pathogenicity

- Non-invasive but produce toxins
- ETEC produces LT enterotoxin (heat-labile; similar to cholera toxin) and ST enterotoxin (heat-stable) causing secretion of fluid and electrolytes
- Large numbers of *E. coli* need to be ingested to cause diarrhoea

Incubation

- 8–44 hours

Clinical

- ETEC causes watery diarrhoea, abdominal cramps, malaise and vomiting; in its most severe form it can cause rice-water faeces with dehydration
- ETEC is the leading bacterial cause of diarrhoea in children in developing areas
- ETEC is the most common cause of traveller's diarrhoea

Duration of symptoms

- The illness may last 3–19 days

Treatment

- Antibiotics can shorten the duration of diarrhoea, but not usually required.
- In severe cases norfloxacin or ciprofloxacin may be used (see Traveller's diarrhoea, p. 402)

3. ENTEROPATHOGENIC *E. COLI* (EPEC)

Pathogenicity

- EPEC is moderately invasive and produces a Shiga toxin

Incubation

- 17–72 hours

Clinical

- More common in young children.
- Watery diarrhoea with mucous, fever, vomiting and abdominal pain

Duration of symptoms

- Illness may be self-limiting or a protracted chronic enteritis; the symptoms usually last for 6 hours to 3 days, although in some children symptoms have been known to last up to 14 days

4. ENTEROINVASIVE *E. COLI* (EIEC)

Pathogenicity

- Highly invasive, but no toxin

Incubation

- 8–24 hours; large amount of bacteria required for the infection

Clinical

- Many patients experience watery diarrhoea (associated with an enterotoxin)
- Some patients develop dysentery (identical to Shigellosis)

EYE PENETRATING INJURY AND ENDOPHTHALMITIS

Endophthalmitis—infection of the intraocular cavities (i.e. the aqueous or vitreous humour). May develop into orbital abscess.

Exogenous endophthalmitis results from direct inoculation as a complication of ocular surgery, foreign bodies and/or blunt or penetrating eye injuries.

Endogenous endophthalmitis results from the haematogenous spread of organisms from a distant source of infection (e.g. endocarditis).

Pathogens

- Streptococci
- Stephylocococci
- Gram-negative bacilli
- Fungi

Clinical

Bacterial endophthalmitis

- Acute pain, redness, eyelid swelling, congested eye and decreased visual acuity
- Some bacteria (e.g. *Propionibacterium acnes*) may cause chronic inflammation with mild symptoms
- *P. acnes* usually inoculated during intraocular surgery and infection may occur months or years after the surgery

Fungal endophthalmitis

- Indolent course over days or weeks
- Blurred vision, pain and decreased visual acuity
- History of penetrating injury with a plant substance or soil-contaminated foreign body

Urgent treatment

- Obtain samples for Gram stain and culture if possible

- Tetanus status assessment (see Tetanus, p. 393) and injection
- Urgent referral to an ophthalmologist for urgent (same-day) intravitreal injection of antibiotics and a pars plana vitrectomy as needed; enucleation may be required to remove a blind and painful eye
- Early admission to hospital
- If there will be significant delay in admission, use:
  - Option 1: vancomycin (IV) **plus** ciprofloxacin (**or** moxifloxacin) (PO)
  - Option 2: cefazolin (IV) **plus** gentamicin (IV)

If soil contamination is suspected
  - **Add** clindamycin (IV)

Topical antibiotics are contraindicated

Dosage of above antibiotics

- Vancomycin 25–30 mg/kg IV for the 1st dose (further dosing see p. 462)
- Ciprofloxacin 750 mg (child: 20 mg/kg up to 750 mg) PO st
- Moxifloxacin 400 mg PO or IV st
- Cefazolin 2 g (child: 50 mg/kg up to 2 g) IV st
- Gentamicin (adult and child) 5 mg/kg IV st
- Clindamycin 600 mg (child: 10 mg/kg up to 600 mg) IV st

FLEA BITES

Pathogens

- Flea (*Pulicidae*), a bloodsucking arthropod

Transmission

- Pets (e.g. cat or dog) spread the fleas

Clinical

- Typical reaction to fleabites—a wheal surrounding each bite site, often grouped in clusters, intense itching
- One individual may react badly to the bites, while other family members seem unaffected

Fleas can cause following medical problems:

- Flea allergy dermatitis (FAD)—papular urticaria, particularly on legs
- Secondary skin infections—after scratching
- Anaemia—due to loss of blood from biting continuously (in extreme cases)
- Transmission of several infectious diseases—such as plague, typhus, Q fever, tapeworm, Lyme disease and *Listeria*
- The only flea-borne disease currently in Australia is Murine typhus; it is transmitted from rats to humans via particular rat fleas

Treatment

Relief of itching and allergic skin reaction

- Carbolated vaseline top PRN
- Crotamiton (e.g. Eurax) cream/lotion top tds
- Calamine lotion top PRN
- Pinetarsol gel/bath oil/solution top PRN
- Corticosteroid cream/oint top
- Antihistamine PO

Treat secondary skin infections

- Alcohol swab to wipe the lesions PRN
- Chlorhexidine (e.g. Savlon Antiseptic) 1% cream top PRN
- Povidone-iodine (e.g. Betadine) cream/oint/lotion/solution top PRN
- Ethanol and iodine (e.g. iodine tincture) top PRN
- Mupirocin* (e.g. Bactroban) 2% cream/oint top tds

---

*Mupirocin is a topical antibiotic; bacteria may develop resistance to it

Prevention

- Apply repellents on outer clothing and exposed skin (do not apply over cuts, wounds or irritated skin, around eyes or mouth or to the hands of young children)
- Regularly vacuum floors, and wash pets and bedding with an insecticidal preparation

FOLLICULITIS

Folliculitis is the inflammation of hair follicles.

Pathogens and risk factors

- *Staphylococcus aureus*—patient is often a chronic carrier of *S. aureus*
- *Pseudomonas aeruginosa*—from contaminated water in hot tubs and spas
- *Malassezia* yeast (formerly known as Pityrosporum)
- *Trichophyton rubrum* (tinea barbae)
- Herpes simplex virus (HSV)
- *Staphylococcus epidermidis*—may be cultured in 'sterile' folliculitis

Eosinophilic folliculitis—a non-infective condition seen in HIV disease

Laboratory

- Swab for bacterial culture or viral culture (if suspect HSV infection)
- If cultures are negative, take a skin biopsy to determine a non-infective cause

Treatment

For mild staphylococcal folliculitis

Use either of following:
  - Chlorhexidine 1% cream (e.g. Savlon Antiseptic) top PRN
  - Alcohol swabs to wipe the lesions PRN
  - Mupirocin 2% oint/cream (e.g. Bactroban) top tds

For more severe staphylococcal folliculitis

  - Flucloxacillin (PO) for 7–10 days
  - Cefalexin (PO) for 7–10 days (if non-immediate penicillin allergy)
  - Roxithromycin (PO) for 7–10 days (if immediate penicillin allergy)

For pseudomonal folliculitis

  - Identify the source (e.g. hot-water tank/spa) and stop contact with it until the water supply has been treated

For fungal folliculitis

  - Topic antifungal treatment (see Tinea, p. 396)

For herpes simplex folliculitis

- Early treatment with:
  - Aciclovir 5% cream top q4h during day time

Dosage of above antibiotics

- Flucloxacillin 500 mg (child: 12.5 mg/kg up to 500 mg) PO q6h
- Cefalexin 500 mg (child: 12.5 mg/kg up to 500 mg) PO q6h
- Roxithromycin 300 mg PO daily (child: 4 mg/kg up to 150 mg PO q12h)

If lesions continue to recur

- Take nasal, axilla and perineal swabs to confirm the *S. aureus* carrier
- Eradication of *S. aureus* for patient, whole family and close contacts (see Staphylococcal skin infection—recurrent, p. 383)

FUNGAL INFECTION

Other names: Mycoses

SUPERFICIAL AND CUTANEOUS FUNGAL INFECTION

1. **Tinea (skin)**

- **Dermatophytes (moulds):** *Epidermophyton*, *Microsporum*, *Trichophyton*—cause: tinea barbae/tinea capitis (kerion), tinea corporis (ringworm), tinea cruris, tinea pedis, tinea unguium/onychomycosis (see Tinea, p. 396)
- **Ascomycota:** *Hortaea*, *Stenella*—cause tinea nigra
- **Asidiomycota:** *Malassezia*—cause *Pityriasis versicolor* (p. 383)

2. **Piedra (hair) (exothrix/endothrix)**

- ***Trichosporon***—cause white piedra
- ***Piedraia***—cause black piedra

SUBCUTANEOUS, SYSTEMIC AND OPPORTUNISTIC FUNGAL INFECTION

1. **Dimorphic fungi**

- ***Coccidioides immitis***—cause coccidioidomycosis
- ***Histoplasma capsulatum***—cause histoplasmosis
- ***Blastomyces dermatitidsis***—cause blastomycosis
- ***Lacazia loboi***—cause Lobo's disease
- ***Paracoccidioides brasiliensis***—cause paracoccidioidomycosis (PCM)
- ***Sporothrix schenckii***—cause sporotrichosis
- ***Penicillium marneffei***—cause penicilliosis

2. **Yeast-like fungi**

- ***Candida***—cause Candidiasis (p. 40)
- ***Pneumocystis***—cause *Pneumocystis jirovecii* pneumonia (p. 173)
- ***Cryptococcus***—cause cryptococcosis

3. Mould-like/filamentous fungi

- *Mitosporic fungi*—cause aspergillosis (p. 11)
- *Zygomycota*—cause zygomycosis
- *Fonsecaea, Phialophora, Cladosporium*—cause chromoblastomycosis
- *Madurella, Exophiala, Pseudallescheria, Acremonium*—cause eumycetoma, maduromycosis

4. Other/unsorted

- *Geotrichum* spp—cause geotrichosis
- *Microsporidia*—cause microsporidiosis (p. 236)

GANGRENE

Other names: necrotising skin and soft-tissue infections, necrotising cellulitis, necrotising fasciitis, myonecrosis.

- Gangrene—death of tissue due to damaged vascular supply
- Dry gangrene—tissue death with no infection
- Wet gangrene—tissue death with infection

Classification of wet gangrene

Necrotising cellulitis

Necrosis is limited to the skin and subcutaneous fat

- Clostridial necrotising cellulitis—*Clostridium* spp
- Synergistic necrotising cellulitis—mixed aerobes and anaerobes

Necrotising fasciitis

Necrosis involving the subcutaneous tissue and fascia

- *Streptococcus pyogenes* necrotising fasciitis
- Polymicrobial necrotising fasciitis—mixed aerobes and anaerobes

Myonecrosis (gas gangrene)

Necrosis of the muscle

- Clostridial myonecrosis—*Clostridium* spp
- Synergistic gangrene—mixed aerobes and anaerobes

Fournier's gangrene

- Synergistic gangrene of genitalia

Pathogens

- *Clostridium* spp (e.g. *C. perfringens*, *C. septicum* and *C. novyi*)
- *Streptococcus pyogenes*
- Mixed aerobe–anaerobe bacterial flora (e.g. *Escherichia coli*, enterococci, staphylococci, streptococci, *Klebsiella*, *Proteus* and *Bacteroides fragilis*)
- *Vibrio* spp (e.g. *Vibrio vulnificus*)
- *Aeromonas* spp (e.g. *Aermonas hydrophila*)—usually water-related infections

Risk factors

- Penetrating or crushing injuries
- Diabetes mellitus
- Water-related wound
- Malignancy ('spontaneous gas gangrene' due to *C. septicum*)
- Genital trauma (e.g. after vaginal delivery)—Fournier's gangrene

- *S. pyogenes* necrotising fasciitis may occur following varicella (chickenpox)

Clinical

- Rapid development (often within hours of injury)
- Intense pain around the wound (the pain in synergistic gangrene is not as pronounced as with clostridial myonecrosis and may delay the presentation)
- Skin vesicles or bullae, necrosis, swelling with bronze or dusky discolouration and a wooden-hard feeling, oedema beyond the margin of erythema, bloody exudates with foul smell from the wound
- Gas in soft tissues (crepitance on palpation or confirmed on x-ray)
- Systemic toxicity (fever, delirium, bacteraemia and toxic shock syndrome)

Laboratory

- Leucocytosis, high CRP and renal failure
- Blood and tissue cultures

Treatment

- Tetanus vaccine booster as indicated (see Tetanus, p. 393)
- Urgent surgical debridement
- Urgent antibiotic therapy
- Hyperbaric oxygen therapy—if available

Empirical therapy

- Meropenem (IV) **plus** clindamycin (IV) **plus** vancomycin (IV)

Duration of IV therapy

Minimum of 5 days
Switch to oral therapy after significant improvement

For clostridial gas gangrene

- Option 1: benzylpenicillin (IV)
- Option 2: metronidazole (IV) (if penicillin allergy)

For *Streptococcus pyogenes* necrotising fasciitis

- Option 1: benzylpenicillin (IV) **plus** clindamycin (IV)
- Option 2: cefazolin (IV) **plus** clindamycin (IV) (if penicillin allergy)
- Option 3: vancomycin (IV) **plus** clindamycin (IV) (if immediate penicillin allergy)
- Normal immunoglobulin (IV) may be added to above regimens (seek expert advice)

Duration of IV therapy

Minimum of 7 days
Switch to oral therapy after significant improvement

For *Staphylococcus aureus* necrotising skin or soft-tissue infection

- Vancomycin (IV) **plus** clindamycin (IV)

Duration of IV therapy
- Minimum of 5 days
- Switch to oral therapy after significant improvement

For polymicrobial necrotising cellulitis/fasciitis/gas gangrene
- Option 1: meropenem (IV) **plus** clindamycin (IV)
- Option 2: piperacillin/tazobactam (IV) **plus** clindamycin (IV)
- Option 3: ticarcillin/clavulanate (IV) **plus** clindamycin (IV)

If immediate penicillin allergy
- Vancomycin (IV) **plus** ciprofloxacin (IV) **plus** clindamycin (IV)

Dosage of above antibiotics

Empirical therapy
- Meropenem 1 g (child: 25 mg/kg up to 1 g) IV q8h
- Clindamycin 600 mg (child: 15 mg/kg up to 600 mg) IV q8h
- Vancomycin 25–30 mg/kg IV for the 1st dose (further dosing see p. 462)

For clostridial gas gangrene
- Benzylpenicillin 2.4 g (child: 50 mg/kg up to 2.4 g) IV q4h
- Metronidazole 500 mg (child: 12.5 mg/kg up to 500 mg) IV q8h

For *Streptococcus pyogenes* necrotising fasciitis
- Benzylpenicillin 1.8 g (child: 50 mg/kg up to 1.8 g) IV q4h
- Clindamycin 600 mg (child: 15 mg/kg up to 600 mg) IV q8h
- Cefazolin 2 g (child: 50 mg/kg up to 2 g) IV q8h
- Vancomycin 25–30 mg/kg IV for the 1st dose (further dosing see p. 462)
- Normal immunoglobulin 1–2 g/kg IV for 1 or 2 doses during the first 72 hours

For *Staphlococcus aureus* necrotising skin or soft-tissue infection
- Vancomycin 25–30 mg/kg IV for the 1st dose (further dosing see p. 462)
- Clindamycin 600 mg (child: 15 mg/kg up to 600 mg) IV q8h

For polymicrobial necrotising cellulitis/fasciitis/gas gangrene
- Meropenem 1 g (child: 25 mg/kg up to 1 g) IV q8h
- Clindamycin 600 mg (child: 15 mg/kg up to 600 mg) IV q8h
- Piperacillin/tazobactam 4 g (child: 100 mg/kg up to 4 g) IV q6h
- Ticarcillin/clavulanate 3 g (child: 50 mg/kg up to 3 g) IV q4–6h
- Vancomycin 25–30 mg/kg IV for the 1st dose (further dosing see p. 462)
- Ciprofloxacin 400 mg IV q8h (child: 10 mg/kg) IV q12h

GASTROENTERITIS

VIRAL GASTROENTERITIS

Pathogens
- Rotavirus, norovirus, adenovirus (serotypes 40 and 41), astrovirus

Transmission

- Faecal–oral route
- Aerosol spread from vomitus (suspected in some rotavirus and norovirus outbreaks)
- Person-to-person transmission has occurred (e.g. norovirus outbreaks)

Incubation

- Rotavirus—1–3 days
- Norovirus—1–2 days
- Astrovirus—3–4 days

Clinical

- Rotavirus infection—the most common cause of severe gastroenteritis in children; common in winter; vomiting and fever for 1–3 days, followed by diarrhoea for 4–5 days; fatal dehydration can occur in infants; infections in adults are usually mild or asymptomatic
- Norovirus infection—the most common cause of gastroenteritis in adults and older children; predominantly vomiting and abdominal cramping with later watery diarrhoea for 2–3 days; commonly causes outbreaks in institutional settings in winter
- Adenovirus—predominantly in infants and young children; fever, vomiting and diarrhoea; generally self-limiting; many infections are asymptomatic; immunocompromised patients may have more severe infection
- Astrovirus—a common cause of diarrhoea in children; diarrhoea lasts for fewer than 5 days with less vomiting

Treatment/prevention

- Supportive and rehydration
- Rotavirus vaccination for young babies

BACTERIAL GASTROENTERITIS

Pathogens

- *Campylobacter jejuni*
- *Salmonella* spp (non-typhoidal)
- *Escherichia coli* (e.g. enterohaemorrhagic *E. coli*)
- *Shigella*
- *Clostridium difficile* (antibiotic-associated diarrhoea)

Transmission

- Faecal–oral route

Clinical

- Abdominal pain, nausea and vomiting; may have fever/rigor
- Bloody diarrhoea is suggestive of bacterial infection
- Returned travellers and immunocompromised patients are at greater risk

Laboratory

- Routine faecal microbiological testing is not required during acute stage of gastroenteritis
- Indication for faecal microbiological testing:
1. Severe disease (e.g. high fever, severe abdominal pain, high-volume diarrhoea with hypovolaemia, bloody diarrhoea)—test for routine pathogens
2. Hospitalised patient >48 hours or recent antibiotic use—test for *Clostridium difficile* + toxin
3. Immunocompromised patient—test for routine pathogens + parasites + cytomegalovirus
4. Recent international (high-risk area) travel—test for routine pathogens + *Salmonella typhi* and *paratyphi* A, B, C)
5. Patient resident in an aged-care facility or a food handler—contact public health authorities and perform faecal microbiological testing for routine pathogens
- Routine faecal microbiological testing—screen for *Campylobacter*, non-typhoidal *Salmonella*, *Shigella* and parasites
- Faecal multiplex PCR testing—screen for multiple organisms (bacteria, parasites); it is fast and sensitive
- Faecal *Clostridium difficile* + toxin

Treatment

- Fluid and electrolyte therapy; symptomatic treatment
- Most bacterial diarrhoea is self-limiting and does not usually require antibiotics
- Child with bloody diarrhoea without fever—do not use antibiotic (potentially precipitate haemolytic uraemic syndrome (HUS) if it is caused by enterohaemorrhagic *E. coli*)
- Indications for antibiotic therapy in acute diarrhoea:
1. Severe diarrhoea that is likely to be bacterial in origin
2. Patient has serious underlying diseases or is immunocompromised
3. Invasive bacterial diarrhoea (bloody diarrhoea and rigors/fevers)
4. Persistent diarrhoea (>1–2 weeks)—a trial of antibiotic therapy may be considered

Antibiotic treatment should be started after collection of faecal samples for testing

Empirical antibiotic therapy

Not appropriate for hospitalised patients
- Option 1: ciprofloxacin (PO) for 3 days
- Option 2: norfloxacin (PO) for 3 days

If the infection is likely acquired from Southeast Asia (quinolone-resistant)
- Azithromycin (PO) for 3 days

If IV therapy is required
- Ceftriaxone (IV) for 3 days

Adjust therapy according to microbiological testing results

Dosage of above agents
- Ciprofloxacin 500 mg (child: 12.5 mg/kg up to 500 mg) PO q12h
- Norfloxacin 400 mg (child: 10 mg/kg up to 400 mg) PO q12h
- Azithromycin 500 mg (child: 10 mg/kg up to 500 mg) PO daily
- Ceftriaxone 2 g (child ≤1 month: 50 mg/kg up to 2 g) IV daily

TOXIN-INDUCED GASTROENTERITIS

Causes

- Toxin produced from *Staphylococcus aureus*
- Toxin produced from *Bacillus cereus*

Incubation

- Several hours

Clinical

- Sudden onset of vomiting, abdominal pain; may be followed by diarrhoea; no fever
- Symptoms usually resolve within 24–48 hours

Treatment

- Symptomatic and supportive treatment

GIARDIASIS

Pathogens

- *Giardia intestinalis* (also known as *Giardia lamblia* or *Giardia duodenalis*)

Transmission

- Faecal–oral—ingestion of contaminated water (cysts remain viable in water for up to 3 months)
- Animals may carry the parasite and pass it to humans

Incubation

- 1–3 weeks

Clinical

- Many infected patients are asymptomatic carriers
- Most commonly infected are infants, young children and adults aged 20–40 years

- Diarrhoea, nausea, abdominal pain and distension, usually lasting a few days, but may continue for weeks or months (associated with flatulence and weight loss)

Laboratory

- Faeces OCP—to see the cysts
- Faecal multiplex PCR testing—sensitivity 98–100%, result available in 24 hours
- Giardia antigen test (faeces, duodenal aspiration)
- Duodenal aspiration/biopsy via gastroscopy—to see the cysts or trophozoites

Exclusion

- Food handlers, childcare workers and healthcare workers with giardiasis must not work
- Child patients must not attend childcare centres or school until symptoms resolve

Treatment

- Asymptomatic passage of giardia cysts—may or may not require treatment

First-line treatment

- Option 1: tinidazole (PO) for 1 to 3 days
- Option 2: metronidazole (PO) for 3 **or** 7 days
- Option 3: nitazoxanide* (PO) for 3 days
- Option 4: paromomycin* (PO) for 7 days (for pregnant women)

For resistant infection

- Option 1: metronidazole + nitazoxanide* + furazolidone* (PO) for 10 days
- Option 2: paromomycin* + nitazoxanide* + furazolidone* (PO) for 14 days

Repeat stool test 4–6 weeks after treatment to determine the eradication

Dosage of above agents

- Tinidazole 2 g (child: 50 mg/kg up to 2 g) PO daily for 1 to 3 days
- Metronidazole 2 g (child: 30 mg/kg up to 2 g) PO daily for 3 days
  or Metronidazole 400 mg (child: 10 mg/kg up to 400 mg) PO tds for 7 days
- Nitazoxanide 500 mg (child 1–3 years: 100 mg; 4–11 years: 200 mg) PO bid for 3 days
- Paromomycin 500 mg (children: 10 mg/kg up to 500 mg) PO tds for 7 days

---

Available via Special Access Scheme <www.tga.gov.au/hp/access-sas.htm> or from compounding chemist

For resistant infection
- Metronidazole 400 mg PO bid
- Nitazoxanide 500 mg PO bid
- Furazolidone 100 mg PO tds
- Paromomycin 500 mg PO tds

GINGIVITIS—ACUTE ULCERATIVE

Other names: Vincent's angina, trench mouth
Gingivitis is an inflammation of the gums.

Pathogens

- *Borrelia vincentii* (a spirochaete)
- *Bacteroides*
- *Fusobacterium*

Clinical

- Most commonly seen in young adult smokers (rarely in children)
- Extremely painful infection of the periodontal tissues
- Punched-out interdental papillae, ulcers (covered with greyish membrane)
- Fetid odour
- Often with systemic symptoms and signs

Treatment

- Debridement under local anaesthesia (may be delayed until less painful)
- Chlorhexidine mouthwash (to improve plaque control)
- Give advice on oral hygiene and smoking cessation
- Antibiotics—when systemic symptoms and signs are present

Mild cases

- Metronidazole (PO) for 5 days
- Chlorhexidine mouthwash for 5 days

More severe or unresponsive cases

- Penicillin V (PO) **or** amoxicillin (PO) **plus** metronidazole (PO) for 5 days

If penicillin allergy
- Clindamycin (PO) **plus** metronidazole (PO) for 5 days

If develop necrotising ulcerative periodontitis (e.g. in HIV patients)
- Refer to a specialist

Dosage of above antibiotics

- Metronidazole 400 mg (child: 10 mg/kg up to 400 mg) PO q12h
- Chlorhexidine 0.2% mouthwash (e.g. Savacol® Alcohol-free Mouth & Throat Rinse) 10 mL rinse in mouth for 1 min q8–12h
  or Chlorhexidine 0.12% mouthwash (e.g. Savacol® Freshmint Antiseptic Mouth & Throat Rinse) 15 mL rinse in mouth for 1 min q8–12h

- Penicillin V 500 mg (child: 10 mg/kg up to 500 mg) PO q6h
- Amoxicillin 500 mg (child: 10 mg/kg up to 500 mg) PO q8h
- Clindamycin 300 mg (child: 5 mg/kg up to 300 mg) PO q8h

GLANDERS

Glanders is a disease of animals such as horses, mules and donkeys. Cases in humans are rare and sporadic. Glanders may be used in biological warfare.

Pathogens

- *Burkholderia mallei* (gram-negative bacillus)

Transmission

- Direct contact between infected animal tissues and broken skin or mucous membranes
- Inhalation of droplets from an infected patient
- Human-to-human transmission has been reported

Incubation

- 1–21 days

Risk groups

- Veterinarians, animal caretakers, abattoir workers and laboratory personnel

Clinical

- **Localised form**—local infection with ulceration, swollen lymph glands
- **Pulmonary form**—pneumonia, pulmonary abscesses and pleural effusions
- **Septicaemia**—affects multiple systems, usually fatal within 7–10 days
- **Chronic form**—multiple abscesses involving liver, spleen, skin or muscles

Laboratory

- Gram stain and culture of sputum, urine and skin lesions
- Complement fixation tests—positive if titre ≥1 : 20

Prevention

- Use isolation room, disposable surgical masks, face shields and gowns to prevent human-to-human transmission

Post-exposure prophylaxis

- Cotrimoxazole 320/1600 mg (child: 8/40 mg/kg up to 320/1600 mg) PO q12h for 3 months

Treatment

Choose one of following antibiotics
  • Ceftazidime (IV) **or** meropenem (IV) **or** imipenem (IV) for at least
    2 weeks
For osteomyelitis and septic arthritis
  • One of above regimens for 4–8 weeks
Eradication after intensive therapy
  • Cotrimoxazole **plus/minus** doxycycline (PO) for a further 3 months
  • Folic acid 5 mg (child: 0.1 mg/kg up to 5 mg) PO daily

Dosage of above antibiotics

  • Ceftazidime 2 g (child: 50 mg/kg up to 2 g) IV q8h
  • Meropenem 1 g (child: 25 mg/kg up to 1 g) IV q8h
  • Imipenem/cilastatin 1 g (child: 25 mg/kg up to 1 g) IV q6h
  • Cotrimoxazole 320/1600 mg (child: 8/40 mg/kg up to 320/1600 mg)
    PO q12h
  • Doxycycline 100 mg (child >8 years: 2.5 mg/kg up to 100 mg) PO
    q12h

GLANDULAR FEVER

Other names: infectious mononucleosis, 'kissing disease'

Pathogens

• Epstein-Barr virus (EBV, human herpes virus type 4)
• Occasionally other viruses

Transmission

• Person-to-person via saliva (e.g. kissing between an uninfected person
  and an EBV-seropositive person who is shedding the virus
  asymptomatically)
• Only about 5% of patients acquire EBV from someone who has acute
  infection
• Blood transfusion may also transmit the virus
• About 15–20% of infected adults become chronic carriers

Incubation

• 4–6 weeks

Clinical

• More common in young children and adolescents
• In most young children, primary EBV infection is asymptomatic
• Fatigue, fever, pharyngitis and lymphadenopathy
• Fatigue may persist for weeks or months, sometimes leading to
  depression
• Severe pharyngitis/tonsillar exudate may resemble streptococcal
  pharyngitis and tonsillitis, but EBV infection usually has posterior

triangle glands enlargement, while streptococcal tonsillitis/pharyngitis causes submandibular glands tenderness

Complications

- Airway obstruction, splenic rupture, thrombocytopenia, haemolytic anaemia, aplastic anaemia, pneumonia, aseptic meningitis, encephalitis, Guillain-Barré syndrome, fulminant liver failure and lymphoma

Laboratory

- Blood film—lymphocytosis with atypical lymphocytes (20% of all WBCs)
- Monospot (heterophil antibody test)—high specificity, low sensitivity
- EBV serology—IgM positive indicates current infection
- CSF PCR for EBV

Treatment

- Usually self-limiting, supportive treatment only, no antibiotics are indicated
- Corticosteroids may be helpful for complications such as impending airway obstruction, severe thrombocytopenia or haemolytic anaemia
- Avoid amoxicillin/ampicillin—frequently precipitate a rash
- Prevent splenic rupture—avoid heavy lifting and contact sports for 1 month
- Antiviral therapy—aciclovir (limited effect) or cidofovir

For severe complications (e.g. pneumonia, viral meningitis, encephalitis)
  - Empirical: aciclovir 10 mg/kg IV q8h for 1–2 weeks
  - Confirmed: cidofovir 5 mg/kg IV weekly for 2 weeks + probenecid

Use aciclovir in suspected viral encephalitis; once EBV encephalitis is confirmed, use cidofovir as an alternative

Prevention

- Minimise contact with saliva
- Vaccines against the major EBV glycoprotein have been effective in animal studies and are undergoing clinical trials

GONOCOCCAL CONJUNCTIVITIS

Other names: hyperacute conjunctivitis

Pathogens

- *Neisseria gonorrhoeae*, a gram-negative intracellular diplococcus
- In central and northern Australia (sporadic)—the bacteria are still penicillin-susceptible
- In other areas of Australia (sporadic)—high penicillin-resistant bacteria

Transmission

- Direct or indirect sexual contact

Incubation

- 2–7 days

Clinical

- Abrupt onset of red eye with foreign body sensation; may be 'glued' shut with copious purulent discharge, eyelid oedema and fever; enlarged preauricular lymph nodes
- Cornea ulceration and perforation can lead to blindness
- In chronic cases, corneal infiltrates lead to marginal ulceration with anterior uveitis
- May be associated with infection of the urethra, cervix and rectum

Laboratory

Conjunctival swab/scraping for:

- Microscopy (detect typical gram-negative intracellular diplococci)
- Immediate *gonorrhoea* culture and sensitivity test
- *Gonorrhoea* PCR testing

Treatment

- Irrigate the eyes with saline several times daily until purulence subsides (particularly for neonates)
- Oral antibiotic only (eye drops/ointments are not required)
- The mother of an infected neonate and her sexual contacts should also be treated
- In an epidemic situation, all household and classroom contacts should be treated

Treat both gonorrhoea and *Chlamydia* at the same time

- Ceftriaxone (**or** cefotaxime*) (IM or IV) st
- Azithromycin (PO) st (coinfection with *Chlamydia trachomatis* is common)

If immediate penicillin allergy

- Seek expert advice

If cornea ulceration occurs

- Immediate referral to an ophthalmologist

Dosage of above antibiotics

- Ceftriaxone 1 g (child: 50 mg/kg up to 1 g) IM** or IV st
- Cefotaxime 1 g (child: 50 mg/kg up to 1 g; neonate: 100 mg/kg) IM or IV st
- Azithromycin 1 g (child: 20 mg/kg up to 1 g) PO st (neonate: 20 mg/kg PO daily for 3 days)

---

*In neonates and pre-terms do not use ceftriaxone (it displaces bilirubin from albumin and increases the risk of bilirubin encephalopathy)

**IM injection of ceftriaxone needs reconstitute with 1% lidocaine (lignocaine)

GONOCOCCAL NEONATE OPHTHALMIA

Pathogen

- *Neisseria gonorrhoeae*, a gram-negative intracellular diplococcus

Transmission

- Acquired when neonate passes through an infected birth canal
- Highly contagious

Incubation

- 2–7 days

Clinical

- Occurs within the first 3–5 days of life
- Sudden onset of severe red eye, which may be 'glued' shut with purulent discharge
- Conjunctival papillae, superficial punctate keratitis and chemosis

It may rapidly lead to perforation of the globe and blindness

Laboratory

Conjunctival swabs for:

- Microscopy—finds typical gram-negative intracellular diplococci
- Culture and sensitivity test for *Neisseria gonorrhoeae*
- PCR for *Neisseria gonorrhoeae*

Treatment

- Urgent treatment is required to save the vision of the neonate
- Start IV antibiotics ASAP (eye drops/ointments are not required)
- Use saline to irrigate the eye several times a day until purulence subsides
- The mother of the neonate should be treated for gonococcal cervicitis (p. 47)
- The mother's sexual contacts should be treated for gonococcal urethritis (p. 419)
  - Cefotaxime* (IV) for 7 days **plus** azithromycin (PO) as a single dose
If penicillin-susceptible (some central and northern areas of Australia)
  - Benzylpenicillin (IV) for 7 days **plus** azithromycin (PO) as a single dose

Dosage of above antibiotics

- Cefotaxime 50 mg/kg IV q6h
- Azithromycin 20 mg/kg PO as a single dose

---

*In neonates and pre-terms do not use ceftriaxone (it displaces bilirubin from albumin and increases the risk of bilirubin encephalopathy)

- Benzylpenicillin 30 mg/kg IV q12h during the 1st week of life, then 30 mg/kg IV q6–8h during the 2nd to 4th weeks of life

GONORRHOEA

Pathogens

- *Neisseria gonorrhoeae*, a gram-negative intracellular diplococcus
- In central and northern Australia (sporadic or epidemic)—the bacteria are still penicillin-susceptible
- In other areas of Australia (sporadic)—high penicillin-resistant bacteria

Transmission

- Sexual transmission (direct or indirect sexual contact)
- Vertical transmission to neonatal during vaginal delivery

Incubation

- 2–7 days

Clinical

Symptoms in male

- Urethral discharge and irritation (early symptoms)
- Dysuria (the most common symptom)
- Tenderness and/or swelling of the epididymis (epididymitis)
- Tenderness and/or swelling of the testis (orchitis, usually one side)
- Tenderness and/or swelling of the prostate (prostatitis, uncommon)

Symptoms in female

- Often asymptomatic
- Vaginal discharge
- Pelvic pain (may occur with sex)
- Mucopurulent or purulent exudate at the endocervix (cervicitis)
- Cervical friability (bleeding with gentle passage of a cotton swab through cervical os—cervicitis)
- Uterine, adnexal or cervical motion tenderness (PID)

Neonatal infection

- Neonate ophthalmia—if untreated, it may rapidly lead to perforation of the globe and blindness
  - Occurs within the first 2–5 days of life
  - Sudden onset of severe red eye with white/yellow discharge; eyes may be 'glued' shut
  - Conjunctival papillae, superficial punctate keratitis and chemosis
  - Subconjunctival haemorrhage and enlarged preauricular lymph nodes
- Neonatal sepsis (include arthritis and meningitis)
- Less severe infections—rhinitis, vaginitis, urethritis and reinfection at a site of fetal monitoring

Other infections

- Pharyngeal gonorrhoea—anterior cervical lymphadenopathy
- Rectal gonorrhoea—anal pruritus, rectal pain, rectal discharge, rectal bleeding, tenesmus
- Gonococcal meningitis—fever, headache, purpuric skin rash, stiff neck, seizures, focal cerebral signs
- Gonococcal arthritis—polyarthralgia
- Gonococcal endocarditis—heart murmur
- Chronic gonococcal eye infection—corneal infiltrates lead to marginal ulceration with anterior uveitis

Complications

- Epididymitis/orchitis (men)
- Chronic pelvic pain (women)
- Ectopic pregnancy (women)
- Tubal infertility (women)
- Infertility (women and men)
- Blindness (neonates)
- Polyarthritis (women and men)
- Meningitis (women, men and neonates)
- Endocarditis (women and men)
- Perihepatic abscesses (women)
- Fitz-Hugh-Curtis syndrome (gonococcal perihepatitis, mimics acute cholecystitis)

Laboratory

- PCR for *N. gonorrhoeae* (first-void urine; urethral, cervical and vaginal swabs; Pap smear; low specificity for pharyngeal and anal swabs)—the most sensitive
- Gram stain (urine, urethral, endocervical, conjunctival swabs, synovial fluid, CSF)—gram-negative intracellular diplococci
- Culture + susceptibility testing for *N. gonorrhoeae* (urethral, endocervical, conjunctival swabs, blood, synovial fluid, CSF, low sensitivity for pharyngeal and anal swabs)—guide antibiotic treatment
- Urinalysis—for urethritis in men, if no urethral discharge

Treatment

For uncomplicated gonorrhoea

A single dose of ceftriaxone

- Ceftriaxone 500 mg in 2 mL 1% lidocaine (lignocaine) IM st **or** 500 mg IV st

In remote Australia where penicillin-resistant *N. gonorrhoeae* is low

- Amoxicillin 3 g **plus** probenecid 1 g PO st

If gonococci is resistant to ceftriaxone, seek expert advice

For disseminated gonococcal sepsis

- Ceftriaxone 1 g IV daily (**or** cefotaxime 1 g IV q8h)

Continue for 48 hours after afebrile, then switch to oral based on culture and susceptibility results

Total duration

- Should be 7 days or 14 days (if symptoms persist)

Treat gonococcal urethritis—see Urethritis (p. 419)
Treat gonococcal epididymitis and orchitis—see Epididymo-orchitis (p. 106)
Treat gonococcal cervicitis—see Cervicitis (p. 47)
Treat gonococcal pelvic infection—see Pelvic inflammatory disease (p. 273)
Treat gonococcal neonate ophthalmia—see Gonococcal neonate ophthalmia (p. 135)
Treat gonococcal endocarditis—see Endocarditis—direct therapy (p. 95)
Treat gonococcal arthritis—see Septic arthritis/bursitis (p. 373)

Note

- Empirical treatment should always cover both *Chlamydia* and gonococci
- As cefalosporin-resistant gonorrhoea emerges, any suggestion of possible treatment failure in gonorrhoea should be reported to public health authorities and advice should be obtained from a sexual health practitioner

HAEMORRHAGIC FEVER—VIRAL

Other names: Crimean-Congo, Ebola, Hantaan, Lassa, Marburg

Viral haemorrhagic fevers (VHFs) refer to a group of illnesses caused by several distinct viruses. They are not endemic in Australia, but may occur in returned travellers.

Haemorrhagic fever viruses include:

- **Non-BSL-4 (biosafety level 4) viruses**—dengue, yellow fever and scrub typhus, which can cause haemorrhagic fever as a severe complication
- **BSL-4 viruses**—exotic agents that pose a high risk of life-threatening disease, which may be transmitted by the aerosol route (see below)

Incubation

- 4–21 days

1. CRIMEAN-CONGO HAEMORRHAGIC FEVER (CCHF)

Pathogen

- Nairovirus—a member of *Bunyaviruses*

Transmission

- Tick-borne
- Direct handling of fresh carcasses of infected animals

Distribution

- Eastern Europe, Mediterranean, north-western China, central Asia, southern Europe, Africa, the Middle East and Indian subcontinent

Treatment

- Ribavirin (adult and child) 30 mg/kg up to 2 g IV for 1st dose, then 16 mg/kg up to 1 g IV q6h for 4 days, then 8 mg/kg up to 500 mg IV q8h for 6 days

2. EBOLA HAEMORRHAGIC FEVER

Pathogen

- Ebola virus—a member of filoviruses

Transmission

- Contact with fruit bats or monkeys
- Human-to-human transmission through broken skin, needle-stick injury or sexual contact

Distribution

- Congo, Côte d'Ivoire, Democratic Republic of Congo, Gabon, Sudan and Uganda

3. HANTAAN HAEMORRHAGIC FEVER WITH RENAL SYNDROME (HFRS)

Pathogen

- Hantavirus

Transmission

- Striped field mouse

Distribution

- Central and Eastern Asia

Treatment

- Ribavirin (adult and child) 30 mg/kg up to 2 g IV for 1st dose, then 16 mg/kg up to 1 g IV q6h for 4 days, then 8 mg/kg up to 500 mg IV q8h for 6 days

4. LASSA FEVER

Pathogen

- Lassa virus—a member of arenaviruses

Transmission

- Inhalation of aerosols from rodent urine, ingestion of rodent-contaminated food or direct contact of broken skin with rodent excreta

Distribution

- Rural areas of West Africa, with areas of hyperendemicity in eastern Sierra Leone, Guinea, Liberia and Nigeria

Treatment

- Ribavirin (adult and child) 30 mg/kg up to 2 g IV for 1st dose, then 16 mg/kg up to 1 g IV q6h for 4 days, then 8 mg/kg up to 500 mg IV q8h for 6 days

5. MARBURG HAEMORRHAGIC FEVER

Pathogen

- Marburg virus—a member of filoviruses

Transmission

- Direct contact with infected monkeys
- Direct contact with infected persons
- Direct contact with contaminated equipment in hospital

Distribution

- Europe and Africa, including parts of Uganda, western Kenya, Democratic Republic of Congo, Angola and possibly Zimbabwe

Treatment

- Ribavirin (adult and child) 30 mg/kg up to 2 g IV 1st dose, then 16 mg/kg up to 1 g IV q6h for 4 days, then 8 mg/kg up to 500 mg IV q8h for 6 days

HAND, FOOT AND MOUTH DISEASE (HFMD)

Pathogens

- *Coxsackievirus* A16 or A10
- *Enterovirus* 71 (EV71) (also causes fatal neurological disease in young children)

Transmission

- Direct contact with the fluid of the blisters, mucus, saliva or faeces of an infected person
- The virus may continue to be excreted in the faeces for many weeks after symptoms develop
- Typically occurs in small epidemics in nursery schools or kindergartens, usually during the summer and autumn months

Incubation

- 3–7 days

Clinical

- Commonly affects children; highly infectious
- Slight fever, sore throat, followed by blisters on the hands and feet and ulcers in the mouth; rash and blisters may also occur on other parts of the body
- ***Enterovirus* 71 (EV71) neurological disease**—occasionally, *Enterovirus* 71 can cause acute flaccid paralysis, meningitis or encephalitis in young children (see *Enterovirus* 71, p. 105)

Laboratory

- HFMD—does not require laboratory testing
- EV71 neurological disease (HFMD with high fever, paralysis, stiff neck or mental status change)—consider and test for:
    - Viral swabs for EV71 virus isolation—from throat, mouth ulcers, skin lesions, faecal samples or CSF specimens
    - Enterovirus serology (IgM)

Treatment

- Symptomatic treatment
- Recovery usually occurs within a week
- Treatment for EV71 neurological disease, see *Enterovirus* 71 (p. 105)

Prevention

- Wash hands with soap and water after going to toilet, before eating and after touching skin lesions
- School exclusion until blisters and ulcers have healed
- EV71 vaccines and antiviral agents are being worked on

HELICOBACTER PYLORI

Helicobacter pylori infects 20–30% of Australians and up to 50% of the populations in many parts of the world.

Pathogen

- *Helicobacter pylori*, a spiral-shaped Gram-negative bacteria, colonises the gastric epithelium under the mucus layer

Transmission

- Person-to-person (oral–oral or faecal–oral)

Clinical

- *H. pylori* causes peptic ulcer disease, gastric cancer and, rarely, MALT lymphoma
- Most infections do not cause significant disease clinically

Laboratory

- Urea breath test (^{13}C)—diagnosis and eradication monitoring
- Faecal *H. pylori* antigen test—diagnosis and eradication monitoring
- *H. pylori* serology (IgG)—diagnosis only (if never treated before)
- Endoscopy with gastric/duodenal biopsy—for rapid urease test, culture and histology

Treatment

- There are multiple strains of *H. pylori* that have different sensitivity to antibiotics
- First-line therapy may eradicate sensitive strains leaving the resistant strains behind
- After first-line therapy, repeat urea breath test or faecal antigen test in 4 weeks to check the eradication status; if still positive, use second-line therapy

1. **First-line therapy (cure rate only 65–80%)**
   - Esomeprazole/omeprazole + clarithromycin + amoxicillin (PO) for 7 days (e.g. Nexium Hp7)
   If penicillin allergy
   - Esomeprazole/omeprazole + clarithromycin + metronidazole (PO) for 7 days

2. Second-line therapy (if first-line therapy fails)

- Option 1: omeprazole + amoxicillin + furazolidone* + colloidal bismuth* (PO) for 14 days
- Option 2: omeprazole + amoxicillin + furazolidone* + rifabutin* (PO) for 14 days

If penicillin allergy

- Omeprazole + furazolidone* + colloidal bismuth* + levofloxacin* + rifabutin* (PO) for 14 days

For child 29–50 kg

- Omeprazole + amoxicillin + rifabutin* (PO) for 14 days

3. Third-line therapy (Marshall therapy)

- Esomeprazole/omeprazole + amoxicillin + ciprofloxacin + rifabutin* (PO) for 14 days

After eradication, followed by

- Esomeprazole/omeprazole 20 mg PO daily for 3–4 weeks

Note

- Take medication with food and avoid drinking alcohol

Dosage of above antibiotics

1. First-line therapy
   - Esomeprazole/omeprazole 20 mg PO bid for 7 days
   - Clarithromycin 500 mg PO bid for 7 days
   - Amoxicillin 1 g PO bid for 7 days

If penicillin allergy

   - Esomeprazole/omeprazole 20 mg PO bid for 7 days
   - Clarithromycin 500 mg PO bid for 7 days
   - Metronidazole 400 mg PO bid for 7 days

2. Second-line therapy

Option 1

   - Omeprazole 20 mg PO bid for 14 days (20 mg × 28)
   - Amoxicillin 1 g PO bid for 14 days (1 g × 28)
   - Furazolidone 200 mg PO bid for 14 days (200 mg × 28)
   - Colloidal bismuth 120 mg PO qid for 14 days (120 mg × 56)

Option 2

   - Omeprazole 40 mg PO tds for 14 days (40 mg × 42)
   - Amoxicillin 1.5 g PO tds for 14 days (500 mg × 126)
   - Furazolidone 100 mg PO tds for 14 days (100 mg × 42)
   - Rifabutin 60 mg PO bid for days 1–2, then 120 mg PO bid for days 3–14 (60 mg × 4; 120 mg × 24)

If penicillin allergy

   - Omeprazole 40 mg PO tds for 14 days (40 mg × 42)
   - Furazolidone 100 mg PO tds for 14 days (100 mg × 42)

---

*Available via Special Access Scheme <www.tga.gov.au/hp/access-sas.htm> or from compounding chemist

- Colloidal bismuth 300 mg, 2 caps PO tds for 14 days (300 mg × 84)
- Levofloxacin 375 mg, 1 cap mane, 2 caps nocte PO for 14 days (375 mg × 42)
- Rifabutin 60 mg PO bid for days 1–2, then 120 mg PO bid for days 3–14 (60 mg × 4; 120 mg × 24)

For child
- Omeprazole 10 mg PO tds for 14 days (10 mg × 42)
- Amoxicillin child 29–39 kg: 420 mg; 40–50 kg: 450 mg PO tds for 14 days (420 mg × 42 or 450 mg × 42)
- Rifabutin 30 mg PO bid for days 1–2, then 60 mg PO bid for days 3–14 (30 mg × 4; 60 mg × 24)

3. Third-line therapy (Marshall therapy)
   - Esomeprazole/omeprazole 40 mg PO tds for 14 days (40 mg × 42)
   - Amoxicillin 1 g PO tds for 14 days (1 g × 42)
   - Ciprofloxacin 500 mg PO bid for 14 days (500 mg × 28)
   - Rifabutin 150 mg PO bid for 14 Days (150 × 28)

HENDRA AND NIPAH VIRUSES

Other names: equine morbillivirus infection
Hendra virus (HeV) was first found in Australia in 1994. New cases still occur in Queensland. Deaths from the infection have been reported.

Pathogens

- Hendra virus together with Nipah virus forms the genus *henipavirus* in the family *Paramyxoviridae*
- Unlike other Paramyxoviruses, which tend to be host-specific, Hendra can infect more than one animal species

Distribution

- Hendra virus is found only in Australia and Papua New Guinea
- Nipah virus is found in Southeast Asia and Indonesia

Transmission

- Fruit bats (flying foxes) are the natural hosts of Hendra and Nipah viruses
- Horses eat infected bat faeces mixed with grass and become infected
- Human infections occur from contact with infected horses (blood, respiratory and nasal secretions, saliva, urine or tissues of the ill horses or during autopsies); the virus gains entry via open wounds or cuts
- No human-to-human transmission

Clinical

- Flu-like illness, fever; may progress to pneumonia or encephalitis

Laboratory

- Serology of HeV—rising antibody titre
- PCR testing for HeV—from blood, nasal secretions, CSF or body tissues

Treatment

- When Hendra virus infection is suspected in animals and potential human exposure occurs, medical advice should be sought
- Early treatment with an antiviral drug (ribavirin) may reduce both the duration and the severity of the disease
- Symptomatic and supportive treatment; may need mechanical ventilation

Prevention

- Vaccine against Hendra virus is under development
- Avoid contact with suspected horses until a veterinarian has investigated and advice for safe handling has been provided
- All those involved in investigating a suspect case must wear full protective clothing: impervious overalls, boots, gloves, respirator mask and face shield
- If contamination occurs, the contaminated skin should be washed thoroughly with soap and water
- Any cuts or abrasions that become exposed or contaminated should be cleansed thoroughly with soap and water and an antiseptic with antivirus action such as povidone-iodine, iodine tincture, aqueous iodine solution or alcohol (ethanol) should be applied after washing
- Ribavirin may be given for 5 days as prophylaxis for a patient's contacts

HEPATITIS A

Pathogen

- Hepatitis A virus (HAV), an RNA picornavirus

Transmission

- Faecal–oral
- HAV is excreted in faeces (infectious) from 2 weeks prior to the onset of symptoms to 1 week after jaundice starts

Incubation

- 2–7 weeks

Clinical

- Fever, jaundice, anorexia, nausea and vomiting, occasionally 'cholestatic form of hepatitis'; rarely, fulminant hepatitis, liver coma and death
- No carrier, no chronic liver disease, no association with liver cancer

Diagnosis

Liver damage plus either:

- HAV serology—anti-HAV IgM positive (without recent HAV vaccination)
- HAV PCR testing

Treatment

- Symptomatic and supportive
- Cholestatic form of hepatitis A—short course of corticosteroid

HAV vaccination

Vaccination is indicated for

- All travellers to endemic areas (including all developing countries)
- Aboriginal and Torres Strait Islander children residing in the Northern Territory, Queensland, South Australia and Western Australia (at 12–24 years)
- Those at occupational risk of exposure to HAV (e.g. childcare and healthcare workers, food handlers, plumbers or sewage workers, and sex workers)
- Male–male intercourse and injecting drug users
- Patients with chronic liver disease, including chronic hepatitis B or C

Monovalent vaccines
  - HAV vaccine (e.g. Avaxim, Havrix, VAQTA®) ≥16 years: 1.0 mL (1–15 years: 0.5 mL) IM, followed by a booster at 6–12 months

Combination vaccines
  - Hep A/hep B (Twinrix) ≥16 years: 1.0 mL (1–15 years: 0.5 mL) IM, at 0, 1, 6 months
  - Hep A/typhoid (Vivaxim) ≥16 years: 1.0 mL IM st, then a booster hep A vaccine (e.g. Havrix 1440, VAQTA® Adult) at 6–36 months

A booster produces antibodies for at least 1 year; the immunity can last for 10 years

Passive immunisation (for people occasionally at risk)
  - Normal immunoglobulin 0.03–0.06 mL/kg IM

One injection of immunoglobulin provides protection for 3–4 months

Prevention

- Wash hands before handling food and after toileting
- While travelling overseas, boil drinking water and fully cook foods

HEPATITIS B

Hepatitis B affects almost 1% of the Australian population.

Pathogen

- Hepatitis B virus (HBV), a DNA virus

Transmission

- Mother-to-neonate at or around the time of birth or through breastfeeding
- Unprotected sex (higher risk with anal intercourse)
- Injecting drug use, tattooing/body piercing, needle-stick injuries
- Child-to-child contact through open sores or wounds
- Household sharing of toothbrush, razor etc with a carrier or patient

Incubation

- 4–20 months

Clinical

- Anorexia, nausea, jaundice, RUQ abdominal pain and fatigue

Prognosis

- The rate of spontaneous virus clear: adults: 95%, children: 30%, infants: 5%
- Fulminant hepatitis: 1%
- Persistent hepatitis and HBV carriers (positive HBsAg >6 months): 1–10%
- Chronic active hepatitis: 25% of carriers

Diagnosis

Acute hepatitis B

- Recent risk factors + ALT (alanine aminotransferase) elevation
- HBsAg positive (recent) + HBcAb (Ig M) positive

Chronic hepatitis B

Acute hepatitis B infection becomes chronic in 5–10%

- Persistent HBsAg positive >6 months
- HBcAb (IgG) positive + HBeAg positive or negative
- Normal or mild ALT elevation

Chronic hepatitis B carriers

- Persistent HBsAg positive >6 months
- HBsAb and HBcAb negative
- Normal ALT

Treatment

Acute hepatitis B

- Symptomatic treatment, stop alcohol, cease oral contraceptive pills
- Acute liver failure (encephalopathy, renal impairment, abnormal prothrombin time)—refer to a liver transplant unit

Chronic hepatitis B

- Long-term suppression of viral replication to improve liver histology and to prevent cirrhosis, liver failure and hepatocellular carcinoma

- Liver biopsy is useful for assessing chronic liver damage in patients with negative HBeAg and lower HBV DNA
1. Normal ALT, positive HBeAg, high HBV DNA (immune tolerance phase)—no treatment, yearly ALT
2. Elevated ALT, positive HBeAg, HBV DNA >2000 IU/mL (immune clearance phase)—treat
3. Normal ALT, negative HBeAg, low HBV DNA (immune control phase)—no treatment, 3-monthly ALT and HBV DNA
   → If ALT becomes abnormal >6 months and HBV DNA increasing—treat
4. Elevated ALT, negative HBeAg, HBV DNA >2000 IU/mL (immune escape phase)—treat

Antiviral therapy

Good response to treatment when the following are present:
- High ALT, low HBV DNA, female and presence of disease activity on liver biopsy

Drugs for hepatitis B virus

1. Nucleoside/nucleotide analogues (entecavir and tenofovir)
- High rate of complete HBV DNA suppression
- Very effective in HBeAg negative disease
- Easy to take (once daily)
- Few adverse effects, safe in cirrhosis and liver failure
- Need for long-term (or life-long) treatment
- Risk of antiviral resistance
- Risk of severe flare of hepatitis and viral rebound after stopping treatment
2. Pegylated interferon (peginterferon)
- No antiviral resistance, long-term durability
- Most suitable for low HBV DNA and high ALT (with no decompensation or cirrhosis)
- Good response for genotype A, poor response for genotypes C and D
- Suitable for women of childbearing age
- Significant adverse effects
- Less effective for patients with mildly elevated ALT and high HBV DNA

Treatment options

- Option 1: entecavir (e.g. Baraclude) adult, child ≥16 years: 0.5 mg PO daily
- Option 2: tenofovir (e.g. Viread) adult: 300 mg PO daily
- Option 3: peginterferon alfa-2a (e.g. Pegasys) 180 mcg SC weekly for 48 weeks

For pregnant women
- Peginterferon alfa-2a (e.g. Pegasys) 180 mcg SC weekly for 48 weeks

---

*HBeAg-negative chronic hepatitis B is more resistant to treatment, and often progressive with a relatively high rate of cirrhosis and hepatocellular carcinoma

Duration of oral therapy (options 1 and 2)

- Continue for 12 months after HBeAg seroconversion
- If no HBeAg seroconversion or HBeAg-negative disease* or with cirrhosis or severe fibrosis—long term (often lifelong) treatment

Monitor patients on entecavir and tenofovir

- Check HBV DNA at 12, 24, 36 and 48 weeks—assess response
- Resistance testing is strongly recommended to guide future treatment

Pregnant women with hepatitis B

- Should not use oral antiviral therapy
- Peginterferon may be used (see treatment options above)
- Baby should receive hep B vaccination + hep B immunoglobulin within 12 hours of birth
- Baby should be tested for HBsAg after 1 year

Prevention

- Safe sex, avoid use of any potentially contaminated instruments for injection, acupuncture, piercing or tattooing

HBV vaccination

Indication for HBV vaccination:

- All children, particularly infants born to hepatitis B-positive mothers
- All sexual and household contacts of acute hepatitis B and chronic hepatitis B carriers
- Chronic liver disease and/or hepatitis C
- At occupational risk of exposure to hepatitis B blood or body fluids
- Impaired immunity (e.g. haemodialysis, HIV)—double the dose
- Men who have sex with men—combined hepatitis A/B may be appropriate
- Travelling to intermediate or high endemic regions

National immunisation program (4-doses schedule)

- Hepatitis B vaccine (e.g. Engerix-B paediatric, H-B-Vax II paediatric) 0.5 mL IM, 4 doses at birth, 2, 4, 6–12 months of age

Catch-up hep B vaccination

Child and adult <20 years

- Hepatitis B vaccine (e.g. Engerix-B paediatric, H-B-Vax II paediatric) 0.5 mL IM, 3 doses at 0, 1, 6 months

Adult >20 years

- Hepatitis B vaccine (e.g. Engerix-B, H-B-Vax II) 1.0 mL IM, 3 doses at 0, 1, 6 months

Child 11–19 years

May use two-dose schedule

- Hepatitis B vaccine (e.g. Engerix-B, H-B-Vax II) 1.0 mL IM, 2 doses at 0, 6 months

Combined hepatitis A/B vaccines (to cover both hep A and B)

- Twinrix (720/20) for child 1–15 years: 1.0 mL IM, 2 doses at 0, 6–12 months

or Twinrix Junior (360/10) 0.5 mL IM, 3 doses at 0, 1, 6 months

- Twinrix (720/20) for child ≥16 years and adult: 1.0 mL IM, 3 doses at 0, 1, 6 months

Rapid schedule (when time is limited before going to endemic area)

- Engerix-B (paediatric) for child <20 years: 0.5 mL IM, 3 doses at 0, 1, 2 months, and a later booster at 12 months
- Engerix-B (adult) for ≥20 years (**or** Twinrix (720/20) for ≥16 years): 1.0 mL IM, at 0, 7, 21 days, and a later booster dose at 12 months

Hepatitis B immunoglobulin (HBIg)

For neonates born to hepatitis B carrier mothers

- Hepatitis B immunoglobulin (HBIg)—neonate: 100 IU (together with Hep B vaccine in the opposite anterolateral thigh) IM, within 12 hours of birth

For occupational exposure to the blood of HBsAg positive person or sexual partners of patients with acute hepatitis B

- Hepatitis B immunoglobulin (HBIg)—400 IU + HBV vaccine IM, ASAP

Surveillance for hepatocellular carcinoma

High-risk groups: cirrhosis, family history of liver cancer, Asians >35 years old and Africans >20 years old
Monitor:

- Serum AFP (alfa-fetoprotein) every 6 months
- Abdominal ultrasound every 6 months

Patient education website: www.hepatitisinfo.com.au

HEPATITIS C

Pathogens

- Hepatitis C virus (HCV)—a RNA virus
- Genotypes 1a, 1b, 2, 3, 4, 5 and 6
- Genotypes 1 and 3—most common in Australia

Transmission

Peak infectivity—just before the onset of acute disease

- Drug injecting, non-sterile tattooing or body piercing
- Blood transfusions before 1991
- Needle-stick injury or non-sterile medical procedures
- Sharing blood-contaminated toothbrushes, razors, sex toys or other items
- Mother-to-baby transmission (2–5%)
- Sexual transmission (<1%)

Incubation

- 1–6 months

1. ACUTE HEPATITIS C

Clinical

- Most of patients with acute hepatitis C have no symptoms
- Some patients have flu-like symptoms, loss of appetite or jaundice

Laboratory

- At risk people should check hep C serology (as part of STI screening)
- Those with abnormal LFT (raised ALT) should check hep C serology
- Those with positive HCV serology (anti-HCV) should check HCV-RNA to confirm the diagnosis
- Once diagnosed, HCV g type should be tested

Treatment

- Not all patients with acute hepatitis C need antiviral treatment
- More than 25% of patients clear the virus spontaneously within 3–6 months; clearance rates are higher in symptomatic patients (up to 40%) and young females
- The optimal timing and regimen for acute hepatitis C is unclear due to a lack of data with combinations of oral direct-acting antiviral (DAA) drugs
- Monitor for spontaneous resolution by checking HCV RNA regularly—if HCV RNA becomes negative, no treatment is required
- If spontaneous clearance has not occurred (continuous positive HCV RNA) by 6 months, treat as for chronic hepatitis C (see Chronic hepatitis C below)
- There is no approved therapy for post-exposure prophylaxis for HCV

2. CHRONIC HEPATITIS C

Clinical

- Following acute hepatitis, about 55–85% of patients develop chronic hepatitis C
- Most of patients have no symptoms
- Some patients have fatigue, loss of appetite, myalgia, arthralgia, RUQ pain
- Some patients (5–20%) develop cirrhosis after 20 years; some may further develop liver failure or liver cancer
- Advanced liver disease—may have jaundice, ascites and spider angiomas

Laboratory

Chronic hepatitis C = anti-HCV positive + detectable HCV RNA for >6 months

- HCV serology (anti-HCV)—screen for patients with abnormal LFT

- HCV-RNA (qualitative)—indicates active viral replication ('viraemia') and confirms the diagnosis
- HCV viral load (quantitative)—indicates severity of infection
- HCV genotype—to guide treatment and predict response to treatment (better response with genotypes 2 and 3)
- Fibroscan—to assess cirrhosis
- APRI score (AST to platelet ratio index)—if Fibroscan is not available:
  - APRI = (AST level/upper limit of normal [IU/L] ÷ platelet count [10^9/L]) × 100
  - APRI online calculator: www.hepatitisc.uw.edu/page/clinical -calculators//apri
  - APRI score >1.0 has a sensitivity of 76% and specificity of 72% for predicting cirrhosis
- Abdominal ultrasound—see changes of cirrhosis and screen for liver cancer

Treatment

Step 1

Confirm diagnosis—HCV RNA (qualitative) positive
Refer patients <18 years to specialist

Step 2

Order baseline tests—LFT, FBC, EUC, FBG, lipids, HCV viral load (quantitative), HCV genotype, hep A serology, HBsAg, HBsAb, HBcAb, HIV serology
Refer genotypes 4, 5, 6 to specialist
Refer HBV, HIV coinfection to specialist
Refer patients with eGFR<50 to specialist

Step 3

Check cirrhosis/liver cancer—Fibroscan (or APRI score) and abdominal ultrasound
Refer patients with cirrhosis or liver cancer to specialist

Step 4

Exclude pregnancy and arrange contraception
Refer patients who may need ribavirin for treatment to specialist

Step 5

Check drug–drug interactions with DDAs using online tool (www.hep-druginteractions.org)
Refer patients on multiple medications to specialist

Step 6

Select treatment regimen

Anti-HCV regimens

Genotype 1a and 1b—response rate 95%
- Option 1: sofosbuvir/ledipasvir (Harvoni®) 400/90 mg PO daily

For 12 weeks—without cirrhosis
For 24 weeks—with cirrhosis

- Option 2: sofosbuvir (Sovaldi®) 400 mg PO daily **plus** daclatasvir (Daklinza™) 60 mg PO daily

For 12 weeks—without cirrhosis
For 24 weeks—with cirrhosis

Genotype 1a—response rate 95%
- Paritaprevir/ritonavir/ombitasvir 75/50/12.5 mg PO daily **plus** dasabuvir 250 mg PO bid **plus** ribavirin (Ibavirin) PO (weight-based dosing)* (Viekira Pak-RBV Combination)

For 12 weeks—without cirrhosis
For 24 weeks—with cirrhosis

Genotype 1b—response rate 95%
- Paritaprevir/ritonavir/ombitasvir (75/50/12.5 mg) 2 PO daily **plus** dasabuvir (VIEKIRA PAK) 250 mg PO bid

For 12 weeks—if no decompensated liver disease

Genotype 2—response rate 93%
- Sofosbuvir (Sovaldi) 400 mg PO daily **plus** ribavirin (Ibavyr) PO (weight-based dosing)*

For 12 weeks—without cirrhosis
For 16–24 weeks—with cirrhosis

Genotype 3—response rate 93–95% (58–76% with cirrhosis)
- Option 1: sofosbuvir (Sovaldi) 400 mg PO daily **plus** daclatasvir (Daklinza) 60 mg PO daily

For 12 weeks—without cirrhosis
For 24 weeks—with cirrhosis

- Option 2: sofosbuvir (Sovaldi) 400 mg PO daily **plus** daclatasvir (Daklinza) 60 mg PO daily **plus** ribavirin (Ibavyr) PO (weight-based dosing)*

For 12 weeks—with or without cirrhosis

- Option 3: sofosbuvir (Sovaldi) 400 mg PO daily **plus** ribavirin (Ibavyr) PO (weight-based dosing)*

For 24 weeks

Genotype 4, 5, 6—response rate >90%
- Sofosbuvir (Sovaldi) 400 mg PO daily **plus** Ibavyr (Ibavyr) PO (weight-based dosing)* **plus** pegiterferon alfa-2a 180 mcg SC weekly

---

*Ribavirin: <65 kg: 400 mg PO bid; 65–75 kg: 400 mg PO mane + 600 mg PO nocte; 75–105 kg: 600 mg PO bid; >105 kg: 600 mg PO mane + 800 mg PO nocte

For 12 weeks—if low viral load and no cirrhosis

Pan-genotypic (effective for all genotypes 1–6)
- Sofosbuvir/valpatasvir (Epclusa®)

Step 7

Monitor and follow up

- Check HCV-RNA at end of treatment and 12 weeks after treatment
  - If undetectable—cure
  - If still detectable—relapse or non-response—refer to specialist
- If patient still at high risk of reinfection—annual HCV-RNA testing
- If LFTs still abnormal—refer to specialist for alternative causes of liver disease
- Minimise or abstain alcohol/cannabis use and lose weight (if overweight)
- All patients with hepatitis C should have hepatitis A and B vaccination if non-immune

HEPATITIS D

Hepatitis D has the highest mortality rate of all hepatitis infections.

Pathogens

- Hepatitis delta virus (HDV)—a defective RNA virus
- HDV is dependent on hepatitis B virus (to provide HBsAg core) for replication

Coinfection—HDV infection via simultaneous infection with HBV
Superinfection—HDV infection via infection of an individual previously infected with HBV

Transmission

- Via blood, saliva; rarely sexual or vertical; no faecal–oral

Incubation

- A few months

Clinical

- High rate of fulminant acute hepatitis when simultaneous coinfection with both HBV and HDV
- High rate of severe chronic hepatitis when HDV superinfection of an HBsAg positive patient, often progressing to cirrhosis and liver failure
- Chronic hepatitis D may lead to the development of liver cancer

Risk group

- Chronic HBV carriers
- Individuals who have not been infected and not been vaccinated against HBV are at risk of HBV infection with simultaneous or subsequent HDV infection

- Intravenous drug users
- People exposed to unscreened blood or blood products

Laboratory

- HBV serology (HBsAg, HBeAg, HBV-DNA and/or HBcAb)
- HDV serology (anti-HDV IgM/IgG)
- Detection of hepatitis D virus on liver biopsy

HBsAg positive migrants should be tested for HDV antibodies

Treatment

- 95% of cases will recover spontaneously and clear both viruses
- Referral to a specialist centre is recommended
- Only interferon alfa (standard or pegylated) has efficacy against HDV
- Liver transplantation may be considered for fulminant and end-stage chronic hepatitis D

Prevention

- Control of HDV infection is achieved by targeting HBV infections; all measures aimed at preventing the transmission of HBV will prevent the transmission of hepatitis D
- Hepatitis B Ig and HBV vaccine do not protect HBV carriers from infection by HDV
- Prevention of HBV-HDV superinfection can be achieved through education to reduce risk factors

Vaccination

- HBV vaccine (to prevent HBV-HDV coinfection)

HEPATITIS E

Hepatitis E virus may cause fulminate hepatitis with high mortality (10–20%) in pregnant women (particularly during the third trimester).

Pathogen

- Hepatitis E virus (HEV)—an RNA virus

Transmission

- Faecal–oral (waterborne or ingestion of raw or uncooked shellfish)
- Possible zoonotic spread (several non-human primates, pigs, cows, sheep, goats and rodents act as reservoirs)
- No blood, sexual or vertical transmission

Incubation

- 3–8 weeks

Clinical

- In general—a self-limiting infection with a mortality rate of 0.5–4%

- In pregnant women (particularly during the third trimester)—fulminate hepatitis occurs more frequently with high mortality (10–20%)
- In children—mostly asymptomatic or a very mild illness without jaundice that is often undiagnosed
- No carrier, no chronic liver disease and no association with liver cancer

Laboratory

- HEV serology (IgM or IgG)
- Detection of hepatitis E virus by nucleic acid testing
- Detection of hepatitis E virus in faeces by electron microscopy

Treatment

- Supportive only, usually self-limited
- Hospitalisation is required for fulminant hepatitis and should be considered for infected pregnant women
- No available therapy is capable of altering the course of acute infection

Prevention

- Good personal hygiene, clean water and proper disposal of sanitary waste
- Travellers to highly endemic areas should avoid drinking water and/or ice of unknown purity and eating uncooked shellfish, uncooked fruits or vegetables
- Healthcare workers, childcare workers and food handlers should remain away from work for at least 7 days after the onset of illness
- Children should not attend school or childcare for 7 days after the onset of symptoms

Vaccination

- No vaccine available, no hyperimmune E globulin available for pre- or post-exposure prophylaxis

HERPANGINA

Other names: mouth blisters

Pathogens

- *Coxsackieviruses* (A1–10, 16 or 22)
- *Enterovirus*
- *Echovirus*

Transmission

Coxsackieviruses and other *enteroviruses* are present in both faeces and respiratory secretions. They can spread through:

- Faecal–oral
- Droplets
- Direct contact

Incubation

- 4–6 days

Clinical

- Most commonly affects infants and young children but can occur at any age
- Typically occurs in the summer
- Acute high fever with small painful blisters (usually 2–6) in the mouth; the blisters are surrounded by red rings and may become ulcers (2–4 mm in size)
- Other symptoms include headache, backache, runny nose, drooling, loss of appetite, vomiting and diarrhoea
- The illness usually lasts 3–6 days

Complications

- Meningoencephalitis (may occur in infants aged 6–11 months)

Diagnosis

- Consider herpangina in a child with high fever and multiple small painful blisters in the mouth
- Laboratory tests are available for the *Coxsackieviruses* and other enteroviruses, but not usually necessary

Treatment

- Supportive: hydration, antipyretics and topical analgesics (e.g. topical lignocaine gel or spray)
- Recovery occurs within a few days

HERPES GENITALIS

Other names: genital herpes (GH)

Pathogens

- Herpes simplex virus (HSV) types 1 or 2 (HSV-1, HSV-2)
- Recurrent genital herpes is usually caused by HSV-2

Transmission

- In adult—sexually transmitted
- In child—anogenital HSV infection can occur via autoinoculation (HSV-1) or from a caregiver with oral or other HSV-2 lesions (non-sexually)
- In neonate—vertical transmission may occur

Primary episode genital herpes—multiple painful vesicles in clusters on an inflamed area, fever, malaise, dysuria, vaginal discharge and tender lymph nodes
Secondary episodes of genital herpes—fewer lesions and less severe symptoms

Clinical

- Majority of HSV infections are undiagnosed due to asymptomatic initial infection
- If symptoms of initial infection occur, they can be severe, with widespread severe painful genital ulcers
- Recurrences are usually less painful and have shorter duration

Laboratory

- HSV PCR and viral culture (swab from de-roofed skin lesions)

Treatment

- Antiviral treatment for HSV is not curative, but it shortens the episode
- Start antiviral treatment within 72 hours of onset

Initial genital herpes

- Option 1: famciclovir 250 mg PO q8h for 5–10 days
- Option 2: valaciclovir 500 mg PO q12h for 5–10 days
- Option 3: aciclovir 400 mg PO q8h for 5–10 days (child <2 years: 100 mg; ≥2 years: 200 mg PO 5 times a day for 10 days)

In severe cases, longer treatment may be required

Infrequent recurrent genital herpes

Episodic therapy
Commence within 1 day of onset

- Option 1: famciclovir 1 g PO q12h for 1 day
- Option 2: valaciclovir 500 mg PO q12h for 3 days
- Option 3: aciclovir 800 mg PO q12h for 2 days **or** 400 mg PO q8h for 5 days (child <2 years: 100 mg; ≥2 years: 200 mg PO 5 times a day for 5 days)

For immunocompromised
- Famciclovir 500 mg PO q12h for 7 days

Frequent, severe recurrent genital herpes

Prophylactic suppression therapy
- Option 1: famciclovir 250 mg PO q12h for 6 months
- Option 2: valaciclovir 500 mg PO daily for 6 months
- Option 3: aciclovir 400 mg PO q12h for 6 months

For pregnant women
- Option 1: valaciclovir 500 mg PO q12h from 36 weeks until delivery
- Option 2: aciclovir 400 mg PO q8h from 36 weeks until delivery

Reassess at 6 months

For immunocompromised patients
- Higher doses of antiviral therapy may be required—seek expert advice

If HSV is resistant to above antiviral agents (laboratory confirmed) and patient has extensive ulcerations
- Foscarnet 40 mg/kg IV q8h for 2–3 weeks or until lesions heal

HERPES LABIALIS

Other names: cold sores

Pathogen
- Herpes simplex virus (HSV)

Cause
- After primary gingivostomatitis, the virus remains in the body, reactivates and causes recurrent mild symptoms

Clinical
- **Primary attack (herpetic gingivostomatitis)**—often in childhood: mouth ulceration with fever, lymphadenopathy, toxicity and difficult to eat and drink (see Herpetic gingivostomatitis, p. 164)
- **Recurrent attacks (cold sores)**—perioral vesical lesions for a few days, triggered by fevers, sunlight or body rundown; the earliest symptoms of a cold sore are tingling, itching or burning

Laboratory
- For severe or prolonged disease—ulcer swab for HSV PCR or rapid immunofluorescence
- Viral culture (may take several days)

Treatment

Minor attacks

Oral ulceration or perioral lesions—use either:
- Famciclovir 1.5 g PO st (**or** 750 mg q12h for 1 day) (at the first sign of symptom)
- Valaciclovir 2 g PO q12h for 1 day (at the first sign of symptom)
- Aciclovir 5% cream topically q4h while awake for 5 days

Other treatment
- Topical anaesthetics (e.g. lignocaine 2% + chlorhexidine 0.05% gel)
- Topical antiseptic mouthwash (e.g. Difflam-C)

More severe primary or recurrent attacks

Use either:
- Famciclovir 125 mg PO q12h for 5 days
- Valaciclovir 500 mg PO q12h for 5 days
- Aciclovir 400 mg (child: 10 mg/kg up to 400 mg) PO q8h for 5 days

If unable to take orally
- Aciclovir 5 mg/kg IV q8h for 5 days

Severe recurrences or chronic lesions (suppressive therapy)

Use either:

- Famciclovir 250–500 mg PO q12h for 6 months
- Valaciclovir 500 mg PO daily for 6 months
- Aciclovir 200 mg (child: 5 mg/kg up to 200 mg) PO q12h for 6 months

If recurs after 6 months, restart longer term suppression
If breakthrough during suppressive therapy, use higher dose therapy

HERPES SIMPLEX ENCEPHALITIS

Other name: herpes viral encephalitis
Herpes simplex encephalitis (HSE) is the most common cause of sporadic viral encephalitis and early aciclovir treatment can reduce the mortality.

Pathogens

- Herpes simplex virus type 1 (HSV-1) (90%)—mainly affects adults
- Herpes simplex virus type 2 (HSV-2) (10%)—mainly affects neonates

Transmission

- Caused by the retrograde transmission of reactivated HSV virus from a peripheral site on the face, along a nerve axon, to the brain
- Can be passed from mother to baby during birth (neonatal herpes simplex encephalitis)
- HSV encephalitis is not infectious to other people

Classification

1. **Adult and child HSE**—brain damage is usually localised to the temporal and frontal lobes
2. **Neonatal HSE**—brain damage is generalised (mainly caused by HSV-2)

Clinical

- **Adult and child HSE**—fever, headache, vomiting, confusion, focal neurological signs, partial paralysis, seizures, hallucinations and personality changes
- **Neonate HSE**—lethargy, irritability, seizures and poor feeding in the first 2 weeks of life
- **In immunocompromised hosts**—presentation may be subacute or atypical
- Without treatment, HSE results in rapid death in approximately 70% of cases
- Most survivors suffer severe neurological damage

Laboratory

- CSF pleocytosis + negative bacteria and fungi
- CSF HSV PCR—confirm diagnosis
- HSV serology (blood or CSF)—only for retrospective diagnosis
- MRI brain—characteristic changes in the temporal lobes
- CT brain—changes in temporal/frontal lobes (less sensitive than MRI)
- Electroencephalography (EEG)—focal abnormalities in temporal/frontal lobes

Treatment

Start aciclovir when HSV encephalitis is suspected:

- Fever + confusion + focal neurological signs +/– personality change +/– seizure
- Early treatment (within 48 hours of onset) improves the chance of recovery

Adult and child HSE

- Aciclovir 10 mg/kg IV q8h for at least 2 weeks

If CSF PCR for HSV is positive
- Repeat CSF PCR in 2 weeks

If the 2nd CSF PCR becomes negative
- Aciclovir may be stopped

Neonate HSE

- Aciclovir 20 mg/kg IV q8h for 3 weeks
- When treated, HSE is still fatal in 30% of cases, and causes moderate or severe neurological deficits in more than 50% of survivors
- Rarely, treated patients can relapse weeks to months later

HERPES SIMPLEX VIRUS INFECTION—NEONATAL

Pathogen

- HSV-2, HSV-1 (15–30%)

Transmission

- Most transmissions occur as neonate passes through birth canal, with primary genital HSV infection during delivery
- Many transmissions occur during the third trimester from maternal asymptomatic primary genital HSV infection
- Some transmissions occur postnatally through contact with oral or skin lesions of infected mother

Clinical

Three subtypes of neonatal HSV infections:

1. Neonatal skin, eye or mouth HSV infection (no mortality)
2. Neonatal HSV encephalitis (15% mortality)

3. Neonatal HSV disseminated infection involving multiple organs, e.g. central nervous system, lung, liver, adrenals, skin, eyes or mouth (57% mortality)

Long-term morbidity (common in infants who survive with encephalitis or disseminated disease)—seizures, psychomotor retardation, spasticity, blindness or learning disabilities

Diagnosis

- Infants often do not have skin lesions; by the time diagnosis is made, many infants will have severe disease and complications
- Neonatal HSV infection should be suspected in all neonates who present in the first month of life with fever, poor feeding, lethargy or seizure
- Any vesicular rash in an infant up to 8 weeks of age should be checked for HSV and antiviral therapy should be commenced immediately pending the results
- HSV PCR or HSV immunofluorescence test (swab from skin lesions or CSF)
- HSV culture and bacterial culture (vesicular lesions, blood, CSF, urine and fluid from eyes, nose and mucous membranes)

Treatment

- Mother's primary and secondary HSV infection near term or at the time of delivery should receive antiviral therapy (see Herpes genitalis, p. 157)
- If active HSV infection is present at the time of delivery—caesarean section
- Early treatment of neonatal HSV infection is important to prevent dissemination

IV therapy

- Aciclovir 20 mg/kg IV q8h (q12h for preterm infant)

Duration of therapy

- For disease limited to skin, eyes and mucous membranes—2-week course
- For central nervous system or disseminated disease—3-week course (until HSV negative in CSF)

Oral suppression therapy (prevent recurrence)

- Aciclovir 50–100 mg PO 3 times a day

HERPES ZOSTER

Other names: shingles

Pathogen

- Varicella zoster virus (VZV), a member of the family *Herpesviridae*

Transmission

- Reactivation of the virus from previous chickenpox infection
- Re-exposure to the virus

- Exposure may cause chickenpox in non-immune contacts
- It is contagious in the vesicular stage

Risk factors of reactivation

- Stress
- Sleep disturbance
- Depression
- Recent weight loss
- Family history
- Prior episodes of zoster

Clinical

- More severe in the elderly and immunosuppressed
- May affect children and can be seen in infants if having history of maternal varicella
- Some patients may have genetic susceptibility to the virus
- Unilateral vesicular or bullous rash in a dermatomal distribution on an erythematous base; thoracic, lumbar/sacral dermatomes and ophthalmic division of trigeminal nerve are most vulnerable
- In immunocompromised patients, the eruption may be multidermatomal
- Pain, fever and malaise
- Lesions erupt over a week and may last for 2 weeks

Complications

- Ophthalmic herpes zoster—corneal damage and anterior uveitis
- Ramsay Hunt syndrome—external ear canal painful vesicles + facial palsy + loss of taste in anterior 2/3 of tongue
- Disseminated zoster—visceral, CNS (encephalitis) and pulmonary involvement
- Post-herpetic neuralgia—pain persisting >4 weeks after vesicles crusted

Diagnosis

Clinical diagnosis is usually sufficient. When the diagnosis is unclear:

- Varicella zoster virus PCR and culture (vesicle fluid, ulcer scrapings)
- Varicella zoster virus serology—a four-fold rise of antibodies in titres
- Skin biopsy—in cases of atypical lesions

Treatment

- Bathe lesions with saline three times a day to remove crusts and exudates
- Cover the lesions with a non-adherent padded dressing
- Analgesia—paracetamol, aspirin, opioids or tricyclic antidepressants

Antiviral treatment

Should be started whin 72 hours of the onset of rash

- Option 1: famciclovir 250 mg PO q8h for 7 days
- Option 2: valaciclovir 1 g PO q8h for 7 days (safe in pregnancy)
- Option 3: aciclovir 800 mg (child: 20 mg/kg up to 800 mg) PO 5 times daily for 7 days (safe in child and pregnancy)

For ophthalmic herpes zoster

If vision is threatened: urgent ophthalmologist referral and use IV aciclovir:

- Aciclovir 10 mg/kg IV q8h for 7–14 days

For immunocompromised (e.g. HIV-infected) adults (even >72 hours)

- Option 1: famciclovir 500 mg PO q8h for 10 days
- Option 2: valaciclovir 1 g PO q8h for 14 days (safe in pregnancy)
- Option 3: aciclovir 800 mg (child: 20 mg/kg up to 800 mg) PO 5 times daily for 14 days (preferred in child and pregnancy)

For disseminated disease or if not tolerated orally

- Aciclovir 10–12.5 mg/kg (child <1 year: 10 mg/kg; 1–5 years: 20 mg/kg; ≥5 years: 15 mg/kg) IV q8h

After significant improvement, switch to oral to complete 7 days (IV + PO) course

Vaccination

- Prevents shingles/post-herpetic neuralgia for old people
- The vaccine's efficacy persists for at least 4 years

Varicella zoster vaccination

- Option 1: Zostavax 0.65 mL SC as a single dose
- Option 2: Shingrix (HZ/su) 2 doses IM 2 months apart

HERPETIC GINGIVOSTOMATITIS

Pathogen

- HSV-1

Transmission

- Often the source of infection is a person with cold sores
- Through contact with saliva that contains the virus (such as on a drinking glass or utensil)

Clinical

- **Primary attack (herpetic gingivostomatitis)**—often affects toddlers and young children: painful mouth with vesicles and ulcers on the lips, gums, tongue and cheeks; red and swollen mucosa and gingivae with

lymphadenopathy, toxicity and difficulty in swallowing; lasts about 14 days
- **Recurrent attacks (cold sores)**—after resolution of primary mouth sores, the virus remains in the body and can recur as cold sores (see Herpes labialis, p. 159)
- **Disseminated herpes simplex**—in children with atopic dermatitis and in immunosuppressed patients, causing generalised eruption and toxicity

Treatment

- Paracetamol or ibuprofen for fever and mouth pain
- Topical anaesthetics (see below)
- Prevent dehydration by drinking plenty of fluids
- Keep hands away from mouth and eyes

Antiviral treatment

Start ASAP within 3 days of development of sores

- Option 1: famciclovir 125 mg PO q12h for 5 days
- Option 2: valaciclovir 500 mg PO q12h for 5 days
- Option 3: aciclovir 400 mg (child: 10 mg/kg up to 400 mg) PO q8h for 5 days (preferred in child and pregnancy)
- Topical anaesthetics (e.g. lignocaine 2% + chlorhexidine 0.05% gel)
- Topical antiseptic mouthwash (e.g. Difflam-C)

If unable to swallow
- Aciclovir 5 mg/kg IV q8h for 5 days

Seek specialist advice

HERPETIC WHITLOW AND PARONYCHIA

Herpetic whitlow—an intense painful infection of a finger or thumb.
Herpetic paronychia—a superficial infection of the lateral aspect of the nail.

Pathogens

- In children—commonly HSV-1
- In adults—most cases caused by HSV-2

Transmission

- In children, the primary source of infection is the oropharyngeal area (e.g. herpes labialis or herpetic gingivostomatitis) and it is transferred by chewing or sucking of the fingers or thumbs
- In adults, it is most often due to autoinoculation from genital herpes
- In healthcare workers (e.g. dentists), infection with HSV-1 is more common and usually is due to unprotected exposure to infected oropharyngeal secretions of patients

Incubation

- 2–20 days

Clinical

- Pain, burning or tingling of the infected finger, followed by erythema, oedema and development of small grouped vesicles over the next 7–10 days; the vesicles may ulcerate or rupture; lymphangitis and lymphadenopathy may occur; lesions usually crust over and heal after 10–14 days
- Primary infection—usually the most symptomatic
- Recurrent infection—usually milder and shorter in duration

Diagnosis

- Characteristic lesions on the affected finger with concurrent cold sore or gingivostomatitis in children or oral or genital herpes lesions in adults

Treatment

- Oral antiviral treatment
- Topical aciclovir is effective in decreasing the duration of symptoms
- Avoid surgical debridement and drainage (may cause a bacterial superinfection or systemic spread and herpes encephalitis)
  - Option 1: famciclovir 250 mg PO q12h for 5–10 days
  - Option 2: valaciclovir 500 mg PO q12h for 5–10 days
  - Option 3: aciclovir 400 mg (child: 10 mg/kg up to 400 mg) PO q8h for 5–10 days (preferred in child and pregnancy)

Topical ointment
  - Aciclovir 3% eye oint (e.g. Zovirax Ophthalmic) top, 5 times daily (q3h during waking hours) for 14 days or until 3 days after healing

HIDRADENITIS SUPPURATIVA

Other names: apocrinitis, Velpeau's disease

Causes

- Hidradenitis suppurativa (HS) is not caused by bacterial infection—infection is secondary
- Dysfunction of apocrine glands is associated with blockage, genetic predisposition, autoimmune conditions and androgen excess
- Aggravating factors: excessive sweating, humid heat, clothing friction and stress

Clinical

- Blackheads, chronic recurrent suppurative abscess of apocrine sweat glands in axillae, groins, buttocks and under the breasts
- Persistent lesions may lead to scarring, formation of sinus tracts and tunnels connecting the abscesses under the skin
- More common in obese women
- HS often goes undiagnosed or misdiagnosed for years
- It may lead to the development of squamous cell carcinoma in affected areas

Staging

- Stage I—single or multiple abscesses only; no sinus tracts or scarring
- Stage II—recurrent abscesses, widely separated; sinus tracts; scarring
- Stage III—entire region involvement; multiple interconnected tracts and abscesses

Treatment

- Smoking cessation, weight loss, avoid squeezing the lesion, avoid dairy products
- Warm compresses, baths (to induce drainage)
- Oral zinc gluconate 30 mg tds
- Topical treatment (see below)
- Intralesional corticosteroid injection (see below)
- Antibiotic treatment (see below)
- Antiandrogen hormonal therapy for females and males (see below)
- Immunosuppressants (e.g. methotrexate 15–20 mg weekly, ciclosporin)
- Biological agents (e.g. TNF-alpha inhibitors: infliximab, adalimumab and etanercept; IL-12/IL-23 pathway inhibitor: ustekinumab)
- Surgical treatment: punch debridement and de-roofing of sinus tracts, local or radical excision (with or without skin grafting)
- Laser excision
- Radiotherapy

Topical (stage I)

- Clindamycin (e.g. Duac, ClindaTech, Dalacin) 1% lotion/gel **plus** benzoyl peroxide (e.g. Benzac, Brevoxyl, Oxy) 2.5–5% gel/cream top bid

Intralesional corticosteroid (stages I, II)

- Triamcinolone 1–5 mg intralesional inj monthly

Oral antibiotic

Stage I
- Option 1: doxycycline 50–100 mg PO bid for 7–10 days
- Option 2: minocycline 50–100 mg PO bid for 7–10 days
- Option 3: clindamycin 300 mg PO bid for 7–10 days
- Option 4: amoxicillin/clavulanate 500–850 mg PO q12h for 7–10 days
- Option 5: moxifloxacin 400 mg PO daily

Stages II, III
- Option 1: doxycycline **or** minocycline 50–100 mg PO bid for weeks to 6 months
- Option 2: clindamycin 300 mg PO bid **plus** rifampicin 600 mg PO daily for 3–6 months

Hormonal therapy (stages I—III)

For women
- OCP with cyproterone (e.g. Brenda-35 ED, Diane-35 ED) 1 tab PO daily for long term

For men
- Finasteride 1 mg PO daily for long term

HIV AND AIDS

HIV (human immunodeficiency virus) infection—acute viral illness (seroconversion), followed by an asymptomatic (latency) period
AIDS (acquired immunodeficiency syndrome)—HIV infection becomes advanced when CD4 count is below 200/mL and opportunistic infections occur

Pathogen

- HIV—a lentivirus (a member of the retrovirus family)

Two strains of HIV

- HIV-1: worldwide, with high transmittability
- HIV-2: mainly in West Africa, with low transmittability

Transmission

- Unprotected sexual intercourse (vaginal or anal)
- Contaminated needles or blood products
- Vertical transmission from mother to baby at birth
- Breast milk

Clinical

1. Acute HIV infection (seroconversion)

- Flu- or mononucleosis-like illness (fever, lymphadenopathy, sore throat/mouth, rash, myalgia, malaise, headache, nausea and vomiting) 2–4 weeks post-exposure
- The duration of symptoms varies; usually lasts at least a week
- Seroconversion occurs 6–8 weeks after exposure, may be delayed up to 3 months ('window period')
- The patient is highly infectious during this period

2. Latency phase

- Varies between 2 weeks and 20 years
- HIV is active within lymphoid organs
- Patients in this phase are still infectious

3. AIDS

- When CD4+ T-cell count declines to $<0.2 \times 10^9$—cell-mediated immunity is lost
- Symptoms—unexplained weight loss, recurring respiratory tract infections, skin rashes, oral ulcerations, opportunistic infections and tumours (Epstein-Barr virus-induced B-cell lymphomas and Kaposi's sarcomas)

Diagnosis

Consent should be obtained from the patient for the testing

- Rapid HIV screen testing (a mouth swab)—gives result within 20 minutes
- HIV serology (screen testing)—repeat the test if positive (to confirm)
- HIV western blot (confirmatory testing)—if western blot result is indeterminate, a second western blot test should be made a month later
- HIV viral PCR testing

Tests before starting HIV treatment:

- CD4 cell count
- HIV RNA (viral load)—may be used during 'window period' and for monitoring
- HIV ARV drug-resistance testing
- HLA-B*5701 before prescribing abacavir
- Hepatitis B and C serology
- FBC, EUC, LFT, phosphate, fasting blood glucose and lipids, and urinalysis

Treatment

- Refer patient to sexual health service or HIV specialist clinic
- Antiretroviral therapy—only those doctors with experience in HIV management should initiate or change antiretroviral therapy
- New treatments include Cre Recombinase and Tre Recombinase (to remove HIV from infected cells)
- Once treatment has been started, it should be continued indefinitely, unless oral therapy cannot be taken or serous toxicity develops

Early antiretroviral therapy

- Early antiretroviral therapy significantly improves survival rates in asymptomatic HIV patients
- Early treatment also reduces toxic side effects of antiretroviral therapy
- Commence antiretroviral therapy as soon as the diagnosis of HIV infection

Antiretroviral drugs

Four classes of antiretroviral drugs for initial therapy:

1. Nucleoside/nucleotide reverse transcriptase inhibitors (NRTIs)
2. Non-nucleoside reverse transcriptase inhibitors (NNRTIs)
3. Protease inhibitors (PIs)
4. Integrase inhibitors (raltegravir)

Reserved drugs for resistant HIV infection:

1. Fusion inhibitors (enfuvirtide T20)
2. Entry inhibitors (maraviroc)

3. Special PIs (tipranavir and darunavir)
4. Special NNRTIs (etravirine)

Initial antiretroviral regimens

Two NRTIs **plus** one NNRTI

- Emtricitabine + tenofovir + efavirenz (Atripla)

Two NRTIs **plus** one PI (if resistance testing result is unavailable)

- Emtricitabine + tenofovir (Truvada) **plus** atazanavir/ritonavir

Two NRTIs **plus** one integrase inhibitor

- Option 1: emtricitabine + tenofovir (Truvada) **plus** dolutegravir
- Option 2: lamivudine + abacavir (Kivexa) **plus** dolutegravir (if HLA-B*5701 negative)
- Option 3: emtricitabine + tenofovir + elvitegravir/cobicistat (Stribild)
- Option 4: emtricitabine + tenofovir (Truvada) **plus** raltegravir

For detailed information on antiretroviral drugs, see www.ashm.org.au/hiv/management-hiv

HIV vaccination

- Clinical phase III trial has shown that an investigational HIV vaccine decreased HIV infections by 30%

HIV AND AIDS—OPPORTUNISTIC INFECTION

1. *CANDIDA ALBICANS* INFECTION

Treatment

Oropharyngeal *Candida*

- Option 1: fluconazole 50 mg PO daily for 10–14 days
- Option 2: itraconazole 100 mg PO daily for 10–14 days
- Option 3: miconazole 2% gel 2.5 mL PO q6h for 10–14 days
- Option 4: nystatin liquid (100,000 units/mL) 1 mL PO q6h for 10–14 days

For frequent recurrences

- Fluconazole 50 mg PO daily or 150 mg PO weekly

Oesophageal *Candida*

See also *Candida* oesophagitis, p. 35

- Option 1: fluconazole 100 mg PO daily for 2 weeks
- Option 2: itraconazole 200 mg PO daily for 2 weeks

For fluconazole- and itraconazole-resistant *Candida*

- Option 1: posaconazole 400 mg PO q12h for 2 weeks
- Option 2: voriconazole 200 mg PO q12h for 2 weeks

2. CRYPTOCOCCUS PNEUMONIA

Pathogens

- *Cryptococcus neoformans*
- *Cryptococcus gattii*

Diagnosis

- Serum cryptococcal antigen test
- Sputum or fine-needle/surgical lung biopsy for microscopy and culture
- Blood culture
- Chest x-ray: lung nodules, consolidation and interstitial changes

Treatment

For *C. neoformans* infection

- Option 1: amphotericin B liposomal (IV) **plus** flucytosine (IV or PO) for at least 2 weeks

If flucytosine is not tolerated

- Option 2: amphotericin B liposomal (IV) **plus** fluconazole (PO) for at least 2 weeks

If improvement after 2 weeks, change to

- Fluconazole 400 mg PO daily for 8 weeks

Maintenance to prevent recurrence

- Fluconazole 200 mg PO daily

Duration of maintenance

For at least 1 year until CD4 cell count >100/µL for ≥3 months with inactive disease and non-detectable or stable low HIV viral load

For *C. gattii* infection

- Amphotericin B liposomal (IV) **plus** flucytosine (IV or PO) for at least 2 weeks

If improvement after 2 weeks, change to

- Fluconazole 400 mg PO daily for 6–12 weeks

Dosage of above agents

- Amphotericin B liposomal 3–4 mg/kg IV daily
- Flucytosine 25 mg/kg IV or PO q6h
- Fluconazole 800 mg PO daily

3. *CRYPTOSPORIDIUM PARVUM* INFECTION (GASTROENTERITIS)

Other names: cryptosporidiosis

Treatment

- Nitazoxanide* 500 mg (child 1–3 years: 100 mg; 4–11 years: 200 mg) PO q12h for 3 days

---

*Available via Special Access Scheme <www.tga.gov.au/hp/access-sas.htm> or from compounding chemist

4. CYTOMEGALOVIRUS (CMV) INFECTION

Treatment

- Option 1: valganciclovir 900 mg PO q12h for 2–3 weeks
- Option 2: ganciclovir 5 mg/kg IV q12h for 2–3 weeks
- Option 3: foscarnet 90 mg/kg IV q12h for 2–3 weeks
- Option 4: cidofovir 5 mg/kg IV weekly for 2 weeks **plus** probenecid

Maintenance to prevent recurrence

- Option 1: valganciclovir 900 mg PO daily
- Option 2: ganciclovir 10 mg/kg IV 3 times weekly **or** 5 mg/kg IV 5 times weekly
- Option 3: foscarnet 90-120 mg/kg/day IV 5 times weekly
- Option 4: cidofovir 5 mg/kg IV fortnightly **plus** probenecid

Cessation of maintenance

When CD4 cell count >100–150/μL for ≥6 months with inactive disease and non-detectable or stable low HIV viral load

5. HERPES SIMPLEX VIRUS INFECTION

Treatment

- Option 1: valaciclovir 500 mg PO q12h for 7–10 days
- Option 2: famciclovir 500 mg PO q12h for 7–10 days
- Option 3: aciclovir 400 mg PO q8h for 7–10 days

For frequent severe recurrences

- Option 1: valaciclovir 500 mg PO q12h
- Option 2: famciclovir 500 mg PO q12h
- Option 3: aciclovir 400 mg PO q12h

6. MYCOBACTERIUM TUBERCULOSIS INFECTION

Treatment

Only by specialists with HIV and TB expertise (complex drug interactions between HIV and TB drugs) (See Tuberculosis, p. 405)

Primary prophylaxis

Treatment of latent TB:

- If tuberculin skin test >5 mm in patient who has had no BCG and no evidence of active TB or interferon-gamma release assay (IGRA) positive, treat with:
  - Isoniazid 300 mg **plus** pyridoxine 25 mg PO daily for 9 months

7. *MYCOBACTERIUM AVIUM* COMPLEX (MAC) INFECTION

Treatment

- Azithromycin (**or** clarithromycin) **plus** ethambutol **plus/minus** rifabutin (PO)

Dosage of above agents

- Azithromycin 500 mg (child: 10 mg/kg up to 500 mg) PO daily
- Clarithromycin 500 mg (child: 12.5 mg/kg up to 500 mg) PO q12h
- Ethambutol (adult and child ≥6 years) 15 mg/kg PO daily
- Rifabutin 300 mg (child: 5 mg/kg up to 300 mg) PO daily

If rifabutin taken with a ritonavir-boosted proteinase inhibitor: 150 mg (child: 2.5 mg/kg up to 150 mg) PO daily
If rifabutin taken with efavirenz: 450 mg (child 7.5 mg/kg up to 450 mg) PO daily

Maintenance to prevent recurrence

- As for above treatment, use 2 to 3 drugs according to tolerance

Cessation of maintenance

When CD4 cell count >100/μL for ≥ 6 months with inactive disease and non-detectable or stable low HIV viral load and after ≥12 months of MAC treatment with no signs or symptoms of MAC

Primary prophylaxis

Commence when CD4 cell count < 50/μL

- Option 1: azithromycin 1.2 g PO weekly
- Option 2: clarithromycin 500 mg PO q12h
- Option 3: rifabutin 300 mg PO daily

Cessation of prophylaxis

When CD4 cell count >100/μL for ≥ 6 months with inactive disease and non-detectable or stable low HIV viral load

8. *PNEUMOCYSTIS JIROVECII* PNEUMONIA

Laboratory

- Bronchial lavage for microscopy and cytological examination

Treatment

Mild to moderate disease

PaO_2 >70 mmHg on room air, A–a gradient <35 mmHg, O_2 sat >94% on room air

- Option 1: cotrimoxazole (PO) for 3 weeks
- Option 2: clindamycin (PO) **plus** primaquine (PO) for 3 weeks
- Option 3: dapsone (PO) **plus** trimethoprim (PO) for 3 weeks
- Option 4: atovaquone (PO) for 3 weeks

Severe disease

PaO_2 <70 mmHg on room air, A–a gradient >35 mmHg, O_2 sat <94% on room air

- Option 1: cotrimoxazole (IV then oral) for 3 weeks
- Option 2: clindamycin (IV or PO) **plus** primaquine (PO) for 3 weeks
- Option 3: pentamidine (IV) for 3 weeks

Concomitant corticosteroids should be used

- Prednisone (PO)

Dosage of above agents

Mild to moderate disease

- Cotrimoxazole 5/25 mg/kg (max 320/1600 mg) PO or IV q8h
- Clindamycin 450 mg PO q8h
- Primaquine 15 mg PO daily
- Dapsone 100 mg PO daily
- Trimethoprim 5 mg/kg PO q8h
- Atovaquone 750 mg PO with fatty food or full-fat milk q12h

Severe disease

- Cotrimoxazole 5/25 mg/kg (max 320/1600 mg) IV q6–8h until improvement, then PO
- Clindamycin 900 mg IV (or 450 mg PO) q6–8h
- Primaquine 30 mg PO daily
- Pentamidine 4 mg/kg up to 300 mg IV daily
- Prednisone 40 mg (child: 1 mg/kg up to 40 mg) PO q12h for 5 days, then daily for 5 days, then 20 mg (child: 0.5 mg/kg up to 20 mg) PO daily for 11 days

Maintenance

- Cotrimoxazole 80/400 mg PO daily **or** 160/800 mg PO 3 times weekly

If cotrimoxazole is not tolerated
- Option 1: dapsone 100 mg PO daily
- Option 2: atovaquone 1.5 g PO with full-fat milk daily
- Option 3: pentamidine 300 mg neb every 4 weeks

Cessation of maintenance

When CD4 cell count >200/μL for ≥ 3 months with inactive disease and non-detectable or stable low viral load

Primary prophylaxis

- Same regimens as for above maintenance therapy

Start primary prophylaxis when CD4 cell count < 200/μL or if CD4 cell less than 14%

9. *TOXOPLASMA GONDII* INFECTION

Treatment

- Option 1: sulfadiazine* (PO or IV) **plus** pyrimethamine (PO) for 6 weeks
  (calcium folinate 15 mg PO daily may reduce the incidence of neutropenia)
- Option 2: clindamycin (IV or PO) **plus** pyrimethamine (PO) for 6 weeks
- Option 3: atovaquone (PO) **plus** pyrimethamine (PO) for 6 weeks

Maintenance

- Option 1: sulfadiazine* (PO) **plus** pyrimethamine (PO)
- Option 2: clindamycin (PO) **plus** pyrimethamine (PO)

Cessation of maintenance

When CD4 cell count >200/μL for ≥6 months with inactive disease and non-detectable or stable low HIV viral load

Primary prophylaxis

- Option 1: cotrimoxazole (PO)
- Option 2: dapsone (PO) **plus** pyrimethamine (PO) (if does not tolerate sulfonamides)

Dosage of above agents

Treatment

- Sulfadiazine 1 g PO or IV q6h
- Pyrimethamine 50 mg PO for the 1st dose, then 25 mg PO daily
- Clindamycin 600 mg IV or PO q6h
- Atovaquone 1.5 g PO q12h

Maintenance

- Sulfadiazine 1 g PO q12h
- Pyrimethamine 25 mg PO daily
- Clindamycin 600 mg PO q8h

Primary prophylaxis

- Cotrimoxazole 80/400 or 160/800 mg PO daily (**or** 160/800 mg PO 3 times weekly)
- Dapsone 100 mg PO 3 times weekly
- Pyrimethamine 50 mg PO weekly

For more detailed information on the treatment of opportunistic infections guidelines, see https://aidsinfo.nih.gov/guidelines

---

*Available via Special Access Scheme <www.tga.gov.au/hp/access-sas.htm>

HIV AND PREGNANCY

This is a highly specialised area and management involves close collaboration between an HIV specialist, an obstetrician and a paediatrician.

Antepartum

- All pregnant women should undergo HIV at the first antenatal visit
- All HIV-infected pregnant women should be offered HIV counselling and antiretroviral therapy regardless of CD4 cell count and HIV viral load
- Discuss pros, cons and uncertainties of treatment with patient
- Perform HIV ARV drug-resistance testing before starting treatment
- If women who have HIV infection are on effective ARV treatment, the regimen should be continued during pregnancy

Intrapartum

- If mother has an undetectable viral load near delivery, intrapartum therapy to prevent mother-to-child transmission (MTCT) is not required
- If mother's viral load is >400 copies/mL or unknown, intrapartum therapy is indicated
- If mother's viral load is <400 copies/mL, intrapartum therapy may be considered
- If mother is on oral zidovudine, change to IV zidovudine during labour
  - Zidovudine* 2 mg/kg IV over 1 hour, 3 hours before anticipated caesarean section or at onset of labour, followed by 1 mg/kg/hour IV until the umbilical cord is clamped

Management of infant

- Avoid breastfeeding
- Start zidovudine as soon as possible after birth (within 6–12 hours)

Antiretroviral prophylaxis

Low risk of MTCT

Mother had undetectable viral load

- Neonate born after 35 weeks: zidovudine 4 mg/kg PO q12h for 4 weeks
- Neonate born at 30–34 weeks: zidovudine 2 mg/kg PO q12h for 2 weeks, then q8h for 2 weeks
- Neonate born at less than 30 weeks: zidovudine 2 mg/kg PO q12h for 4 weeks

High risk of MTCT

Mother had detectable viral load or viral load was unknown, or mother did not receive antepartum ARV therapy

- Zidovudine (dose as above) **plus** lamivudine 2 mg/kg PO q12h for 4 weeks **plus** nevirapine 2 mg/kg PO daily for 1 week, then 4 mg/kg

---

*Available via Special Access Scheme <www.tga.gov.au/hp/access-sas.htm>

PO daily for 1 week (if mother has been taking nevirapine over the last 3 days or more: 4 mg/kg PO daily for 2 weeks)

For more detailed information on perinatal HIV guideline, see www.asid.net.au/resources/clinical-guidelines

HORDEOLUM

Other names: stye, meibomianitis, meibomian abscess, meibomian cyst, chalazion, tarsal cyst

Hordeolum is an acute focal infection involving either the gland of Zeis (external hordeolum, or stye) or, less frequently, the meibomian gland (internal hordeolum, or meibomianitis).

Pathogen

- *Staphylococcus aureus*

1. EXTERNAL HORDEOLUM (STYE)

- Small staphylococcal abscess of the sebaceous glands associated with eyelash follicle

Treatment

- Usually self-limiting, spontaneously resolves in 1–2 weeks
- Non-antibiotic management is usually sufficient
  - Warm compresses until the stye points and discharges spontaneously
  - Removal of the eyelash involved is usually helpful

Topical or oral antibiotics are usually not required

2. INTERNAL HORDEOLUM (MEIBOMIANITIS, MEIBOMIAN ABSCESS)

- Infection of the meibomian gland (meibomianitis) may progress to an abscess (meibomian abscess) and can leave a residual swelling (meibomian cyst, also called a tarsal cyst or chalazion) when acute inflammation subsides

Treatment

- For meibomian cyst (tarsal cyst or chalazion)—repeated warm compresses, usually resolve within 1 month
- For persistent meibomian cyst or recurrent meibomian abscess—refer to ophthalmologist for surgical incision and curettage
- For meibomianitis and meibomian abscess—warm compresses and antibiotic treatment
  - Flucloxacillin (PO) for at least 5 days

If non-immediate penicillin allergy
  - Cefalexin (PO) for at least 5 days

If immediate penicillin allergy
  - Option 1: doxycycline (PO) for at least 5 days
  - Option 2: clindamycin (PO) for at least 5 days

Dosage of above antibiotics

- Flucloxacillin 500 mg (child: 12.5 mg/kg up to 500 mg) PO q6h
- Cefalexin 500 mg (child: 12.5 mg/kg up to 500 mg) PO q6h
- Doxycycline 100 mg (child >8 years: 2 mg/kg up to 100 mg) PO daily
- Clindamycin 300 mg (child: 10 mg/kg up to 300 mg) PO q8h

HUMAN PAPILLOMAVIRUS

Other names: cervical intraepithelial neoplasia (CIN), squamous intraepithelial lesions (SIL), cervical dysplasia

Pathogens

Human papillomavirus (HPV)

- High-risk (oncogenic) genotypes—HPV 16, 18, 31, 33, 35, 39, 45, 51, 52, 56, 58, 59, 68
- Low-risk genotypes—HPV 6 and 11

Transmission

- Direct contact, sexually or non-sexually

Clinical

HPV infection is usually asymptomatic, but HPV can cause warts and cancers:

- Cervical cancer—70% caused by HPV 16, 18 and 45, 30% caused by other genotypes
- Anal cancer (particularly in HIV-infected men who have sex with men)—HPV 16 and 18
- Penile cancer—HPV 16 and 18
- Vaginal cancer—HPV 16 and 18
- Vulvar cancer—HPV 16 and 18
- Oropharyngeal cancer—HPV 16 (over 90% cases)
- Genital warts (condylomata acuminate)—HPV types 6 and 11 (>90% of genital warts)

Laboratory

- HPV-DNA testing (cervical swab or Pap smear with liquid cytology specimen)—to detect HPV infection
- Pap smear to find cervical cell changes (CINs)
- Colposcopy and cervical lesion biopsy—to confirm the cancer

Australian National Cervical Screening Program (NCSP)

Five-yearly primary HPV DNA test on cervical swab (for women >30 years of age)

- If swab test positive for HPV 16 or 18, refer to a gynaecologist for colposcopy

- If swab test positive for other 11 high-risk genotypes, perform Pap smear for liquid-based cytology

HPV-related changes of cervical cells
- CIN1 (= LSIL = low-grade dysplasia)
- CIN2 or CIN3 (= HSIL = high-grade dysplasia)

Treatment
- Treat cellular changes on cervix (e.g. laser, loop excision, cone biopsy or hysterectomy)

Prevention
- Male circumcision reduces the incidence of HPV infection

HPV vaccination
- 2vHPV vaccine (e.g. Cervarix)—against HPV 16 and 18
- 4vHPV vaccine (e.g. Gardasil®)—against HPV 16, 18, 6 and 11 (protect more than 70% cervical cancer)
- 9vHPV vaccine (e.g. Gardasil®9)—against 9 genotypes, including HPV 16, 18, 6 and 11 (protect more than 90% cervical cancer)

HPV vaccination is recommended for following groups:

- Female 9–45 years—for prevention of cervical cancer, other cancers and genital warts
- Male 9–26 years—for prevention of anal and penile cancers, genital warts
  - 2vHPV vaccine (e.g. Cervarix) 0.5 mL IM, 3 doses at 0, 1 and 6 months
  - 4vHPV vaccine (e.g. Gardasil®) 0.5 mL IM, 3 doses at 0, 2 and 6 months
  - 9vHPV vaccine (e.g. Gardasil®9) 0.5 mL IM, 2 doses at 0, and 6–12 months

HUMAN T-CELL LYMPHOTROPIC VIRUS TYPE I

Pathogen
- Human T-cell lymphotropic virus type I (HTLV-I)—a human RNA retrovirus, a distant relative of the human immunodeficiency viruses (HIV)

It causes:

- Adult T-cell leukaemia/lymphoma (ATLL)
- HTLV-I associated myelopathy/tropical spastic paraparesis (HAM/TSP)

Transmission
- Mother to child—primarily through breastfeeding (20–50% of babies born to infected mothers will become carriers)

- Blood transfusion
- Sexual transmission (more risk from males to females)
- Sharing of contaminated needles

Distribution

- Endemic in Japan, the Caribbean, central Africa, Iran, Iraq, southern India, China, the Seychelles, Papua New Guinea, the Solomon Islands and Australia
- In Australia, the virus occurs in many Aboriginal populations

Laboratory

- HTLV-I antibody (blood, semen)—screen test
- HTLV-I western blot—confirmatory test

Clinical

- ATLL (5% of HTLV-I infected patients)
- HTLV-I associated myelopathy/tropical spastic paraparesis (HAM/TSP) (0.25–3% of HTLV-I infected patients)
- Other diseases less clearly associated with HTLV-I: opportunistic lung diseases, chronic lung diseases, certain cancers, eye inflammation, infective dermatitis, crusted (Norwegian) scabies and chronic low-grade immunosuppression

Treatment

- No treatment for chronic HTLV-I infection
- Conventional combination chemotherapy has generally proved disappointing
- No specific treatment for HAM/TSP

Prevention

- Bottle-feed infants of infected mothers
- HTLV-I infected persons should refrain from donating blood and tissues
- HTLV-I infected persons should use condoms to prevent sexual transmission
- Healthcare workers caring for HTLV-I infected persons need to be aware of the risk of percutaneous exposure to HTLV-I contaminated blood
- When needle-stick injuries occur in some inland Aboriginal populations with a higher prevalence of HTLV-I infection, HTLV-I antibodies should be tested

HYDATID DISEASE

Other names: echinococcosis, hydatid cysts

Pathogen

- Dog tapeworm (*Echinococcus granulosus*)

Transmission

- After the person eats dog faeces-contaminated food or water, the larvae penetrate the intestinal mucosa, enter the portal system and deposit in various organs where they grow into cysts
- In Australia, it is prevalent in areas where dogs are used in the herding of sheep

Clinical

- Slow-growing cysts in liver (60%), lungs (20%), kidneys (3%) or brain (1%)
- Symptoms from pressure, leakage or rupture of the cysts depend on the location
- Sudden rupture of the cyst may cause fatal anaphylaxis and dissemination of infectious protoscolices

Diagnosis

Do not attempt to do diagnostic aspiration of the cyst

- Ultrasound or CT scan—to locate the cyst
- Plain x-ray—may show calcification (a calcified cyst may still have active infection)
- Hydatid serology—supports the clinical diagnosis
- Macroscopic appearance on surgically removed cysts—diagnostic
- If a cyst ruptures—examination for protoscolices, brood capsules and cyst wall in sputum, vomitus, faeces or urine (depends on the location of the cyst)
- Peripheral eosinophilia elevation (30%)

Treatment

- If asymptomatic—observation
- Small lung cysts—may respond to albendazole treatment alone
- Liver cysts—**PAIR**: **P**ercutaneous **A**spiration under ultrasound guidance → **I**ntra-cyst injection of hypertonic saline or ethanol → **R**e-aspiration after 15 minutes, followed by prolonged high dose of oral albendazole (see below)
- Symptomatic cysts—surgical removal of cysts with oral albendazole +/– praziquantel

Oral therapy adjunct to surgery

Albendazole alone or with praziquantel

- Albendazole (PO) starting 1 week before surgery, continuing for 4 weeks after surgery, may repeat after 2 weeks for up to 3 cycles
- Praziquantel (PO) starting 1 week before surgery, if spillage at surgery, continuing for 2 weeks after surgery

If cyst spillage from trauma

- Praziquantel (PO) for 2 weeks after spillage, followed by albendazole for 4 weeks, may repeat after 2 weeks for up to 3 cycles

Dosage of above agents

- Albendazole 400 mg (adult <60 kg, child >6 years: 7.5 mg/kg up to 400 mg) PO (with fatty food) q12h
- Praziquantel 30 mg/kg PO q4h for 1st day, then q8h or 20 mg/kg q12h for 2 weeks

Alveolar hydrated disease (AHD)

- Caused by *Echinococcus multilocularis*
- Characteristic budding appearance of the cysts
- Management is complex—seek expert advice

IMPETIGO

Other names: school sores

Pathogens

- *Staphylococcus aureus*—the most common
- *Streptococcus pyogenes*—common in remote Indigenous communities

Types of impetigo

1. **Crusted or non-bullous impetigo**—yellow crusts and erosions, itchy or irritating but not painful (less acute)
2. **Bullous impetigo**—mild irritating blisters that erode rapidly and form brown crusts

Laboratory

- Skin swabs for culture + susceptibility if severe or no response to empirical treatment
- Skin viral swabs for herpes simplex virus PCR if painful or no response to treatment

Treatment

- Treat any underlying dermatitis, scabies (see Scabies, p. 358) or head lice (see Lice, p. 203)
- Antibiotic therapy—treat as *Staphylococcus aureus* infection

Mild or localised impetigo

- Remove crusts with soap and water **or** saline **or** aluminium acetate **or** potassium permanganate solution q8h
- Mupirocin 2% cream/oint (e.g. Bactroban) top q8h for 7 days

Widespread or recurrent infections

Topical antiseptics
- Option 1: triclosan 1% solution (e.g. PHisoHex) wash daily
- Option 2: chlorhexidine 2% solution (e.g. Microshield 2) wash daily

Antibiotics
- Option 1: flucloxacillin (PO) for up to 10 days
- Option 2: cefalexin (PO) for up to 10 days (non-immediate penicillin allergy)
- Option 3: cotrimoxazole (PO) for 5 days (immediate penicillin allergy)

In remote Indigenous communities in central and northern Australia
- Option 1: benzathine penicillin (IM) st
- Option 2: cotrimoxazole (PO) for 5 days

Dosage of above agents

- Aluminium acetate 13% (Burow's) solution diluted 1:20 to 1:40 before use

- Potassium permanganate (Condy's crystals) 0.1% solution diluted 1 : 10 before use (it is caustic and will stain; handle carefully)
- Flucloxacillin 500 mg (child: 12.5 mg/kg up to 500 mg) PO q6h
- Cefalexin 500 mg (child: 12.5 mg/kg up to 500 mg) PO q6h
  or Cefalexin 1 g (child: 25 mg/kg up to 1 g) PO q12h
- Cotrimoxazole 160/800 mg (child >1 month: 4/20 mg/kg up to 160/800 mg) PO q12h
- Benzathine benzylpenicillin 900 mg (child 3–6 kg: 225 mg; 6–10 kg: 337.5 mg; 10–15 kg: 450 mg; 15–20 kg: 675 mg; ≥20 kg: 900 mg) IM as a single dose
- Cotrimoxazole 160/800 mg (child >1 month: 4/20 mg/kg up to 160/800 mg) PO q12h
  or Cotrimoxazole 320/1600 mg (child >1 month: 8/40 mg/kg up to 320/1600 mg) PO daily

Recurrent impetigo

Total body eradication for patient, whole family and close contacts
Commence total body eradication after all acute lesions have healed

- To eradicate nasal carriage—use either of the following:
  - Mupirocin 2% nasal oint (e.g. Bactroban) intranasally q8h for 5 days
  - Chlorhexidine 0.3% nasal cream (e.g. Nasalate) intranasally q6–8h for 5 days
- To eradicate skin colonisation (antiseptic total bodywash)—wash whole body daily for at least 5 days with one of the following:
  - Triclosan 1% solution (e.g. Microshield T) or soap (e.g. Cetaphil Antibacterial Bar)
  - Chlorhexidine 2% solution (e.g. Microshield 2)
  - Chlorhexidine 0.05% and cetrimide 0.5% irrigation solution
- Pay particular attention to hair-bearing areas
- Wash clothes, towels and sheets in hot water (>60˚C) on 2 separate occasions

INFLUENZA

Pathogens

- Influenza A and B viruses
- Novel influenza A strains—H5N1, H7N9 (see Avian influenza, p. 13) and H1N1 2009 (see Swine influenza, p. 387)

Transmission

- Droplets from coughing and sneezing

Incubation

- 1–3 days

Laboratory

- Nasal/throat swabs for influenza virus PCR or viral antigen detection
- Influenza serology
- Nasal/throat swabs for viral culture

High-risk groups

- ≥65 years old (Aboriginal ≥50 years)
- Children <5 years old
- Chronic diseases (especially asthma and COPD)
- The immunosuppressed
- Pregnant women
- The morbidly obese
- Aboriginal and Torres Strait Islander peoples >15 years old
- Nursing home residents
- Homeless people

Treatment

- High-risk group—treat, even if the onset of symptoms has been >48 hours
- Severe influenza (e.g. pneumonitis)—treat, regardless of duration of illness or risk group
- Low-risk group with mild symptoms—only treat if onset of symptoms is <48 hours

Neuraminidase inhibitors

Preferably use within 48 hours after onset

- Option 1: oseltamivir (e.g. Tamiflu) (PO) for 5 days (category B1)
- Option 2: zanamivir (e.g. Relenza) (inh) for 5 days (category B1)

For severe influenza requiring ventilation

- Option 1: oseltamivir 150 mg PO q12h
- Option 2: zanamivir (IV)*
- Option 3: peramivir (IV)*

Dosage of above agents

- Oseltamivir (e.g. Tamiflu) 75 mg (child >1 year and <15 kg: 30 mg; 15–23 kg: 45 mg; 23–40 kg: 60 mg; >40 kg: 75 mg) PO q12h
- Zanamivir (e.g. Relenza) adult, child >5 years: 10 mg inh via device provided q12h

Prevention

1. Post-exposure prophylaxis

- For close contacts of proven cases, particularly if the contacts are in high-risk group

---

*IV zanamivir and peramivir are available via Special Access Scheme <www.tga.gov.au/hp/access-sas.htm>

- For healthcare workers with unprotected exposure
- For hospital inpatients or aged care residents—to control influenza outbreaks
- For control of major outbreak of novel strains of influenza in community

Ideally use within 48 hours after exposure

- Option 1: oseltamivir (e.g. Tamiflu) (PO) for 10 days (category B1)
- Option 2: zanamivir (e.g. Relenza) (inh) for 10 days (category B1)

Longer course for repeated exposure

Dosage of above agents

- Oseltamivir (e.g. Tamiflu) 75 mg (child >1 year and <15 kg: 30 mg; 15–23 kg: 45 mg; 23–40 kg: 60 mg; >40 kg: 75 mg) PO daily
- Zanamivir (e.g. Relenza) adult, child >5 years: 10 mg inh via device provided daily

2.   Influenza vaccination—annually before winter

Influenza vaccination is strongly recommended for

- All people ≥65 years of age
- All children aged 6 months to 5 years old
- All Aboriginal and Torres Strait Island peoples ≥15 years old
- Chronic illness sufferers and the immunocompromised
- Chronic steroid use or long-term aspirin therapy in children (6 months to 10 years)
- Pregnant women, people with Down syndrome or obesity
- Residents and staff of nursing homes and other long-term care facilities
- Healthcare providers
- Poultry workers during an avian influenza outbreak

National immunisation program

- Protection is usually achieved within 10–14 days
- Protection after vaccination may begin to wane after 3–4 months

Quadrivalent influenza vaccines

Children aged 6 months to 3 years old

- FluQuadri Junior—0.5 mL IM, 2 doses at least 4 weeks apart, then 1 dose annually

Children aged 3 years and older

- FluQuadri—0.5 mL IM annually
- Fluarix Tetra —0.5 mL IM annually

People aged 18 years and older

- Afluria Quad—0.5 mL IM annually

ISOSPORA BELLI GASTROENTERITIS

Other names: isosporiasis

Pathogen

- *Isosora* (*Cystoisospora*) *belli*—a protozoan

Distribution

- Worldwide, especially in tropical and subtropical areas

Transmission

- Faecal–oral

Incubation

- 3–14 days

Clinical

- Infection often occurs in immunocompromised individuals, notably AIDS patients
- Profuse, watery, offensive-smelling diarrhoea with abdominal cramps
- The diarrhoea can last for weeks and result in malabsorption and weight loss
- In immunosuppressed patients and in infants and children, the diarrhoea can be severe

Diagnosis

- Peripheral eosinophilia—an important clue
- Faeces OCP with modified acid-fast stain or ultraviolet autofluorescence microscopy—identify the large oocysts (may need repeated examinations with concentration procedures because the oocysts may be passed in small amounts and intermittently)
- Duodenal aspirate or string test (Enterotest)—if negative faeces examination

Treatment

- In immunocompetent patients—self-limiting gastroenteritis—no treatment
- In immunocompromised patients (e.g. AIDS)—treat
  - Cotrimoxazole (PO) for 7–10 days, then 3 times weekly for maintenance

Dosage of above agent

- Cotrimoxazole 160/800 mg (child >2 months: 4/20 mg/kg up to 160/800 mg) PO q6h, then 3 times weekly

J

JAPANESE ENCEPHALITIS

Japanese encephalitis (JE) is very uncommon in travellers but can lead to death or serious disability.

Pathogen

- Japanese encephalitis virus (JEV), a mosquito-borne flavivirus

Distribution

- Indian subcontinent, Southeast Asia and China; also in the Torres Strait Islands and northern Australia

Transmission

- From wading bird to pigs, and then to humans by various mosquito vectors
- Humans are an incidental host

Clinical

- Most infections are asymptomatic
- Gastrointestinal symptoms may be prominent
- Acute neurological syndrome (1 in 200 cases)—headache, fever, focal neurological signs, central hyperpnoeic breathing, extrapyramidal signs, convulsions, confusion and coma

Laboratory

- JEV isolation—from blood during the 1st week of illness
- JEV PCR testing
- JEV-specific IgM in CSF or blood—in the absence of IgM to MVE, Kunjin and dengue viruses and with no recent vaccination for JE or yellow fever (confirmation of laboratory result by a second arbovirus reference laboratory is required if the case appears to have been acquired in Australia)
- JEV-specific IgG seroconversion or a ≥four-fold rise in titre (with no recent vaccination for JE or yellow fever)
- CT or MRI—bilateral thalamic lesions with haemorrhage; the basal ganglia, putamen, pons, spinal cord and cerebellum may also show abnormalities

Treatment

- Supportive
- Suramin and diethyldithiocarbamate have shown reasonably good antiviral efficacy against JEV in vitro
- A novel intervention using a plant lignan called arctigenin has shown complete protection against experimental JE in a mouse

Vaccination

JE vaccination is recommended for:

- Travellers spending ≥1 month in rural areas of Asia or the Western Province of Papua New Guinea, particularly during the wet season
- Travellers spending ≥1 year in urban areas of Asia (except for Singapore)
- All residents of the outer Torres Strait Islands and all non-residents who will live in the region for ≥1 month during the wet season (December–May)
- All research laboratory personnel who may be exposed to the virus
- Consider vaccination for short-term travellers in the wet season where there is considerable outdoor activity, or the accommodation is not mosquito-proof
  - JE vaccine (Jespect) – adult ≥18 years: 0.5 mL IM, 2 doses on days 0 and 28 (the last dose is best given at least 35 days before travelling)

Protection may last up to 2–3 years
JE vaccine is safe for pregnant women

K

KAWASAKI DISEASE

Other names: mucocutaneous lymph node syndrome
Kawasaki disease is an acute febrile illness that involves the skin, mouth, eyes and lymph nodes and most often affects children under 5 years of age. Early diagnosis and aspirin treatment can reduce cardiac complications.

Pathogens

- Clinically appears similar to an infection, but no infective agent has been isolated
- There is no evidence of person-to-person transmission

Clinical

- Persistent high fever (≥39°C); conjunctivitis; sore throat; enlarged cervical lymph nodes; polymorphous rash on chest, abdomen or genital area; red, dry, cracked lips; purple-red and swollen palms of the hands and soles of the feet, with subsequent peeling of the fingers and toes
- The child may have joint pain, diarrhoea, vomiting and abdominal pain

Complications

If untreated, it can lead to serious heart complications:

- Vasculitis (can affect the coronary arteries)
- Myocarditis, endocarditis and pericarditis
- Arrhythmias

Diagnosis

- Blood test: very high ESR and increased platelet count
- Diagnosis is made by evaluating the symptoms and ruling out other conditions

Criteria of diagnosis

A fever lasting ≥5 days plus at least 4 of the following:

- Conjunctivitis (both eyes)
- Lips, tongue or mouth—red, dry and cracked
- Fingers and toes—swelling, discolouration or peeling
- Hands and feet—red, swollen palms and soles
- Rash in the trunk or genital area
- Enlarged cervical lymph nodes

Treatment

- **Aspirin**—should be started ASAP, within 10 days of development of fever
- Normal immunoglobulin

- Monitor ECG and echocardiogram
  - Aspirin 10 mg/kg PO q8h until fever settles, then 3–5 mg/kg PO daily
  - Normal immunoglobulin (e.g. Sandoglobulin NF) 2 g/kg IV over 6–8 hours

Prognosis

- Symptoms often disappear within 2 days of treatment
- If treated within 10 days of onset, heart complications usually do not develop

KERATITIS

Other names: corneal infection, microbial keratitis, bacterial keratitis, fungal keratitis, amoebic keratitis, viral keratitis, herpes keratitis

Pathogens

- Bacteria (common)—*Staphylococcus epidermidis*, *S. aureus*, *Pseudomonas aeruginosa*, *Streptococcus* spp, *Moraxella* spp, *Neisseria gonorrhoeae*, mycobacterium
- Viruses (the most common)—herpes simplex virus type 1 (HSV-1), varicella zoster virus, adenovirus
- Fungi—*Aspergillus* spp, *Candida* spp, *Fusarium* spp
- Parasites—*Acanthamoeba*, *Microsporidia*

Risk factors

- Contact lenses
- Ocular trauma (especially involving vegetative matter)
- Corneal surgery or prior corneal transplantation
- Eye surface diseases—severe dry eye, Stevens-Johnson syndrome, cicatricial pemphigoid, atopic keratoconjunctivitis, ocular rosacea, radiation and chemical injury
- Topical ocular corticosteroid use—can cause rapid corneal melting and perforation
- Systemic diseases—malnutrition, diabetes, autoimmune and vascular diseases, alcoholism
- Immunosuppression—cancer, HIV/AIDS

1. BACTERIAL KERATITIS

Clinical

- Rapid onset of pain, photophobia, reduced vision (does not clear with blinking) and conjunctival injection
- A small white spot often seen on cornea

Laboratory

- Corneal scraping for Gram stain and culture (by ophthalmologist)

Treatment

- Increasing pain and progressive deterioration should prompt urgent referral to an ophthalmologist
- If patient can see an ophthalmologist straight away, do not use topical antibiotic
- If unable to see an ophthalmologist straight away, start topical treatment without delay
    - Option 1: ciprofloxacin 0.3% eye drops 1–2 drops top every 15 min for 6 hours, then hourly for 48 hours, then q4h until healed
    - Option 2: ofloxacin 0.3% eye drops 1–2 drops top every 15 min for 6 hours, then hourly for 48 hours, then q4h until healed
    - Option 3: cefalotin 5% plus gentamicin 0.9% eye drops* 1–2 drops top hourly for 48 hours, then reduce frequency until healed

If scleral or intraocular extension of infection exist
    - **Add** ciprofloxacin 500 mg PO q12h

2.   HERPES SIMPLEX KERATITIS

Herpes simplex keratitis (dendritic ulcer) is the most common keratitis and the most frequent cause of infectious blindness in the Western world.

Pathogen

- Herpes simplex virus type 1 (HSV-1)

Transmission

- Direct contact with virus-laden lesions or secretions
- Reactivation of the virus in the trigeminal ganglion, which migrates down the nerve axon to produce a lytic infection in ocular tissue

Clinical

- Typically presents as a unilateral 'red eye' with pain, irritation, photophobia and epiphora; vision may or may not be affected; pain may be less severe than the eye signs
- Herpes simplex keratitis in children is marked by a disproportionate risk of binocular disease, a high recurrence rate and amblyopia

Diagnosis

- Always suspect HSV infection if the unilateral red eye appears worse on examination than the patient feels
- Corneal fluorescein staining + slit lamp examination—dendritic ulcer (suggest diagnosis)
- HSV PCR (ocular swab or corneal scraping)
- Bacterial culture (ocular swab or corneal scraping)

---

*Cefalotin plus gentamycin eye drops require extemporaneous preparation

Treatment

- HSV infection must be managed aggressively and quickly to prevent deeper penetration
- Topical steroid use without antiviral cover is dangerous
- When suspected, start antiviral treatment within 72 hours of onset
- Consult or referral to an ophthalmologist if keratitis has been >72 hours
- Child patients may need hospital admission
  - Option 1: famciclovir 250 mg PO q8h for 7 days
  - Option 2: valaciclovir 1 g PO q8h for 7 days
  - Option 3: aciclovir 800 mg (child: 20 mg/kg up to 800 mg) PO 5 times daily for 7 days (q3h during waking hours) (preferred in child and pregnancy)

Treatment may be supplemented with topical aciclovir
  - Aciclovir 3% eye oint (e.g. Zovirax Ophthalmic) top 5 times daily for 14 days or for 3 days after healing

Avoid topical steroids

If sight is threatened:

Urgent ophthalmologist referral and hospital admission

  - Aciclovir 10–12.5 mg/kg (child <5 years: 20 mg/kg; >5 years: 15 mg/kg) IV q8h for 7 days

For recurrent herpes simplex keratitis (prophylaxis)
  - Aciclovir 400 mg PO daily for 6–12 months

3. HERPES ZOSTER KERATITIS (TRIGEMINAL NERVE SHINGLES)

Pathogen

- Varicella zoster virus

Transmission

- Reactivation of the virus from previous chickenpox infection
- Re-exposure to the virus

Clinical

- Red eye with skin lesion of trigeminal nerve shingles; eye discharge, photophobia and visual loss
- Corneal ulcers are prone to prolonged healing times and may perforate

Treatment

- Consult or referral to an ophthalmologist in all cases of trigeminal nerve shingles

- Child patients are recommended to be admitted to hospital
- Analgesia—paracetamol, aspirin, opioids or tricyclic antidepressants
- Antiviral treatment should be started within 72 hours of the onset of rash
  - Option 1: famciclovir 250 mg PO q8h for 7 days
  - Option 2: valaciclovir 1 g PO q8h for 7 days
  - Option 3: aciclovir 800 mg (child: 20 mg/kg up to 800 mg) PO 5 times daily for 7 days (preferred in child and pregnancy)

If vision is threatened:

Refer to ED and use IV aciclovir

  - Aciclovir 10–12.5 mg/kg (child <5 years: 20 mg/kg; >5 years: 15 mg/kg) IV q8h for 7–14 days

4. FUNGAL KERATITIS

Risk factors

- Contact lenses
- Ocular trauma (especially involving vegetative matter)
- Topical ocular corticosteroids use

Clinical

- Subacute onset with initial foreign-body sensation for several days and slow onset of increasing pain

Laboratory

- Confocal microscopy—may identify fungal hyphae (by ophthalmologist)

Treatment

- Referral to an ophthalmologist
- Prolonged and intensive topical and systemic antifungal therapy
- Surgical intervention may be required

5. AMOEBIC KERATITIS

Pathogen

- *Acanthamoeba*

Clinical

- A chronic contact lens-related infection
- The most characteristic sign—radial perineuritis (under slit-lamp examination)

Laboratory

- Confocal microscopy—may identify *Acanthamoeba* cyst (by ophthalmologist)

Treatment

- Referral to an ophthalmologist
- Treatment before deep infiltration usually gets excellent outcome

KUNJIN VIRUS

Pathogen

- Kunjin virus (KUNV)—a flavivirus

Distribution

- Kunjin virus infection has occurred over wide areas of Australia, infecting humans, and wild and domestic animals (cattle, sheep and horses)

Transmission

- The virus is endemic in the tropical north of Australia and Malaysia, where there are cycles of infection between birds and mosquitoes in enzootic foci
- Human transmission occurs via mosquitoes
- Water birds are vertebrate host and mosquito *Culex annulirostris* is major vector
- No person-to-person transmission

Clinical

1. **Mild disease**—fever, lymphadenopathy, lethargy and rash, sometimes with muscle weakness and fatigue
2. **Encephalitic disease**—acute febrile meningoencephalitis characterised by focal neurological disease or impaired consciousness, abnormal CT or MRI scan or EEG and presence of pleocytosis in the CSF
3. **Asymptomatic disease**

- Fatalities are rare or absent
- Infection confers lifelong immunity

Laboratory

- KUNV serology—IgG seroconversion or a significant rise (a four-fold rise in titre) of KUNV-specific IgG in two blood specimens taken 7–10 days apart
- Isolation of KUNV from clinical material
- Detection of KUNV RNA in clinical material
- KUNV-specific IgM detected in CSF or serum (in the absence of IgM to MVE, JE or Dengue viruses) (only for encephalitic illnesses)

Confirmation of laboratory result by a second arbovirus reference laboratory is required to differentiate from WNV and MVEV if the case occurs in areas of Australia with no enzootic/endemic activity or regular epidemic activity

Treatment

- Symptomatic and supportive

Prevention

- No vaccine is available
- Avoidance of mosquito-prone areas
- Avoidance of mosquito contact and biting times at dusk and dawn
- Personal protection (long sleeves, long trousers, mosquito repellent)
- Reduction of the vector mosquito population

LARYNGITIS AND LARYNGEAL ABSCESS

1. ACUTE LARYNGITIS

Causes

- Infections—usually viral; bacterial or fungal infection may also occur
- Overuse of the vocal cords
- Excessive coughing
- Excessive alcohol consumption or smoking
- Gastro-oesophageal reflux

Clinical

- Raspy hoarseness or loss of voice
- Dry and sore throat
- Coughing
- Difficulty swallowing
- Cold or flu-like symptoms, fever and cervical lymphadenopathy

Treatment

- Usually viral and self-limiting, no antibiotics are indicated
- If persistent hoarseness or loss of voice >2 weeks, referral to an ENT specialist
- If it is due to bacterial or fungal infection, antibiotics or anti-fungal medication

If second infection with streptococci or staphylococci
- Option 1: flucloxacillin (PO) for 7 days
- Option 2: cefalexin (PO) for 7 days

Dosage of above antibiotics
- Flucloxacillin 500 mg (child: 25 mg/kg up to 500 mg) PO q6h
- Cefalexin 500 mg (child: 25 mg/kg up to 500 mg) PO q6h

2. LARYNGEAL ABSCESS

- A serious and potentially fatal problem requiring urgent treatment

Causes

- Associated with malignancy, airway instrumentation or a pre-existing laryngocele

Pathogens

- *Staphylococcus*, *Pseudomonas* or *Proteus*

Clinical

- Severe sore throat, fever, pain on swallowing; may present with stridor, cervical lymphadenopathy and painful lateral movement of the larynx

Treatment

- If stridor, immediate tracheotomy
- IV antibiotics
- Refer for surgical drainage if no response in 24 hours
  - Flucloxacillin (IV) **plus** gentamicin (IV)

Dosage of above antibiotics

- Flucloxacillin 2 g (child: 50 mg/kg up to 2 g) IV q6h
- Gentamicin 4–7 mg/kg (child: 7.5 mg/kg up to 320 mg) IV for the 1st dose (further dosing, see p. 459)

LEGIONELLA

Other names: Legionnaires' disease, Legionellosis, *Legionella* pneumonia, Pontiac fever

Pathogens

- *Legionella pneumophila*, a Gram-negative rod-shaped bacterium that thrives in warm environments (25–45°C), causes Legionnaires' disease
- *Legionella longbeachae* and other *Legionella* spp cause Pontiac fever

Transmission

Legionella pneumophila—inhalation of mist droplets containing the bacteria

- Common sources of *Legionella pneumophila*: cooling towers, air-conditioning systems, evaporative coolers, wellness centres with saunas and whirlpool spas, domestic hot-water systems, showers, architectural fountains, room-air humidifiers, ice-making machines, misting equipment and similar disseminators that draw upon a public water supply
- Natural sources of *Legionella pneumophila*: freshwater ponds and creeks
- The disease is particularly associated with hotels, cruise ships and hospitals with old, poorly maintained pipework and cooling systems

Legionella longbeachae—inhalation of garden dust

- Common sources of *Legionella longbeachae*: potting mix and garden soil
- No person-to-person transmission

Incubation

- 2–10 days (usually 5–6 days).
- Symptoms may appear 5–6 hours after exposure to the *Legionella* bacteria

Clinical

Legionellosis has two distinct forms:

- **Legionnaires' disease/*Legionella* pneumonia**—should be suspected if patient has dry cough, high fever, mental confusion, bronchial pneumonia (bilateral consolidation) on chest x-ray, hyponatraemia, abnormal renal and liver function, and proteinuria; the disease tends to affect the immunocompromised, smokers, those with chronic lung disease and the elderly
- **Pontiac fever**—a milder respiratory illness resembling acute influenza: fever, headache, cough and muscle aches without pneumonia; commonly occurs in healthy people; generally recover in 2–5 days

Risk factors

- Diabetes
- Immunosuppression
- High-dose corticosteroid therapy
- Malignancy
- End-stage renal failure
- History of smoking
- Excessive alcohol use
- Known local prevalence of hospital-acquired disease

Diagnosis

- *Legionella* urinary antigen test—aids early diagnosis; simple, quick and reliable; detects the commonest *Legionella pneumophila* type 1 (cannot be used to match the patient with the environmental source of infection)
- *Legionella* culture (special media)—sputum, pleural fluid, bronchial brush, wash or bronchoalveolar lavage
- *Legionella* PCR—sputum, pleural fluid, bronchial brush, wash or bronchoalveolar lavage
- *Legionella* serology (IgM)—two blood samples obtained 3–9 weeks apart (retrospective diagnosis)
- PCR or rapid immunological assays—to detect *Legionella* in water samples

Treatment

- **For Pontiac fever**—no specific antibiotic treatment
- **For Legionnaires' disease/*Legionella* pneumonia**—start antibiotic therapy ASAP when suspected; delay in giving the appropriate antibiotic leads to higher mortality

Antibiotic therapy for *Legionella* pneumonia
  - Option 1: azithromycin (PO) for 5 days
  - Option 2: doxycycline (PO) for 10–14 days

For severe cases requiring ICU care
- Azithromycin (IV or PO) (**or** erythromycin [IV]) **plus** ciprofloxacin (**or** rifampicin) (IV or PO)

Duration of therapy for severe cases

- For immunocompetent patients: 1–2 weeks
- For immunocompromised patients: 2–3 weeks

Dosage of above antibiotics

- Azithromycin 500 mg (child: 10 mg/kg up to 500 mg) PO daily
- Doxycycline 100 mg (child >8 years: 2.5 mg/kg up to 100 mg) PO q12h
- Azithromycin 500 mg (child: 10 mg/kg up to 500 mg) IV daily, then 500 mg (child: 10 mg/kg up to 500 mg) PO daily
- Erythromycin 1 g IV (preferably through a central line) q6h
- Ciprofloxacin 400 mg IV q12h, then 750 mg PO q12h (for obese patient: 400 mg IV q8h)
- Rifampicin 300 mg (child: 5–10 mg/kg up to 300 mg) IV or PO q12h

LEPROSY

Other names: Hansen's disease
Leprosy remains a leading cause of deformity and permanent physical impairment in many countries

Pathogen

- *Mycobacterium leprae*

Transmission

- By close contact (but only 1% of contacts develop the disease)
- Other potential sources: soil, armadillos and possibly bedbugs and mosquitoes

Incubation

- 2–6 years (from a few months to 20 years)

Clinical

- **Tuberculoid leprosy**—localised disease: a few well-defined hypopigmented anaesthetic maculas with raised edges; loss of sensation and nerve enlargement; the lesions usually heal spontaneously
- **Lepromatous leprosy**—generalised disease: widely scattered small skin lesions progressing into nodular lesions with skin thickening on face and ears ('leonine faces'); later, loss of sensation leads to loss of fingers and toes; muscle weakness results in finger clawing and foot dropping; eyes, testes and bones may also be involved
- **Borderline leprosy**—lesions are intermediate between tuberculoid and lepromatous and consist of maculas, papules and plaques with anaesthesia

- **Lepra reactions** (during treatment):
1. Non-lepromatous reaction (type I)—inflammation in pre-existing skin lesions
2. Erythema nodosum leprosum (type II)—painful red papules or nodules with fever, arthralgia and iridocyclitis

Laboratory

Consult pathologist prior to collecting specimens

- Smear (from nasal mucosa, skin lesions or excision biopsies) or tissue fluid (from nasopharynx or skin lesions) for microscopy—view the characteristic acid-fast bacilli
- PCR for *M. Leprae* DNA (in tissue samples)
- Skin or nerve biopsy—compatible with leprosy examined by a laboratory experienced in leprosy diagnosis
- Culture of *M. leprae* (in footpads of mice)

Prevention and treatment

- Isolation is unnecessary—leprosy is contagious only in the untreated lepromatous form and even then the disease is not easily transmitted to others
- BCG vaccine—offers some protection against leprosy; should be given to all child contacts of lepromatous patients (given by specially trained staff)
- Multi-drug therapy (MDT)—stops progression, but does not reverse the damage

Multi-drug therapy regimens

FOR PAUCIBACILLARY (BORDERLINE/TUBERCULOID) LEPROSY

Child 0–9 years
- Dapsone 25 mg PO daily **plus** rifampicin 300 mg PO monthly for 6 months

Child 10–14 years
- Dapsone 50 mg PO daily **plus** rifampicin 450 mg PO monthly for 6 months

Adult
- Dapsone 100 mg PO daily **plus** rifampicin 600 PO monthly for 6 months

FOR MULTIBACILLARY (BORDERLINE/LEPROMATOUS) LEPROSY

Child 0–9 years
- Dapsone 25 mg PO daily **plus** rifampicin 300 mg PO monthly **plus** clofazimine* 50 mg PO twice a week + 100 mg PO monthly for 24 months

---

*Available via Special Access Scheme <www.tga.gov.au/hp/access-sas.htm>

Child 10–14 years
- Dapsone 50 mg PO daily **plus** rifampicin 450 mg PO monthly **plus** clofazimine 50 mg PO alternate days + 150 mg PO monthly for 24 months

Adult
- Dapsone 100 mg PO daily **plus** rifampicin 600 PO monthly **plus** clofazimine 50 mg PO daily **plus** clofazimine 300 mg PO monthly for 2 years (should be under supervision)

SECOND-LINE DRUGS (IF ABOVE DRUGS HAVE SEVERE SIDE EFFECTS)
- Minocycline 100 mg PO daily **or** 100 mg PO monthly depends on the regimen
- Ofloxacin* 400 mg PO daily **or** 400 mg PO monthly depends on the regimen

Treatment of lepra reactions
Lepra reaction in borderline patients
- Prednisone 40–60 mg PO daily, reduce gradually over 2–6 months

Erythema nodosum leprosum
- Thalidomide 100 mg PO nocte, increase by 100 mg weekly to max 400 mg

If thalidomide is contraindicated
- Prednisone 40–60 mg PO daily, reduce gradually over 6–9 months
- Increase clofazimine to 200 mg PO daily for a few weeks
- Leprosy website <www.who.int/lep/>

LEPTOSPIROSIS

Pathogens
- A spirochaete *Leptospira interrogans*
- It can survive for many days in warm fresh water and for 24 hours in seawater

Transmission
- Leptospires are excreted in animal (e.g. rat) urine and enter the human body through skin abrasions or intact mucous membranes, or by ingestion of contaminated water

Incubation
- 7–14 days

Clinical
- More than 90% of infections are subclinical with only mild fever
- Leptospiraemic phase—headache, fever, malaise, anorexia and myalgia; may have meningism

*Available via Special Access Scheme <www.tga.gov.au/hp/access-sas.htm>

- In severe disease—hepatic and renal failure, haemolytic anaemia, shock, heart failure and pulmonary haemorrhage may occur

Laboratory

- *Leptospirosis* serology—specific IgM may be positive at the end of the first week
- *Leptospirosis* agglutination—a ≥ four-fold rise in titre between acute and convalescent phase sera obtained at least 2 weeks apart
- Culture of blood, CSF or urine for *Leptospira* spp (requires specific media and takes several weeks) (consult with pathologist)

Treatment

- Mild cases—may not require treatment
- More severe cases—antibiotic treatment
- When the disease is suspected—early antibiotic treatment
- If patient becomes afebrile before the diagnosis is confirmed—antibiotic is not required

Mild infection/empirical therapy
  - Option 1: doxycycline (PO) for 7 days
More severe infection
  - Option 2: benzylpenicillin (IV) for 7 days
  - Option 3: ceftriaxone (IV) for 5–7 days

Dosage of above antibiotics

  - Doxycycline 100 mg (child >8 years: 2 mg/kg up to 100 mg) PO q12h
  - Benzylpenicillin 1.2 g (child: 50 mg/kg up to 1.2 g) IV q6h
  - Ceftriaxone 1 g (child >1 month: 50 mg/kg up to 1 g) IV daily

LICE

Other names: pediculosis

1. HEAD LICE AND BODY LICE

Pathogens

- Head lice—*Pediculus humanus capitis*
- Body lice—*Pediculus humanus corporis*

Clinical

- Common in school children, acquired by head-to-head contact
- Most cases are asymptomatic
- Itch and secondary bacterial infection with lymphadenopathy may occur

Treatment

Tropical treatment
  - Option 1: maldison 0.5% lotion top, leave for 8 hours, repeat in 7 days (for child >6 months)

- Option 2: malathion 1% foam top, leave for 30 min, repeat weekly for up to 12 weeks (for child >6 months)
- Option 3: permethrin 1% (e.g. Quellada) top, leave for 10 min, repeat in 7 days
- Option 4: pyrethrins + piperonyl butoxide (e.g. Banlice Mousse) top, leave for 10 min, repeat in 7 days
- Option 5: bioallethrin + piperonyl butoxide (e.g. Paralice)

Wet comb after each treatment to check for any live lice (resistant lice)

For resistant lice—suffocation method or LouseBuster
- Hair conditioner: apply to dry hair then fine comb every night for at least 2 weeks
- LouseBuster device: dry out head lice and eggs with heat and pressure

Oral therapy (if unresponsive to topical treatment)
- Ivermectin (e.g. Stromectol) (adult and child ≥15 kg) 200 mcg/kg PO with fatty food st, repeat in 7 days

Note

- Family members should be examined and treated if infested
- Clothing, linen and towels should be washed in hot water (>60°C) or high-heat dried
- Items that cannot be washed may be stored in a sealed plastic bag for 4 weeks
- School should be notified
- Community control (regular rotation of topical preparations)

2. PUBIC LICE (CRAB LICE)

Pathogen

- Mite *Phthirius pubis*

Transmission

- Common in adults, acquired by close contact, often sexual contact
- In children, sexual abuse should be considered, but is not invariable

Clinical

- Itching with the louse and eggs visible on hairs (pubic, axillaries, beard, eyebrows)

Treatment

- Treatment is as for head lice (see above)
- Eyelash infestation—apply a thick layer of white soft paraffin to eyelashes twice a day for 8 days (to suffocate the lice)
- Sexual partners need treatment as well
- Contact tracing is essential

LISTERIOSIS

Other names: listerial infection

Pathogen

- *Listeria monocytogenes*—a Gram-positive bacillus in soil and decayed matter with an unusual ability to multiply at low temperatures

Transmission

- Ingestion of contaminated foods (e.g. cold meats, seafood, unpasteurised soft cheeses or raw vegetables)
- Person-to-person spread has not been reported

Incubation

- Could take up to 70 days

Clinical

- In pregnant women—septic abortion, premature delivery or stillbirth
- In elderly and immunocompromised—pneumonia, meningitis, encephalitis or septicaemia
- In healthy adults—food-born gastroenteritis outbreaks

Diagnosis

Listeriosis is difficult to diagnose quickly

- Culture of blood, CSF, placenta, amniotic fluid, expelled products of conception (vaginal and rectal swabs do not help)

Treatment

- May need to treat on suspicion, particularly for pregnant women
- Antibiotic therapy:
  - Benzylpenicillin (IV)
If allergic to penicillin
  - Cotrimoxazole (IV then PO)

Duration of therapy

- Usually—3 weeks
- Immunocompromised—6 weeks

Dosage of above antibiotics

  - Benzylpenicillin 2.4 g (child: 60 mg/kg up to 2.4 g) IV q4h
  - Cotrimoxazole 160/800 mg (child: 4/20 mg/kg up to 160/800 mg) IV q6h, then PO q12h

Prevention

- Avoid eating pre-prepared foods, chilled seafood
- Eat fresh foods
- Thoroughly cook poultry, meat and seafood
- Wash raw fruits and vegetables before eating

LIVER ABSCESS—PYOGENIC

Pathogens

- *Klebsiella pneumoniae* infection alone—primary liver abscess
- A mixture of aerobic and anaerobic bowel flora—common, secondary liver abscess
- *Streptococcus anginosus/milleri* group alone—occasional
- *Staphylococcal aureus*—common in children

Clinical

- Primary liver abscess—caused by *Klebsiella pneumoniae*; diabetes is a significant risk factor; can also cause endophthalmitis, meningitis and discitis
- Secondary liver abscess—following spread from an intra-abdominal infection (e.g. diverticulitis or biliary tract infection)

Laboratory

- Ultrasound scan—to exclude hydatid disease
- Pus for culture (needle aspiration or drainage)
- If culture-negative—16S rRNA gene sequencing
- Serology testing—if the aetiology is not clearly pyogenic:
  - *Entamoeba histolytica* serology (hepatic amoebiasis)
  - *Echinococcus granulosus* serology (hydatid disease)
  - *Fasciola hepatica* serology (hepatic distomiasis)

Treatment

- Surgical drainage (not necessary for amoebic liver abscess)
- Partial hepatectomy may be considered
- Antibiotic treatment

Triple therapy

  - Ampicillin (IV) **plus** gentamicin (IV) **plus** metronidazole (IV)

After 3 days of gentamicin or for non-immediate penicillin allergy

  - Ceftriaxone (**or** cefotaxime) (IV) **plus** metronidazole (IV)

If immediate penicillin allergy, seek expert advice

  - Option 1: gentamicin (IV) **plus** metronidazole (IV)
  - Option 2: ciprofloxacin (IV) **plus** metronidazole (IV)
  - Option 3: aztreonam (IV) **plus** metronidazole (IV)

When culture results are available, modify the therapy
After clinical improvement, change to oral therapy

Duration of therapy

- Total of 4–6 weeks
- Serial CRP and liver ultrasounds help assess the response to therapy

Dosage of above antibiotics

- Ampicillin 2 g (child: 50 mg/kg up to 2 g) IV q6h
- Gentamicin 4–7 mg/kg (child: 7.5 mg/kg up to 320 mg) IV 1st dose (further dosing, see p. 459)
- Metronidazole 750 mg (child: 15 mg/kg up to 750 mg) IV q8h
- Ceftriaxone 2 g (child: 50 mg/kg up to 2 g) IV daily
- Cefotaxime 2 g (child: 50 mg/kg up to 2 g) IV q8h
- Ciprofloxacin 400 mg (child: 10 mg/kg up to 400 mg) IV q12h
- Aztreonam 2 g (child: 50 mg/kg up to 2 g) IV q6–8h

LUDWIG'S ANGINA

Other names: submandibular abscess
Ludwig's angina is cellulitis of the sublingual and submandibular spaces, usually a complication of dental infection including tooth extraction. It is potentially life-threatening.

Clinical

- Toxic, rapidly swelling cellulitis of the sublingual and submaxillary spaces; may cause trismus and airway obstruction (potentially life-threatening)

Treatment

- CT scan to define the extent and severity
- Hospitalisation
- Airway protection (intubation may be needed)
- Intravenous antibiotics
- Surgical drainage and removal of the tooth, if unresponsive to antibiotics

Empirical therapy

- Metronidazole (IV) **plus** benzylpenicillin (**or** ampi(amoxi)cillin) (IV)

If non-immediate penicillin allergy

- Metronidazole (IV) **plus** cefazolin (IV)

If immediate penicillin allergy

- Metronidazole (IV) **plus** clindamycin (IV)

After improvement, change to oral regimen

- Amoxicillin/clavulanate (PO) for 5 days

If penicillin allergy

- Clindamycin (PO) for 5 days

Dosage of above antibiotics

- Metronidazole 500 mg (child: 12.5 mg/kg up to 500 mg) IV q12h
- Benzylpenicillin 1.2 g (child: 30 mg/kg up to 1.2 g) IV q6h
- Ampi(amoxi)cillin 2 g (child: 50 mg/kg up to 2 g) IV q6h

- Cefazolin 1 g (child: 25 mg/kg up to 1 g) IV q8h
- Clindamycin 450 mg (child: 10 mg/kg up to 450 mg) IV q8h
- Amoxicillin/clavulanate 875 mg (child: 22.5 mg/kg up to 875 mg) PO q12h
- Clindamycin 300 mg (child: 7.5 mg/kg, max 300 mg) PO q8h

LYME DISEASE

Although Lyme disease is not endemic in Australia, it may present in returned travellers or overseas visitors.

Pathogen

- A spirochaete *Borrelia burgdorferi* (a zoonosis of deer and other wild mammals)

Distribution

- Eastern states of North America, Europe, former Soviet Union, Japan and China

Transmission

- *Ixodes* tick bite

Incubation

- 3–20 days

Clinical

- Recently visited North America or Europe (infections occur mainly in the northern hemisphere summer months)
- Skin rash (erythema chronicum migrans) with headache, fever, malaise, myalgia, arthralgia and lymphadenopathy; may persist or intermittently occur
- Early complications—neurological (muscle twitches, muscle weakness, tingling, numbness, meningitis, Bell's palsy or radiculopathy) and heart block
- Late complications—recurrent large joint arthritis, polyneuropathy, encephalopathy or persistent fatigue
- Less common complications—eye inflammation and hepatitis

Laboratory

- Lyme *Borrelia* serology (IgM and IgG)—for suspected patient (may be negative until 4–8 weeks after tick bite); positive test (IgG) may be due to past exposure (the serology test also measures antibodies to other spiral bacteria; a western blot may be used to confirm Lyme disease)
- Lyme *Borrelia* PCR (CSF or synovial fluid)—adds confirmatory information in seropositive patients; a positive result does not prove active infection; a negative result does not exclude Lyme disease

Treatment

The sooner the treatment starts, the quicker and more complete the recovery

- Option 1: amoxicillin (PO) for 3 weeks
- Option 2: doxycycline (PO) for 3 weeks

For severe cases or recurrent arthritis
- Option 1: ceftriaxone (IV) for 2–4 weeks
- Option 2: benzylpenicillin (IV) for 2–4 weeks

Seek expert advice

Dosage of above antibiotics
- Amoxicillin 500 mg (child: 15 mg/kg up to 500 mg) PO q8h
- Doxycycline 100 mg (child >8 years: 2.5 mg/kg up to 100 mg) PO q12h
- Ceftriaxone 1 g (child: 25 mg/kg up to 1 g) IV daily
- Benzylpenicillin 1.2 g (child: 30 mg/kg up to 1.2 g) IV q6h

LYMPHOGRANULOMA VENEREUM

Pathogen
- *Chlamydia trachomatis* serovars L1–3

Transmission
- Sexual—particularly among men who have sex with men
- Non-sexual personal contact and laboratory accidents—the organism enters skin or mucous membranes through breaks and abrasions
- The aerosols of the organism have been associated with lung infection

Incubation
- 3–21 days

Clinical

Three stages (the primary and secondary stages may go undetected):

- **Primary stage**—a painless papule, shallow erosion, ulcer or grouping of lesions with a herpetiform appearance at the site of inoculation
- **Secondary stage**—enlarged tender regional lymph nodes known as buboes with associated constitutional symptoms; homosexual men and women who are receptive to anal sex may have perirectal and pelvic lymph node involvement; oral sex may cause submandibular and cervical chain lymphadenopathy; inhalation of *C. trachomatis* may cause mediastinal lymphadenopathy
- **Tertiary stage**—proctocolitis, elephantiasis of genitalia, perirectal or ischiorectal abscesses, rectovaginal or anal fistulas and rectal stricture

Diagnosis

- Clinical findings of large fluctuant buboes or draining sinuses (suggestive)
- Swabs from sores or ulcers/aspirate—for *Chlamydia trachomatis* PCR
- Serovar-specific LGV testing—if swab is positive for *Chlamydia trachomatis* PCR
- *Chlamydia trachomatis* serotypes L1, L2 or L3

Treatment

- Investigate and treat other sexually transmitted infections
- Aspiration of fluctuant buboes may prevent spontaneous rupture
- Antibiotic therapy for at least 3 weeks
- Sexual contacts should be evaluated and treated
  - Option 1: doxycycline 100 mg PO q12h for 3 weeks
  - Option 2: azithromycin 1 g PO weekly for 3 weeks

Prophylaxis

- Azithromycin 1 g PO st

MALARIA—PROPHYLAXIS

The ABC of malaria prevention

- **A**wareness of risk—pregnant women and post-splenectomy patients should not travel to malaria-endemic areas
- **B**ite avoidance—travellers to malaria-endemic areas are advised to wear light-coloured long clothes that cover as much of the skin as possible, use insect repellent on exposed parts of the body, sleep in screened accommodation or use insecticide-impregnated bed nets and use insecticide spray indoors
- **C**hemoprophylaxis and stand-by emergency treatment

Bite avoidance

- Personal insect repellent and insecticide (for indoor use)
- Light-coloured long trousers and long-sleeved shirts (in the evening)
- Screened accommodation or mosquito nets + /– pyrethroid impregnation
- Avoid outdoor activities between dusk and dawn
- Avoid using perfume and aftershave

Chemoprophylaxis

- Chemoprophylaxis is not always effective
- Any fever while overseas or after return warrants urgent medical attention and investigation
    - Option 1: atovaquone/proguanil (e.g. Malarone) (PO) daily for up to 3 months
    - Option 2: doxycycline (PO) daily for up to 6 months
  Areas without mefloquine-resistant malaria (areas other than parts of Southeast Asia)
    - Option 3: mefloquine (PO) weekly for up to 1 year

Dosage of above agents

  - Atovaquone/proguanil
    Adult formulation (250/100 mg) (e.g. Malarone) adult, child >40 kg: 1 tab PO with fatty food or full-fat milk, daily (starting 1–2 days before entering and continuing until 7 days after leaving malarious area)
    Paediatric formulation (62.5/25 mg) (e.g. Malarone Junior) child 11–20 kg: 1 tab; 21–30 kg: 2 tab; 31–40 kg: 3 tab PO with fatty food or full-fat milk, daily (starting 1–2 days before entering and continuing until 7 days after leaving malarious area)
  - Doxycycline 100 mg (child >8 years: 2 mg/kg up to 100 mg) PO daily (starting 1–2 days before entering and continuing until 4 weeks after leaving malarious area)
  - Mefloquine 250 mg (child 5–15 kg: 62.5 mg [= 1/4 tab]; 16–30 kg: 125 mg [= 1/2 tab]; 31–45 kg: 187.5 mg [= 3/4 tab]; >45 kg: 250 mg

[= 1 tab]) PO weekly (starting 1 week before entering and continuing until 2 weeks after leaving malarious area)

Stand-by emergency treatment

- Travellers who elect not to use chemoprophylaxis can be given a stand-by treatment
- Start treatment once fever develops and medical care is not available within 24 hours
- Travellers should be warned to seek medical attention, even if the stand-by treatment has been taken (to exclude other febrile diseases)
  - Option 1: artemether + lumefantrine (e.g. Riamet) (PO) for 6 doses
  - Option 2: atovaquone + proguanil (e.g. Malarone)* (PO) for 3 days

For pregnant women or children
  - Quinine sulfate (PO) **plus** clindamycin (PO) for 7 days

Dosage of above antimalarials

- Artemether + lumefantrine (e.g. Riamet) (20 + 120 mg tablet)
  Adult and child >34 kg: 4 tab (child 5–14 kg: 1 tab; 15–24 kg: 2 tab; 25–34 kg: 3 tab) PO with fatty food or full cream milk, 6 doses at 0, 8, 24, 36, 48 and 60 hours
- Atovaquone + proguanil (e.g. Malarone) (250 + 100 mg adult formulation)
  Adult and child >40 kg: 4 tab (child 11–20 kg: 1 tab; 21–30 kg: 2 tab; 31–40 kg: 3 tab)
  PO with fatty food or full cream milk, daily
- Quinine sulfate 600 mg (<50 kg: 450 mg) (child: 10 mg/kg up to 600 mg) PO q8h
- Clindamycin 300 mg (child: 5 mg/kg up to 300 mg) PO q8h

MALARIA—TREATMENT

Pathogens

Protozoan parasites of the genus *Plasmodium*:

- *P. falciparum*—the most pathogenic and resistant to standard antimalarials
- *P. vivax*
- *P. malariae*
- *P. ovale*
- *P. knowlesi*

Incubation

- 1 week to 4 months (rarely, longer)

---

*Atovaquone + proguanil (e.g. Malarone) should not be used in patients who have taken this medication as prophylaxis

Clinical

• Consider malaria in any febrile patient who has visited a malarious area

Laboratory

• Malaria antigen test (particularly *P. falciparum* antigen test)
• Thick and thin blood films—on three separate occasions
• A single negative antigen test or blood film does not exclude malaria infection, particularly if antimalarials or antibiotics (e.g. tetracyclines, fluoroquinolones or cotrimoxazole) have been taken recently
• PCR for malaria—more sensitive and accurate
• Red cell parasite count—if falciparum malaria is suspected

Treatment

1. **Uncomplicated *P. falciparum* malaria**
   • Option 1: artemether + lumefantrine (e.g. Riamet) (PO) for 6 doses
   • Option 2: atovaquone + proguanil (e.g. Malarone)* (PO) for 3 days
   • Option 3: quinine sulfate (PO) **plus** doxycycline (**or** clindamycin) (PO) for 7 days

For pregnant women or children <8 years
   • Quinine sulfate (PO) **plus** clindamycin (PO) for 7 days

If *P. falciparum* responds poorly to artemether + lumefantrine, switch to:
   • Quinine sulfate (PO) **plus** doxycycline (**or** clindamycin) (PO) for 7 days

To prevent *P. falciparum* transfer to mosquitoes, add:
   • Primaquine (PO) as a single dose (exclude G6PD deficiency)

Dosage of above antimalarials
   • Artemether + lumefantrine (e.g. Riamet) (20 + 120 mg tablet) Adult and child >34 kg: 4 tab (child 5–14 kg: 1 tab; 15–24 kg: 2 tab; 25–34 kg: 3 tab) PO with fatty food or full cream milk, 6 doses at 0, 8, 24, 36, 48 and 60 hours
   • Atovaquone + proguanil (e.g. Malarone) (250 + 100 mg adult formulation) Adult and child>40 kg: 4 tab (child 11–20 kg: 1 tab; 21–30 kg: 2 tab; 31–40 kg: 3 tab) PO with fatty food or full cream milk, daily
   • Quinine sulfate 600 mg (<50 kg: 450 mg; child: 10 mg/kg up to 600 mg) PO q8h

---

*Atovaquone + proguanil (e.g. Malarone) should not be used in patients who have taken the medication as prophylaxis

- Doxycycline 100 mg (child >8 years: 2 mg/kg up to 100 mg) PO q12h, start on day 2
- Clindamycin 300 mg (child: 5 mg/kg up to 300 mg) PO q8h
- Primaquine 15 mg (child: 0.25 mg/kg up to 15 mg) PO as a single dose

2. Severe *P. falciparum* malaria

Indications for urgent treatment:

- Severe clinical conditions: altered consciousness, vomiting, acidosis, renal failure, jaundice, hypoglycaemia or severe anaemia
- Parasite count >100,000/mm^3 (parasitised red blood cells >2%)
    - Artesunate* (IV) until oral therapy is tolerated, then artemether + lumefantrine (e.g. Riamet) (PO) for 6 doses

If artesunate (IV) is not immediately available

- Quinine dihydrochloride (IV) until improvement, then quinine sulfate (PO) **plus** doxycycline (PO) for 7 days

For pregnant women or children <8 years

- Quinine dihydrochloride (IV) until improvement, then quinine sulfate (PO) **plus** clindamycin (PO) for 7 days

Dosage of above antimalarials

- Artesunate (adult and child) 2.4 mg/kg IV on admission, repeat at 12 hours and 24 hours, then once daily until oral therapy is possible
- Artemether + lumefantrine (e.g. Riamet) (20 + 120 mg tablet) Adult and child >34 kg: 4 tab (child 5–14 kg: 1 tab; 15–24 kg: 2 tab; 25–34 kg: 3 tab) PO with fatty food, 6 doses at 0, 8, 24, 36, 48 and 60 hours
- Quinine dihydrochloride loading dose (adult and child) 20 mg/kg IV infusion over 4 hours, followed by 10 mg/kg IV infusion over 4 hours, q8h
  Initial loading dose can be omitted if patient has received ≥3 doses of quinine or quinidine in previous 48 hours or mefloquine prophylaxis in 24 hours, or a mefloquine treatment dose in previous 3 days; monitor BP and blood glucose (quinine stimulates insulin secretion and can cause hypoglycaemia); cardiac monitoring is advised if patient has pre-existing heart disease
- Quinine sulfate 600 mg (<50 kg: 450 mg) (child: 10 mg/kg up to 600 mg) PO q8h
- Doxycycline 100 mg (child >8 years: 2 mg/kg up to 100 mg) PO q12h, start on day 2
- Clindamycin 300 mg (child: 5 mg/kg up to 300 mg) PO q8h

---

*Artesunate is available via Special Access Scheme <www.tga.gov.au/hp/access-sas .htm>

3. Other forms of malaria

For *P. vivax* (acquired **outside** Indonesia, Timor-Leste or Pacific Island
  nations) and for *P. malariae* and *P. ovale*
  • Chloroquine (PO) for 4 doses
For *P. vivax* (acquired in Indonesia, Timor-Leste or Pacific Island nations)
  and for less severe *P. knowlesi*
  • Option 1: artemether + lumefantrine (e.g. Riamet) (PO) for
    6 doses
  • Option 2: mefloquine (PO) for 2 doses

If cannot tolerate oral therapy, treat as *P. falciparum* malaria

To eliminate liver forms of *P. vivax* infections, **add**
  • Primaquine* 30 mg (child: 0.5 mg/kg up to 30 mg) PO daily with
    food for 14 days

To eliminate liver forms of *P. ovale* infections, **add**
  • Primaquine* 15 mg (child: 0.25 mg/kg up to 15 mg) PO daily with
    food for 14 days

If relapse after above treatment, seek expert advice

Dosage of above antimalarials

  • Chloroquine adult: 4 tab (620 mg) (child: 10 mg/kg up to 620 mg)
    PO, then 2 tab (310 mg) (child: 5 mg/kg up to 310 mg) PO 6 hours
    later and on days 2 and 3 (10 tablets in 4 doses)
  • Artemether + lumefantrine (e.g. Riamet) (20 + 120 mg tablet)
    Adult and child >34 kg: 4 tablets (child 5–14 kg: 1 tab; 15–24 kg:
    2 tab; 25–34 kg: 3 tab) PO with fatty food, 6 doses at 0, 8, 24, 36,
    48 and 60 hours
  • Mefloquine 1st dose: 750 mg (child: 15 mg/kg up to 750 mg) PO;
    2nd dose: 500 mg (child: 10 mg/kg up to 500 mg) PO 6–8 hours
    later (do not use it if patient took it as prophylaxis)

MASTITIS

Pathogen

• *Staphylococcus aureus*

Risk factors

• Lactation—poor infant positioning and milk stasis
• Presence of cracks or sores on the nipples
• Tight clothing or ill-fitting bra

---

*Prior to the use of primaquine, exclude G6PD deficiency; if the patient is G6PD
deficient, seek expert advice

Clinical

- Puerperal mastitis—in lactating women; mild cases are often called breast engorgement
- Non-puerperal mastitis—in non-lactating women; less common
- Mastitis in men—very rare

Differential diagnosis

- Inflammatory breast cancer has symptoms very similar to mastitis
- Keratinising squamous metaplasia of lactiferous ducts may mimic non-puerperal subareolar abscess

Treatment

- Early mastitis—increasing breastfeeding on the affected side and gentle milk expression to empty the breast may prevent progression of the infection
- If systemic symptoms develop—early antibiotics to prevent abscess formation
- If abscess formed—aspiration or incision and drainage (send swab for culture)
- Antibiotic treatment

Mild-to-moderate infection

  - Flucloxacillin 500 mg PO q6h for 5–10 days
If non-immediate penicillin allergy
  - Cefalexin 500 mg PO q6h for 5–10 days
If immediate penicillin allergy
  - Clindamycin 450 mg PO q8h for 5–10 days

Severe infection

  - Flucloxacillin 2 g IV q6h
If non-immediate penicillin allergy
  - Cefazolin 2 g IV q8h
If immediate penicillin allergy
  - Option 1: vancomycin IV daily (monitor blood levels and adjust dose, p. 462)
  - Option 2: clindamycin 600 mg IV q8h

Change to oral therapy (above) when significantly improved

MEASLES

Other names: rubeola

Pathogen

- A paramyxovirus, genus *Morbillivirus*

Transmission

- By direct contact with airway fluids or through droplets/aerosol

Incubation

- 6–19 days
- Infectious from 2 days before prodrome illness to 5 days after onset of the rash

People at risk

- Infants and children who have not been fully vaccinated against measles (MMR at 12 months and 18 months)
- Aboriginal and Torres Strait Islander children
- Adults born during or since 1966 who have never had measles vaccination
- Unimmunised or under-immunised travellers returned from endemic areas

Clinical

- 2–4 days of flu-like symptoms with fever, cough and conjunctivitis
- Maculopapular rash begins on the face and neck, becoming generalised for 4–7 days
- Koplik spots may be seen on buccal mucosa

Complications

- Measles encephalitis, subacute sclerosing panencephalitis (SSPE)
- Secondary bacterial infections (acute otitis media, bronchopneumonia and conjunctivitis)

Diagnosis

Diagnosis is usually clinical

- Measles virus PCR—nasopharyngeal aspirate or nose/throat viral swab
- Measles virus culture—nasopharyngeal aspirate or nose/throat viral swab
- Measles serology—IgM (should have no measles-containing vaccine within 8 days to 8 weeks)
- Measles urine immunofluorescence test—first pass urine (~50 mL)
- CSF—measles antibodies and immunoglobulin studies (oligoclonal bands)

Treatment

- Isolate suspected cases until 5 days after the onset of rash
- Immediately notify local public health unit
- Antibiotics for secondary bacterial complications

Normal human immunoglobulin (NHIG)

Should be given (within 7 days of exposure) to:

- Infants <6 months of age when the mother is the person infected
- Infants <6 months of age who were born before 28 weeks' gestation

- Infants 6–9 months of age if contact was within the last 7 days
- All persons >9 months who are at risk and for whom measles vaccine is contraindicated
- Immunocompromised persons who have been exposed to measles
- Persons who have never received a measles vaccine
  - NHIG 0.2 mL/kg (0.5 mL/kg for immunity impaired) up to 15 mL, deep IM

Vaccination during an outbreak

  - MMR **or** MMRV vaccine 0.5 mL IM given early (on the discretion of public health authorities) to infants 6–12 months of age, followed by the scheduled MMR **or** MMRV at 12 months of age or 4 weeks after the first dose, whichever is the latter
  - Further scheduled dose of MMR **or** MMRV will be at 18 months of age

MEDIASTINITIS

Causes and pathogens

- After cardiac surgery—*Staphylococcus aureus* and *Staphylococcus epidermidis*
- Descending infection following surgery of the head and neck, great vessels or vertebrae—*S. aureus* and streptococci
- Direct extension of perioral/parapharyngeal infection (e.g. Ludwig's angina)—mixed anaerobic and aerobic bacteria, streptococci or *Haemophilus* spp
- Rupture of the oesophagus following severe vomiting or due to carcinoma—polymicrobial infection involving oral organisms and *Candida* spp
- Mediastinal extension of lung infection—respiratory tract pathogens
- Iatrogenic (e.g. following oesophageal dilation, oesophageal variceal sclerotherapy, nasogastric tube insertion, endotracheal intubation, oesophageal/paraoesophageal surgery, transoesophageal echocardiography)—polymicrobial infection involving oral organisms and *Candida* spp
- Following median sternotomy in cardiac surgery—*S. aureus*, enteric gram-negative bacteria (e.g. *Enterobacter* spp) and *P. aeruginosa*

Clinical

- Sternal pain, sternal instability (click), the Hamman sign (a crunching sound heard with a stethoscope over the praecordium during systole), tachycardia and fever
- Systemic signs of sepsis strongly suggest mediastinal involvement
- The mortality rate can be up to 20%

Diagnosis

- Blood, sternal drainage, mediastinal pacing wire—for culture
- CT chest—air-fluid levels, pneumomediastinum, sternal separation and substernal fluid collections
- Chest x-ray—some patients may be asymptomatic and present with an isolated mediastinal mass on chest x-ray
- Local wound exploration is the predominant method of distinguishing between superficial wound infection and deep sternal wound infection

Treatment

- Operative exploration includes reopening the previous sternotomy and debridement of necrotic and infected tissue
- Antibiotic therapy

Skin source infection

- Option 1: flucloxacillin (IV)
- Option 2: cefazolin (IV)

If immediate penicillin allergy

- Option 1: vancomycin (IV)
- Option 2: clindamycin (IV)

Polymicrobial infection

- Option 1: piperacillin/tazobactam (IV)
- Option 2: ticarcillin/clavulanate (IV)

If penicillin allergy

- Ciprofloxacin (IV) **plus** clindamycin (IV)

Adjust antibiotic according to culture results

Dosage of above antibiotics

Skin source infection

- Flucloxacillin 2 g (child: 50 mg/kg up to 2 g) IV q6h
- Cefazolin 2 g (child: 50 mg/kg up to 2 g) IV q8h
- Vancomycin 25–30 mg/kg IV for the 1st dose (further dosing, see p. 462)
- Clindamycin 600 mg (child: 15 mg/kg up to 600 mg) IV q8

Polymicrobial infection

- Piperacillin/tazobactam 4 g IV q8h
- Ticarcillin/clavulanate 3 g IV q6h
- Ciprofloxacin 400 mg (child: 10 mg/kg up to 400 mg) IV q12h
- Clindamycin 900 mg IV q8h (slow infusion)

Prevention

- Prophylactic intranasal mupirocin and total body eradication of *S. aureus* for carriers (this may reduce the rate of overall surgical site infections by *S. aureus* after cardiac surgery)

MELIOIDOSIS

Other names: Whitmore disease
Melioidosis may occur in northern Australia and in parts of the Asia–Pacific region. It may present in returned travellers.

Pathogens

- *Burkholderia pseudomallei* (a soil saprophyte)
- It may be used as an agent of biological warfare

Transmission

- Direct skin contact with contaminated soil or water (via skin sores or cuts)
- Ingestion of contaminated water
- Inhalation of contaminated dust
- Person-to-person transmission has been reported

Incubation

- Natural infection: days to months to years
- Aerosol attack: 1–21 days

Clinical

- The mortality rate can be 20%
- Symptoms may occur months or years after exposure
- Local infection—skin ulcers or abscesses, swollen lymph glands
- Pneumonia, sepsis, lung abscesses, pleural effusions and multiple abscesses (e.g. spleen)
- High-risk people—people who abuse alcohol and people with diabetes, cystic fibrosis or renal failure

Diagnosis

- Microscopy and culture for *Burkholderia* (blood, sputum, urine, wound swab, throat swab, rectal swab or tissue biopsy)
- Melioidosis serology (*B. pseudomallei* antibodies)
- PCR for *B. pseudomallei* (various samples)

Treatment

- Patients should be masked in isolation rooms; use disposable surgical masks, face shields and gowns to prevent person-to-person transmission

Initial intensive therapy

For non-neurological melioidosis
- Option 1: ceftazidime (IV) **plus** cotrimoxazole (PO) **plus** folic acid (PO) for 2 weeks
- Option 2: meropenem[1] (IV) **plus** cotrimoxazole (PO) **plus** folic acid (PO) for 2 weeks

For neurological melioidosis (higher dose meropenem)
- Meropenem[2] (IV) **plus** cotrimoxazole (PO) **plus** folic acid (PO) for 4–8 weeks

For septicaemic melioidosis, consider to **add**
- Granulocyte colony-stimulating factor (G-CSF)

Eradication after initial therapy
- Cotrimoxazole (PO) **plus** folic acid (PO) for a further 3 months

If cotrimoxazole is contraindicated or not tolerated, seek expert advice
- Option 1: doxycycline (PO)
- Option 2: amoxicillin/clavulanate (PO)

Post-exposure prophylaxis for melioidosis
- Cotrimoxazole (PO) for 3 weeks

Dosage of above antibiotics
- Ceftazidime 2 g (child: 50 mg/kg up to 2 g) IV q6h
- Cotrimoxazole 320/1600 mg (adult 40–60 kg: 240/1200 mg; child >1 month: 6/30 mg/kg up to 240/1200 mg) PO q12h
- Folic acid 5 mg (child: 0.1 mg/kg up to 5 mg) PO daily
- Meropenem[1] 1 g (child: 25 mg/kg up to 1 g) IV q8h
- Meropenem[2] 2 g (child: 50 mg/kg up to 2 g) IV q8h
- Doxycycline 100 mg (child >8 years: 2 mg/kg up to 100 mg) PO q12h
- Amoxicillin/clavulanate 875/125 mg (child: 22.5/3.2 mg/kg up to 875/125 mg) PO q12h

MENINGITIS—EMPIRICAL THERAPY

Pathogens

- Neonates—*Streptococcus agalactiae* (group B streptococci), *Escherichia coli*
- Infants—*Neisseria meningitides, Haemophilus influenzae, S. pneumoniae*
- Children—*N. meningitides, S. pneumoniae*
- Non-vaccinated young children—*H. influenzae*
- Adults—*S. pneumoniae, N. meningitides, H. influenzae*
- Adults >50 years of age who are immunocompromised—*Listeria monocytogenes*

Management prior to hospital transfer

- Cough and abdominal pain may help to rule out meningitis as they are less frequent in meningitis
- Photophobia and neck stiffness are classic features of meningitis, but they are absent in many cases presenting to GPs (Fig. 13.1)

> GP suspects meningococcal meningitis
> (fever, neck stiffness, petechial rash, drowsiness)
>
> ↓
>
> Give an immediate dose of antibiotic (below)
> (if possible take blood cultures, aspirates or
> swabs from punctured skin petechial rash
> prior to antibiotic and send with the patient)
>
> ↓
>
> Urgently transfer patient to hospital

FIGURE 13.1

GP management prior to hospital transfer

Immediate antibiotic
  • Benzylpenicillin (IV) or (IM) st
If penicillin allergy or hospital transfer will be delayed >6 hours
  • Ceftriaxone (IV) or (IM) st
If immediate penicillin allergy or cefalosporin allergy
  • Ciprofloxacin (**or** moxifloxacin) (IV) st

Dosage of above agents

  • Benzylpenicillin 2.4 g (child: 60 mg/kg up to 2.4 g) IV or IM st
  • Ceftriaxone 2 g (child: 50 mg/kg up to 2 g) IV or IM* st
  • Ciprofloxacin 400 mg (child: 10 mg/kg up to 400 mg) IV st
  • Moxifloxacin 400 mg (child: 10 mg/kg up to 400 mg) IV st

Early hospital management

• Blood cultures
• Procalcitonin test (blood)—helps in differentiating bacterial from viral infection
• Pneumococcal antigen assay (urine or CSF)—aids rapid diagnosis of pneumococcal meningitis
• Meningococcal PCR (blood or CSF)—not affected by prior antibiotic treatment
• Skin lesions (punctured)—swabs or aspirates for microscopy, culture and meningococcal PCR
• CT brain (for adult)—may be used to assess the risk of lumbar puncture
• Lumbar puncture (without contraindications below)—CSF for microscopy, biochemistry, culture, meningococcal PCR, pneumococcal antigen assay, or viral PCR (negative CSF culture does not exclude meningococcal meningitis)

Contraindications for lumbar puncture

• Bleeding diathesis or on anticoagulant therapy
• Local spine infection
• Focal neurological signs
• Papilloedema

---

*IM injection of ceftriaxone needs to be reconstituted with 1% lidocaine (lignocaine)

- Impaired consciousness
- Immunosuppression

CSF findings (Table 13.1)

TABLE 13.1

CSF FINDINGS

	WBC	Differential	Glucose	Protein	Gram stain
Normal	<5	<1 polymorph	Normal	Normal	Negative
Bacterial	>500	Polymorphs	Low	High	Positive
Viral	<500	Monocytes	Normal	Normal	Negative

Early treatment

1. Corticosteroid

Commence before or with the 1st dose of antibiotics—only for baby >3 months

- Dexamethasone (**or** hydrocortisone) (IV) for 4 days

Note
- Antibiotics should not be delayed if corticosteroids are not available
- If patient has received a dose of benzylpenicillin or ceftriaxone prior to hospital, do not give corticosteroid
- Stop dexamethasone if a cause other than *Haemophilus influenzae* type b (Hib) or *S. pneumoniae* is confirmed

Dosage of above agents

- Dexamethasone 10 mg (child >3 months: 0.15 mg/kg up to 10 mg) IV q6h (start before or with the 1st dose of antibiotics)
- Hydrocortisone 200 mg (child >3 months: 4 mg/kg up to 200 mg) IV (start before or with the 1st dose of antibiotics, only for initial dose when dexamethasone is temporally not available, change to dexamethasone as soon as it is available)

2. Empirical antibiotic treatment

ASAP within 30 min after arrival

Neonates and infants ≤3 months
- Ampi(amoxi)cillin (IV) **plus** cefotaxime (IV) vancomycin (IV)*

Children >3 months and adults ≤50 years
- Ceftriaxone (**or** cefotaxime) (IV) **plus** vancomycin (IV)*

Adults >50 years, immunocompromised or pregnant (to cover *Listeria*)

---

*Add vancomycin if penicillin-resistant *S. pneumoniae* or staphylococci are suspected:
- Gram-positive diplococci or cocci resembling staphylococci are seen on Gram stain
- Pneumococcal antigen assay of urine or CSF is positive
- Patient has known otitis media or sinusitis
- Patient has been treated with a beta lactam
- CSF test is not possible

Add

- Benzylpenicillin (IV)

If immediate penicillin allergy (to cover *Listeria*) or cefalosporin allergy
- Option 1: vancomycin (IV) **plus** ciprofloxacin (IV)
- Option 2: moxifloxacin (IV)
Neurosurgery, head trauma or CSF shunt
- Vancomycin (IV)* **plus** ceftazidime (IV)

Duration of empirical treatment

- Treat until the organism is identified and susceptibility results are available
- If no organism is identified, continue empirical therapy for at least 10 days

Cease vancomycin once resistant *S. pneumoniae* or staphylococci are ruled out

Dosage of above agents

Neonates and infants ≤3 months

- Ampi(amoxi)cillin 50 mg/kg IV q6h
- Cefotaxime 50 mg/kg IV q6h
- Vancomycin 30 mg/kg IV for the 1st dose (further dosing, see p. 462)

Children >3 months and adults

- Ceftriaxone 4 g (child: 100 mg/kg up to 4 g) IV daily **or** 2 g (child: 50 mg/kg up to 2 g) IV q12h
- Cefotaxime 2 g (child: 50 mg/kg up to 2 g) IV q6h
- Vancomycin 25–30 mg/kg IV for the 1st dose (further dosing, see p. 462)
- Benzypenicillin 2.4 g (child: 60 mg/kg up to 2.4 g) IV q4h
- Ciprofloxacin 400 mg (child: 10 mg/kg up to 400 mg) IV q8h
- Moxifloxacin 400 mg (child: 10 mg/kg up to 400 mg) IV daily
- Ceftazidime 2 g (child: 50 mg/kg up to 2 g) IV q8h

MENINGITIS—DIRECT THERAPY

1. MENINGOCOCCAL MENINGITIS

Pathogens

- *Neisseria meningitidis* (or meningococcus), a gram-negative diplococcus
- Globally, serogroups A, B, C, W135 and Y can cause the disease
- In Australia, serogroups B and C occur most frequently (more than 99%)

---

*Add vancomycin if penicillin-resistant *S. pneumoniae* or staphylococci are suspected:
- Gram-positive diplococci or cocci resembling staphylococci are seen on Gram stain
- Pneumococcal antigen assay of urine or CSF is positive
- Patient has known otitis media or sinusitis
- Patient has been treated with a beta lactam
- CSF test is not possible

Transmission

- Respiratory droplets, mouth-to-mouth contact or indirect contact
- 5–10% people are carriers

Incubation

- 2–10 days, most commonly 3–4 days

Clinical

- The leading cause of bacterial meningitis in children and young adults
- The reported mortality rate for *N. meningitidis* meningitis is 3–13%

Antibiotic treatment

- Option 1: benzylpenicillin (IV) for 5 days (child 5–7 days)
- Option 2: ceftriaxone (**or** cefotaxime) (IV) for 5 days (child 5–7 days)

If immediate penicillin allergy or cefalosporin allergy
- Option 1: ciprofloxacin (IV) for 5 days (child 5–7 days)
- Option 2: chloramphenicol for 5 days (child 5–7 days)

Dosage of above antibiotics

- Benzylpenicillin 1.8 g (child: 60 mg/kg up to 1.8 g) IV q4h
- Ceftriaxone 4 g (child >1 month: 100 mg/kg up to 4 g) IV daily **or** 2 g (child >1 month: 50 mg/kg up to 2 g) IV q12h
- Cefotaxime 2 g (child: 50 mg/kg up to 2 g) IV q6h
- Ciprofloxacin 400 mg (child: 10 mg/kg up to 400 mg) IV q8h
- Chloramphenicol 1 g (child: 25 mg/kg up to 1 g) IV q6h

Antibiotic prophylaxis

- For close contacts and patients who have received only benzylpenicillin
- Commence within 24 hours of the index case becoming ill
  - Option 1: ciprofloxacin (PO) st (preferred for women taking OCP)
  - Option 2: ceftriaxone (IM*) st (preferred for pregnant women)
  - Option 3: rifampicin** (PO) for 2 days (preferred for children)

Dosage of above antibiotics

- Ciprofloxacin 500 mg (child <5 years: 30 mg/kg up to 125 mg; 5–12 years: 250 mg) PO st
- Ceftriaxone 250 mg (child >1 month: 125 mg) IM* st
- Rifampicin 600 mg (neonate: 5 mg/kg; child: 10 mg/kg up to 600 mg) PO q12h

Post-infection vaccination for patients with meningococcal disease

- MenCCV **or** 4vMenCV 0.5 mL IM st **or** 4vMenPV 0.5 mL SC st (given on discharge from hospital, or when the patient recovers from the infection)

---

*IM injection of ceftriaxone needs to be reconstituted with 1% lidocaine (lignocaine)
**Rifampicin is associated with multiple drug interactions and is contraindicated in pregnancy, alcoholism and severe liver disease

2. PNEUMOCOCCAL MENINGITIS

Pathogen

- *Streptococcus pneumoniae* (pneumococcus)

Transmission

- Respiratory droplets
- About 5–70% people are carriers

Incubation

- 1–3 days

Clinical

- The most common bacterial cause of meningitis
- The highest mortality rate among bacterial meningitis
- Risk factors—asplenia, hypogammaglobulinaemia, multiple myeloma, corticosteroid therapy, complement (C1–C4) defect, diabetes, chronic renal and liver disease, alcoholism and malnutrition
- All isolated cases of *S. pneumoniae* should have MIC tested for penicillin and ceftriaxone
- Use of corticosteroids (dexamethasone) with early empirical therapy has significant benefit in reducing mortality and neurological sequelae

Treatment

If penicillin susceptible (MIC <0.125 mg/L)
  - Benzylpenicillin (IV)

If penicillin resistant (MIC ≥0.125 mg/L) but ceftriaxone susceptible (MIC <1.0 mg/L)
  - Ceftriaxone (**or** cefotaxime) (IV)

If penicillin resistant (MIC ≥0.125 mg/L) and ceftriaxone resistant (MIC 1.0-2.0 mg/L)
  - Ceftriaxone (**or** cefotaxime) (IV) **plus** vancomycin (IV)

If high-level ceftriaxone resistant (MIC >2.0 mg/L) or immediate penicillin allergy
  - Option 1: vancomycin* (IV) (**or** rifampicin [PO]) **plus** ciprofloxacin (IV)
  - Option 2: moxifloxacin (IV)

Seek expert advice

Duration of treatment

- 10–14 days (longer if severe)

Dosage of above antibiotics

  - Benzylpenicillin 2.4 g (child: 60 mg/kg up to 2.4 g) IV q4h

---

*Dexamethasone could decrease vancomycin CSF penetration; when dexamethasone is used, an alternative for vancomycin is rifampicin, or use moxifloxacin as a single medication

- Ceftriaxone 4 g (child >1 month: 100 mg/kg up to 4 g) IV daily **or** 2 g (child >1 month: 50 mg/kg up to 2 g) IV q12h
- Cefotaxime 2 g (child: 50 mg/kg up to 2 g) IV q6h
- Vancomycin 25–30 mg/kg IV for the 1st dose (further dosing, see p. 462)
- Rifampicin 600 mg (neonate <1 month: 5 mg/kg; child: 10 mg/kg up to 600 mg) PO q12h
- Ciprofloxacin 400 mg (child: 10 mg/kg up to 400 mg) IV q8h
- Moxifloxacin 400 mg (child: 10 mg/kg up to 400 mg) IV daily

3. *HAEMOPHILUS INFLUENZAE* MENINGITIS

Pathogen

- *Haemophilus influenzae* type b, a gram-negative coccobacillus

Transmission

- Respiratory droplets

Incubation

- 2–4 days

Clinical

- Mortality rate for *H. influenzae* meningitis is 3-6%
- Risk factors: paranasal sinusitis, otitis media, alcoholism, CSF leak, asplenia and hypogammaglobulinaemia

Treatment

If susceptible to penicillin
  - Benzylpenicillin (IV) for 7 days
If resistant to penicillin
  - Ceftriaxone (**or** cefotaxime) (IV) for 7 days
If immediate penicillin or cefalosporin allergy
  - Option 1: ciprofloxacin (IV) for 7 days
  - Option 2: chloramphenicol (IV) for 7 days

Dosage of above antibiotics

- Benzylpenicillin 2.4 g (child: 60 mg/kg up to 2.4 g) IV q4h
- Ceftriaxone 4 g (child >1 month: 100 mg/kg up to 4 g) IV daily or 2 g (child >1 month: 50 mg/kg up to 2 g) IV q12h
- Cefotaxime 2 g (child: 50 mg/kg up to 2 g) IV q6h
- Ciprofloxacin 400 mg (child: 10 mg/kg up to 400 mg) IV q8h
- Chloramphenicol 1 g (child: 25 mg/kg up to 1 g) IV q6h

Close contacts prophylaxis

- Option 1: rifampicin (PO) for 4 days
- Option 2: ceftriaxone (IM or IV) for 2 days (preferred for pregnant women)

Dosage of above antibiotics
- Rifampicin 600 mg (neonate: 10 mg/kg; child: 20 mg/kg up to 600 mg) PO daily
- Ceftriaxone 1 g (child >1 month: 50 mg/kg up to 1 g) IM* or IV daily

Vaccination
- If index case <2 years of age—a full course of Hib vaccination ASAP after recovery regardless of any previous Hib vaccination
- Unvaccinated contacts <5 years of age—a full course of Hib vaccination ASAP

4.   *LISTERIA MONOCYTOGENES* MENINGITIS
Pathogen
- *Listeria monocytogenes*, a small gram-positive bacillus

Clinical
- Most cases are food-borne
- Mainly occur in the immunocompromised
- High mortality rate (15–29%)
- Risk factors: pregnant women, infants and children, elderly (>60 years), alcoholics, immunosuppressed, chronic liver and renal disease, diabetes and iron overloading (e.g. haemochromatosis or transfusion-induced iron overload)
- *L. monocytogenes* is resistant to cefalosporins, but sensitive to penicillin

Treatment
- Benzylpenicillin (IV)

If allergic to penicillin
- Cotrimoxazole (IV) then (PO)

Duration of therapy
- Usually—3 weeks
- Immunocompromised—6 weeks (3 weeks IV therapy + 3 weeks oral therapy)

Note: when *Listeria* infection is confirmed, stop dexamethasone therapy

Dosage of above antibiotics
- Benzylpenicillin 2.4 g (child: 60 mg/kg up to 2.4 g) IV q4h
- Cotrimoxazole 160/800 mg (child >1 month: 4/20 mg/kg up to 160/800 mg) IV q6h, then PO q12h

5.   GROUP B STREPTOCOCCAL MENINGITIS (*STREPTOCOCCUS AGALACTIAE*)
Pathogen
- *Streptococcus agalactiae* (group B streptococci), a gram-positive coccus that is isolated from the lower gastrointestinal tract

---

*IM injection of ceftriaxone needs to be reconstituted with 1% lidocaine (lignocaine)

Clinical

- The most common (70%) cause of neonatal meningitis
- Also affects individuals >60 years
- Overall mortality rate in adults is 34%
- Risk factors in adults: diabetes, pregnancy, alcoholism, hepatic failure, renal failure and corticosteroid treatment

Treatment

For neonate
- Benzylpenicillin 60 mg/kg IV (neonate 0–7 days: q12h; 8–28 days: q6h) for 2–3 weeks

For child and adult
- Benzylpenicillin 2.4 g (child: 60 mg/kg up to 2.4 g) IV q4h for 2–3 weeks

Note: when *S. agalactiae* infection is confirmed, stop dexamethasone therapy

6. *STREPTOCOCCUS SUIS* MENINGITIS

- The most common cause of adult meningitis in Southeast Asia (pork-consuming countries)
- Characterised with hearing loss

Pathogen

- *Streptococcus suis*

Transmission

- Through broken skin (occupational exposure to pigs or pork)
- Ingestion of uncooked infected pork has been suggested
- No evidence of person-to-person transmission

Incubation

- A few hours to 3 days

Clinical

- Early severe sensory deafness (>50%), vertigo and ataxia (30%), arthritis and uvetitis
- May also have septic arthritis, endocarditis, pneumonia and sepsis

Laboratory

- Blood culture
- CSF examination and CSF PCR for *S. suis*

Treatment

- Use of dexamethasone (at early empirical therapy) has significant benefit in reducing mortality and neurological sequelae

If penicillin susceptible
- Benzylpenicillin (IV)

If penicillin allergy
- Ceftriaxone (**or** cefotaxime) (IV)

If ceftriaxone resistant or immediate penicillin allergy, seek expert advice
- Option 1: vancomycin* (IV) (**or** rifampicin [PO]) **plus** ciprofloxacin (IV)
- Option 2: moxifloxacin (IV)

Duration of treatment
- 10–14 days (longer if severe)

Dosage of above antibiotics
- Benzylpenicillin 2.4 g (child: 60 mg/kg up to 2.4 g) IV q4h
- Ceftriaxone 4 g (child >1 month: 100 mg/kg up to 4 g) IV daily **or** 2 g (child >1 month: 50 mg/kg up to 2 g) IV q12h
- Cefotaxime 2 g (child: 50 mg/kg up to 2 g) IV q6h
- Vancomycin 25–30 mg/kg IV for the 1st dose (further dosing, see p. 462)
- Rifampicin 600 mg (neonate <1 month: 5 mg/kg; child: 10 mg/kg up to 600 mg) PO q12h
- Ciprofloxacin 400 mg (child: 10 mg/kg up to 400 mg) IV q8h
- Moxifloxacin 400 mg (child: 10 mg/kg up to 400 mg) IV daily

7. CRYPTOCOCCAL MENINGITIS

Commonly seen in immunocompromised patients (HIV or organ transplant recipients).

Pathogens

- *Cryptococcus neoformans*—particularly in immunocompromised patients
- *Cryptococcus gattii*—in patients with normal immunity

Laboratory

- Blood cultures
- CSF culture for *C. neoformans*
- CSF India ink preparation—highly diagnostic, but only 50% sensitivity
- CSF cryptococcal antigen test—sensitivity >90%
- When India ink result is negative in clinically suspected patient, the CSF specimen may be sent to a reference laboratory for CSF cryptococcal antigen test to confirm the diagnosis
- Monitoring the titre of cryptococcal antigen may help gauge the response to treatment
- CSF examination and culture—within 2 weeks after commencing treatment

---

*Dexamethasone could decrease vancomycin CSF penetration; when dexamethasone is used, an alternative for vancomycin is rifampicin, or use moxifloxacin as a single medication

Management

- Cryptococcal meningitis is frequently complicated with increased intracranial pressure (ICP), so measure the opening pressure during the lumbar puncture
- To reduce ICP, may need to repeat the lumbar puncture, or lumbar drainage or shunt; IV mannitol may also help

Antifungal therapy

- Consultation with an expert experienced in the management of cryptococcal meningitis is essential
- For more detailed information, see Australian and New Zealand antifungal guidelines

Induction therapy

  - Amphotericin B* (IV) plus flucytosine (IV or PO*)

Duration of induction

- *C. neoformans*—2 weeks; CSF culture at 2 weeks, if culture positive, continue therapy for 2 or more weeks
- *C. gattii*, patients with cerebral cryptococcomas or neurological dysfunction—4–6 weeks

Consolidation therapy (CSF culture negative)

Switch to

  - Fluconazole (PO) for ≥8 weeks

Eradication (suppression) therapy

  - Fluconazole (PO)

Duration of eradication

- *C. neoformans*—6–12 months
- *C. gattii* or patients with cerebral cryptococcomas—6–18 months
- Persistent immunosuppression—even longer period

For HIV-infected patients with mild disease

  - Fluconazole 800–1200 mg PO or IV daily **plus** flucytosine 25 mg/kg IV or PO*q6h for 2 weeks

CSF culture after 2 weeks, then

  - Fluconazole 400 mg PO daily for 8 weeks (consolidation)

Then

  - Fluconazole 200 mg PO daily for 12 months and until CD4 count >100 cells/mcl for >3 months

---

*Amphotericin B desoxycholate and oral flucytosine are available via Special Access Scheme <www.tga.gov.au/hp/access-sas.htm>

Dosage of above agents

Induction therapy
- Amphotericin B 0.7–1 mg/kg IV daily
  or amphotericin B liposomal 3–4 mg/kg IV daily
  or amphotericin B lipid complex 5 mg/kg IV daily
- Flucytosine 25 mg/kg IV or PO q6h (monitor plasma levels)

Consolidation therapy

- Fluconazole 800 mg (child: 12 mg/kg up to 800 mg) PO for the 1st dose, then 400–800 mg (child: 6 mg/kg up to 400 mg) PO daily

Eradication (suppression) therapy

- Fluconazole 400–800 mg (child: 6–12 mg/kg up to 400-800 mg) PO daily

MENINGITIS—POST TRAUMA OR NEUROSURGERY

Clinical

- Meningitis may develop post cranial trauma, post neurosurgery, post spinal surgery or post insertion of an intracranial device
- Meningitis may occur spontaneously in patients with CSF shunts

Pathogens

- **Intracranial manipulation, neurosurgery**—*Staphylococcus aureus*, coagulase-negative staphylococci, aerobic gram-negative bacilli, including *Pseudomonas aeruginosa*
- **Basilar skull fracture**—*S. pneumoniae*, *H. influenzae*, group A streptococci
- **CSF shunts**—coagulase-negative staphylococci, *S. aureus*, aerobic gram-negative bacilli and *Propionibacterium acnes*

Management

- Removal of intracranial shunt and other devices
- CFS Gram stain and culture
- Antibiotic empirical therapy (treat until bacteria are isolated):
  - Option 1: ceftazidime (IV) **plus** vancomycin (IV)
  - Option 2: meropenem (IV) **plus** vancomycin (IV)

Modify therapy according to Gram stain and CSF culture and susceptibility results

Duration of therapy

- For 14 days after last positive CSF culture
Intraventricular therapy (if intracranial shunt/catheter cannot be removed)
  - Option 1: vancomycin 10–20 mg intraventricular daily (if CSF Gram stain: G+)

- Option 2: gentamicin 4–8 mg intraventricular daily (if CSF Gram stain: G–)
- Option 3: amikacin 30 mg intraventricular daily (if CSF Gram stain: G–)

Seek expert advice

Dosage of above antibiotics

- Ceftazidime 2 g (child: 50 mg/kg up to 2 g) IV q8h
- Vancomycin 25–30 mg/kg IV for the 1st dose (further dosing, see p. 462)
- Meropenem 2 g (child: 40 mg/kg up to 2 g) IV q8h (has lower risk of seizure)

MENINGITIS—VIRAL

Pathogens

1. **Enterovirus**—e.g. *Polioviruses* (3 serotypes), *Coxsackievirus* A (23 serotypes), *Coxsackievirus* B (6 serotypes), *Echovirus* (31 serotypes) and *Enterovirus* serotypes 68–71
2. **Herpesvirus**—e.g. HSV-1, HSV-2 (causes recurrent benign lymphocytic meningitis), EBV (HHV-4), CMV (HHV-5), varicella zoster virus (HHV-3), CMV, HHV-6 and HHV-7
3. **Arthropod-borne viruses**—e.g. St Louis encephalitis virus (a flavivirus), California encephalitis virus (*Bunyavirus* group, including La Crosse encephalitis virus), tick-borne encephalitis virus and Japanese encephalitis virus (JEV)
4. **Lymphocytic choriomeningitis (LCM) virus**
5. **Human immunodeficiency virus (HIV)**
6. **Other viruses**—e.g. mumps virus, adenovirus (serotypes 1, 6, 7, 12 and 32)

Clues of some viral meningitis

- Vesicular and ulcerative genital lesions—HSV infection
- Diffuse maculopapular rash—enterovirus infection
- Oropharyngeal thrush and cervical lymphadenopathy—HIV infection
- Asymmetric flaccid paralysis—West Nile virus infection
- Swollen parotid gland—mumps

Laboratory

- Rapid serum procalcitonin test—may help distinguish viral meningitis from bacterial meningitis (elevated in bacterial infections but low in viral infections)
- Throat and faeces enterovirus cultures—may implicate enterovirus as the cause

- CSF enterovirus culture (sensitivity 65–70%)
- CSF enterovirus PCR—more sensitive than culture and 94–100% specific
- CSF herpes simplex virus and other herpesvirus PCR
- Virus serology—four-fold rise in serology of certain viruses
- LCM virus blood culture (early in disease) or urine culture (later in disease)

Management

- Viral meningitis is generally benign and self-limiting—supportive care only
- Antiviral therapy or immunoglobulin may be used in the following infections

Herpes meningitis (HSV-1, HSV-2)—if associated encephalitis is present

- Aciclovir 10 mg/kg (child: 500 mg/m^2) IV q8h

Recurrent benign lymphocytic meningitis (HSV-2)

Episodic therapy (infrequent recurrence)

- Option 1: valaciclovir 500 mg PO q12h for 3 days
- Option 2: famciclovir 500 mg PO 1st dose, then 250 mg q12h for 3 doses

Suppression therapy (frequent recurrence)

- Option 1: valaciclovir 500 mg PO daily for 6–12 months
- Option 2: famciclovir 250 mg PO q12h for 6–12 months

CMV meningitis (in immunocompromised patients)

- Option 1: ganciclovir 5 mg/kg IV q12h for 3 weeks, then 5 mg/kg IV q24h for maintenance
- Option 2: foscarnet 60 mg/kg IV q8h for 3 weeks, then 100 mg/kg IV q24h for maintenance

Chronic enterovirus meningitis (in immune deficient patients)

- Immunoglobulin 0.4–0.6 g/kg IV q3–4 weekly

MENINGOCOCCAL DISEASE—PROPHYLAXIS

Antibiotic prophylaxis

- For close contacts and patients who have received only benzylpenicillin
- Commence within 24 hours of the index case becoming ill
  - Option 1: ciprofloxacin (PO) st (preferred for women taking OCP)
  - Option 2: ceftriaxone (IM*) st (preferred for pregnant women)
  - Option 3: rifampicin** (PO) for 2 days (preferred for children)

---

*IM injection of ceftriaxone needs to be reconstituted with 1% lidocaine (lignocaine)

**Rifampicin is associated with multiple drug interactions and is contraindicated in pregnancy, alcoholism and severe liver disease

Dosage of above antibiotics
- Ciprofloxacin 500 mg (child <5 years: 30 mg/kg up to 125 mg; child 5–12 years: 250 mg PO st
- Ceftriaxone 250 mg (child >1 month: 125 mg) IM* st
- Rifampicin 600 mg (neonate: 5 mg/kg; child: 10 mg/kg up to 600 mg) PO q12h

Post-infection vaccination

For patients with meningococcal disease

- MenCCV **or** 4vMenCV 0.5 ml IM **or** 4vMenPV 0.5 ml SC st (given on discharge from hospital, or when patient recovers from the infection) (4vMenCV is better than 4vMenPV)

Prophylactic vaccination

National Immunisation Program
- MenCCV (Hib-MenCCV) 1 dose at 12 month—for C
- 4vMenCV 1 dose at 17–18 (school program)—for A, C, W135 and Y

Prevention of meningococcal B (≥6 weeks of age)
- MenBV (Bexsero) 6 weeks to 5 months: 4 doses at 6 weeks, 4, 6, 12 months; 6–11 months: 3 doses 8 weeks apart; >12 months: 2 doses 8 weeks apart

Infants 6 weeks to 6 months with high risk**
- 4vMenCV 3 doses 8 weeks apart, then at 12 months, then 3 years after, then every 5 years

Children 7 months to 23 months with high risk**
- 4vMenCV 2 doses 12 weeks apart, then 3 years after, then every 5 years

Children 2–6 years with high risk**
- 4vMenCV 2 doses 8 weeks apart, then 3 years after, then every 5 years

Children >7 years with high risk**
- 4vMenCV 2 doses 8 weeks apart, then every 5 years

Close contacts of meningococcal C disease (≥6 weeks of age)
- MenCCV single dose

Close contacts of meningococcal A, W135 or Y disease (≥9 months of age)
- 4vMenCV single dose

Laboratory personnel who frequently handle *N. meningitidis*
- 4vMenCV single dose, then every 5 years (if continue to be at risk)

Travellers (aged ≥9 months) to area with epidemic of A, W135 or Y disease
- 4vMenCV single dose, then every 5 years (if continue visiting the area)

Pilgrims who go to Saudi Arabia require a valid certificate of vaccination
- 4vMenCV single dose

---

*IM injection of ceftriaxone needs to be reconstituted with 1% lidocaine (lignocaine)
**High-risk conditions: asplenia (functional or anatomical), complement component disorders, eculizumab treatment, post-HSCT

MICROSPORIDIOSIS

Other names: microsporidiasis, *Microsporidia* infection
Microsporidiosis is an opportunistic infection primarily seen in immunocompromised individuals (e.g. HIV/AIDS) that can cause chronic diarrhoea and systemic infections.

Pathogens

- *Microsporidia* spp—more fungal than protozoal
- Worldwide distribution
- The most prevalent species causing microsporidiosis in humans include:
  - *Encephalitozoon (Septata) intestinalis*
  - *Enterocytozoon bieneusi*
  - *Encephalitozoon cuniculi*

Transmission

- Water-borne or person-to-person

Clinical

- Often seen in patients with HIV infection or in organ transplant recipients
- Chronic diarrhoea (non-bloody), cholangitis
- Central nervous system infection
- Respiratory tract infection, sinusitis
- Eye infection (microsporidial keratoconjunctivitis)
- Myositis
- Nodular skin lesions
- Disseminated infection

Diagnosis

- Faeces microscopy—the most rapid diagnosis
- Modified trichrome stain (chromotrope 2R)—to detect microsporidia in urine, faeces and mucus
- Cytological and histological examinations (e.g. punch biopsy of skin lesion, small-bowel endoscopy and biopsy)
- Conjunctival scraping or swab (keratoconjunctivitis)—for microscopy, PCR
- *Microsporidia* PCR—to diagnose infection with *E. bieneusi, V. corneae* or *Nosema* spp

Treatment

- In immunocompetent patients with self-limiting diarrhoea, no need for specific treatment
- For immunocompromised patients with infection, treatment is required
For *E. (Septata) intestinalis*
  - Albendazole 400 mg (child <10 kg: 200 mg) PO q12h for 3 weeks

For *E. bieneusi*
  • Fumagillin* 20 mg PO q8h for 2 weeks
For microsporidial keratoconjunctivitis
  • Fumagillin* eye drops/ointment, topically

MOLLUSCUM CONTAGIOSUM

Pathogens

• *Molluscum contagiosum* virus subtypes I, II, III and IV

Transmission

• In children—usually skin-to-skin contact with affected persons, sharing towels, baths or swimming pools
• In adults—usually an STI, primarily acquired through sexual contact with an affected partner

Incubation

• 2–7 weeks, but may extend to 6 months

Clinical

• Small, pearly or skin-coloured pimples or papules with a central dimple and white core on the skin; may have cauliflower-like appearance on genital skin
• In children, lesions typically occur on the chest, arms, trunk, legs and face
• In healthy adults, few lesions are limited to genitals, perineum, lower abdomen, buttocks and inner thighs; the average duration of an untreated lesion is 6–9 months
• In immunocompromised and HIV patients, lesions may number in the hundreds and are generally larger (can be >2 cm in diameter) and more deformed

Laboratory

• Skin lesion biopsy—may be obtained to confirm the diagnosis
• Squash preparation—the cellular material in the central umbilication may be manually extracted and examined microscopically

Treatment

Children with few lesions

• No treatment—spontaneous resolution (may take up to 2 years)

Adults

• Cryotherapy
• Pricking the lesion with a pointed stick soaked in 1% or 3% phenol
• Application of 30% trichloroacetic acid

---

*Available via Special Access Scheme <www.tga.gov.au/hp/access-sas.htm> or from compounding chemist

- Electrocautery or diathermy
- Painting with clear nail polish

If widespread lesions interfere with lifestyle and function

- Parents may squeeze and pop out the core of 2–3 lesions each night
- Extract the core with a large needle or curette the lesions and apply 10% povidone-iodine solution (child may require general anaesthesia)

Prevent spreading

- Avoid heated swimming pools
- Shower rather than bathe

MUMPS

Other names: epidemic parotitis, acute viral parotitis

Pathogen

- A paramyxovirus

Incubation

- 12–25 days

Transmission

- Droplets
- Direct contact
- Through fomites

Infectious period

- From 6 days before to 9 days after parotid swelling

Clinical

- Primarily a disease of school-aged children and young adults, uncommon before the age of 2 years
- Non-specific prodromal symptoms, followed by painful swelling of the parotid gland, may be bilateral
- Painful testicular swelling and rash may also occur
- Aseptic meningitis may mimic bacterial meningitis

Complications

- Aseptic meningitis
- Encephalitis
- Epididymo-orchitis
- Infertility or subfertility
- Pancreatitis
- Oophoritis
- Myocarditis
- Mastitis

- Hepatitis
- Thyroiditis

Diagnosis

- Based on clinical features
- Mumps serology—for doubtful cases
- Mumps virus PCR (saliva, throat swab, urine or CSF)—for doubtful cases
- Mumps virus culture (saliva, throat swab, urine or CSF)—for doubtful cases

Treatment

- Supportive, analgesics
- Avoid fruit juice or any acidic foods

Vaccination

- MMR or MMRV vaccine (does not provide immediate protection after exposure)
  - Priorix® (MMR) **or** Priorix Tetra® (MMRV) 0.5 mL IM/SC 2 doses at 12 months and 18 months (**or** 2 doses at any age >18 months at least 4 weeks apart)
- Normal human immunoglobulin (NHIG) has not been shown to be of value in post-exposure prophylaxis for mumps

MURRAY VALLEY ENCEPHALITIS

Other names: Australian encephalitis (AE)

Pathogen

- Murray Valley encephalitis (MVE) virus

Distribution

- Human infections occur in all mainland states of Australia

Transmission

- Mosquito-borne virus, maintained in a bird-mosquito-bird cycle
- Humans get the infection from a mosquito bite
- Water birds act as the vertebrate host and the mosquito *Culex annulirostris* is the major vector
- There is an association between outbreaks and heavy rainfall and widespread flooding

Clinical

- There is no difference clinically between MVE and KUN viral infections
- High-risk groups: babies, young children and tourists

- Most infections are subclinical
- Approximately 1 in 500 infected people become noticeably ill
- Cases vary from mild to severe to fatal
- Symptoms: sudden onset of fever; headache, anorexia, nausea, vomiting, diarrhoea and dizziness; brain dysfunction after a few days with irritability, drowsiness, confusion, convulsions, neck stiffness, delirium, coma and death
- Recovery from encephalitic syndrome is usually associated with residual neurological deficits (50%)

Diagnosis

- MVE virus-specific IgM (blood or CSF)—in the absence of IgM to Kunjin, Japanese encephalitis or dengue viruses (confirm laboratory result by a second arbovirus reference laboratory if the case occurs in areas not known to have established endemic or regular epidemic activity)
- MVE virus PCR
- MVE virus isolation (blood or CSF)

Treatment

- Supportive

Prevention

- Prevent bites from mosquitoes (wear long-sleeved shirts and pants)
- Apply active mosquito control
- Avoid known mosquito-infested areas
- Avoid going out at dawn and dusk
- Use insect repellents

MYCOBACTERIUM AVIUM COMPLEX

Pathogens

Mycobacterium avium complex (MAC)—a group of *Mycobacterium* bacteria, including:

- *Mycobacterium avium hominis* (MAH)—causes most MAC diseases in humans
- *Mycobacterium avium paratuberculosis* (MAP)—causes paratuberculosis, or Johne's disease

Transmission

- Inhalation or ingestion of MAC bacteria (common in the environment)
- Indoor swimming pools
- Raw or partially cooked fish or shellfish
- Via bronchoscopy

Laboratory

- Blood and sputum cultures
- Bone marrow culture may yield an earlier diagnosis (but not an initial step)
- Clarithromycin susceptibility testing of MAC isolates should be done before starting treatment

1. PULMONARY MAC

- Cavitary and fibrotic upper lobe disease (similar to TB)—often in old men with pre-existing lung disease (e.g. COPD)
- Progressive bronchiectasis—productive cough, interstitial or nodular x-ray changes; most common in old women (Lady Windermere syndrome)
- Hypersensitive pneumonitis—follows inhalation of aerosols generated by spas that are colonised with MAC ('hot tub lung'); antibiotic treatment is not required

Treatment

- Focal disease or a solitary nodule—may need surgical resection

Daily regimen

- Azithromycin (**or** clarithromycin) **plus** ethambutol **plus** rifampicin (**or** rifabutin) (PO)

Three-times-weekly regimen (not for moderate or severe disease, or cavitary disease)

- Azithromycin (**or** clarithromycin) **plus** ethambutol **plus** rifampicin (PO) 3 times weekly

For macrolide-resistant cases

- Ethambutol **plus** rifampicin (**or** rifabutin) (PO) daily (full course) **plus** amikacin (**or** streptomycin) (IM) 3 times weekly for first 2 months
- Interferon gamma (SC) 3 times weekly (may be used as adjuvant treatment)

Duration of treatment

- Continue until the patient remains culture-negative for at least 12 months
- The patient needs close monitoring as the treatment may be poorly tolerated

Dosage of above agents

Daily regimen

- Azithromycin 250 mg (child: 5 mg/kg up to 250 mg) PO daily
- Clarithromycin 500 mg (adult <50 kg or >70 years: 250 mg; child: 12.5 mg/kg up to 500 mg) PO q12h
- Ethambutol (adult and child) 15 mg/kg PO daily
- Rifampicin 600 mg (adult <50 kg: 450 mg; child <50 kg: 10 mg/kg up to 450 mg; child >50 kg: 600 mg) PO daily
- Rifabutin 300 mg (child: 5 mg/kg up to 300 mg) PO daily

Three-times-weekly regimen

- Azithromycin 500 mg (child: 10 mg/kg up to 500 mg) PO 3 times weekly
- Clarithromycin 500 mg (child: 12.5 mg/kg up to 500 mg) PO twice a day, 3 days weekly
- Ethambutol (adult and child) 25 mg/kg PO 3 times weekly
- Rifampicin (adult and child) 15 mg/kg up to 600 mg PO 3 times weekly

For macrolide-resistant cases

- Ethambutol (adult and child) 15 mg/kg PO daily
- Rifampicin 600 mg (adult <50 kg: 450 mg; child <50 kg: 10 mg/kg up to 450 mg; child >50 kg: 600 mg) PO daily
- Rifabutin 300 mg (child: 5 mg/kg up to 300 mg) PO daily
- Amikacin 25 mg/kg IM 3 times weekly (dose adjustment for renal impairment)
- Streptomycin 25 mg/kg IM 3 times weekly (available via Special Access Scheme <www.tga.gov.au/hp/access-sas.htm>)
- Interferon gamma 1.5 mcg/kg (3×10^4 units/kg) (body surface area >0.5 m^2: 50 mcg/m^2 [1×10^6 units/m^2]) SC 3 times weekly

2. DISSEMINATED MAC

- Most commonly seen in advanced HIV infection

Treatment

- Azithromycin (**or** clarithromycin) **plus** ethambutol **plus** rifabutin (PO)

Dosage of above agents

- Azithromycin 500 mg PO daily
- Clarithromycin 500 mg PO q12h
- Ethambutol 15 mg/kg PO daily
- Rifabutin 300 mg PO daily

If rifabutin taken with a ritonavir-boosted proteinase inhibitor: 150 mg (child: 2.5 mg/kg up to 150 mg) PO daily

If taken with efavirenz: 450 mg (child 7.5 mg/kg up to 450 mg) PO daily

3. CERVICAL LYMPHADENITIS DUE TO *M. AVIUM*

- Most common in children
- Enlarged cervical lymph nodes without abnormality of immune system
- Treatment—surgery
- Anti-mycobacterial therapy—only for those who cannot have surgery
  - Azithromycin (**or** clarithromycin) **plus** rifabutin (PO) for 18–24 months

Dosage of above antibiotics

- Azithromycin 500 mg (child: 10 mg/kg up to 500 mg) PO daily
- Clarithromycin 500 mg (child: 12.5 mg/kg up to 500 mg) PO q12h
- Rifabutin 300 mg (child: 5 mg/kg up to 300 mg) PO daily

MYCOBACTERIUM—NON-TUBERCULOUS

Non-tuberculous mycobacteria (NTM) are environmental acid-fast bacilli that occasionally cause respiratory, skin and disseminated disease.

Important NTM

- MAC—see p. 240
- *M. abscessus*, *M. chelonae*, *M. fortuitum*—see below
- *M. kansasii*—causes lung infection, see below
- *M. ulcerans*—causes necrotising skin ulcer, see below
- *M. leprae*—causes leprosy (see Leprosy, p. 200)
- *M. marinum*—causes water-related skin granuloma (see Wound infection—water related, p. 451)

Transmission

- Injections of substances contaminated with the bacterium
- Through contaminated medical equipment or material at invasive medical procedure
- Wound contaminated by soil
- Very low risk of transmission from person-to-person

Diagnosis

Diagnosis needs the following three:

- Symptoms
- CXR changes
- At least two positive sputum cultures or a single positive bronchial lavage/wash

Treatment

Should be under an experienced specialist

M. ABSCESSUS, *M. CHELONAE*, *M. FORTUITUM*

- Rapid-growing mycobacteria
- Cause skin infections, respiratory infections, infections of prosthetic material, eye infections associated with contact lenses and ocular surgery, and occasionally disseminated infections

Treatment

- Drug choice should be guided by susceptibility testing results
- Duration of treatment
    - Skin and soft-tissue infections—minimum 4 months
    - Bone infections (with prosthetic material)—at least 6 months
    - Respiratory infections with *M. fortuitum* or *M. chelonae*—use 2 oral drugs (e.g. doxycycline, ciprofloxacin or cotrimoxazole), continue until 12 months of negative sputum cultures

- Respiratory infections with *M. abscessus* are very difficult to treat; need periodic multidrug therapy with a macrolide and one or more injectable medications (e.g. amikacin, cefoxin or imipenem); surgical treatment may be required

M. KANSASII

- Similar to pulmonary tuberculosis
- Resistant to pyrazinamide
- Needs longer course of treatment

Treatment

- Isoniazid **plus** rifampicin **plus** ethambutol (PO) daily for 18 months with at least 12 months of negative sputum cultures

Dosage of above agents

- Isoniazid 300 mg (child: 10 mg/kg up to 300 mg) PO daily
- Rifampicin 600 mg (adult <50 kg: 450 mg; child <50 kg: 15 mg/kg up to 450 mg; child ≥50 kg: 600 mg) PO daily
- Ethambutol (adult and child) 15 mg/kg PO daily

M. ULCERANS

- Causes a necrotising skin ulcer (known as Buruli, Bairnsdale or Daintree ulcer)
- Occur in coastal Victoria and far north Queensland and less commonly in Capricorn coast of Queensland

Treatment

- Surgical treatment (repeated debridement, excision of the ulcer) is usually required with antibiotic therapy
- Clinical deterioration during antibiotic treatment can be caused by a paradoxical reaction to the treatment; the treatment should be continued
- Adjuvant thermotherapy (direct application of heat to the ulcer or wound after resection for several hours per day for 4 weeks) may be useful to reduce the risk of relapse

For adults

- Rifampicin **plus** ciprofloxacin (PO) for 8 weeks

For children

- Rifampicin **plus** clarithromycin (PO) for 8 weeks

Very severe cases **add**

- Amikacin (IV)

Dosage of above agents

- Rifampicin 600 mg (adult <50 kg: 450 mg; child <50 kg: 15 mg/kg up to 450 mg; child ≥50 kg: 600 mg) PO daily
- Ciprofloxacin 500 mg (child: 12.5 mg/kg up to 500 mg) PO q12h

- Clarithromycin child: 12.5 mg/kg up to 500 mg PO q12h
- Amikacin 15 mg/kg IV daily 5 times a week

For detailed information on NTM diseases, see: An official ATS/IDSA statement: diagnosis, treatment, and prevention of nontuberculous mycobacterial diseases. *Am J Respir Crit Care Med* 2007;175(4): 367–416

MYCOPLASMA—GENITAL TRACT INFECTION

Pathogens

- Belong to *Mollicutes* class and *Mycoplasmataceae* family
- Four species can affect human genital tract:
  - *Mycoplasma genitalium*
  - *Mycoplasma fermantans*
  - *Mycoplasma primatum*
  - *Mycoplasma hominis*

Prevalence

- Men with acute non-specific urethritis—10–38%
- Men with persistent or recurrent non-specific urethritis—12–41%
- Women with urethritis—4–9%
- Women with cervicitis—8–27%
- Women with PID—3.6–6.5%

Transmission

- Primarily acquired through sexual contact

Incubation

- 2–35 days

Clinical

- Urethritis (acute and chronic, both sexes)—mucopurulent discharge, urinary burning
- Cervicitis (females)—vaginal discharge, PV bleeding after sex
- Pelvic inflammatory disease (females)—pelvic pain, fever, pain on intercourse
- Pregnancy complications—spontaneous miscarriage, stillbirth, chorioamnionitis, preterm rupture of membranes, preterm labour and postpartum infection
- Neonate and fetus—may cause spontaneous abortion, stillbirth, premature delivery, low-birth-weight baby, neonatal pneumonia, neonatal sepsis or neonatal meningitis
- A co-factor in HIV transmission
- May play a role in the development of prostate cancer, ovarian cancer and lymphoma

Laboratory

Testing is recommended for symptomatic patients and sexual contacts of infected persons

- PCR test for *Mycoplasma genitalium* (urine, urethral swab, cervical swab, anal swab)

Treatment

- Option 1: azithromycin 500 mg PO daily for 4 days
- Option 2: doxycycline 100 mg PO q12h for 10 days

If above treatment fails

- Moxifloxicin 400 mg PO daily for 7 days

For chronic PID not responding to standard therapy

- Moxifloxacin 400 mg PO daily for 14 days
- Azithromycin-resistant *M. genitalium* infection has been reported
- Sex partners should be treated at the same time to prevent reinfection
- A test of cure 1 month after treatment is recommended

Prevention

- Safe sex with condom use
- No unprotected sex until antibiotic treatment is completed for patient and partners (to prevent reinfection)

NEEDLE-STICK INJURIES AND BLOOD EXPOSURE

Type of injuries

- Needle-stick injuries
- Cuts with contaminated sharp objects
- Contact of mucous membrane or non-intact skin (e.g. chapped, abraded or affected by dermatitis) with blood, tissue or potentially infectious body fluids

Pathogens may be exposed

- Hepatitis B virus (HBV)
- Hepatitis C virus (HCV)
- Human immunodeficiency virus (HIV)
- Syphilis
- Malaria
- Cytomegalovirus (CMV)
- Agent of Creutzfeldt-Jacob disease

Management

- Immediate treatment:
  - Contaminated skin wound—encourage bleeding from the wound and wash with copious amounts of soapy water or skin disinfectant
  - Contaminated eyes—rinse the eyes with saline or water
  - Contaminated mouth—spit out any fluid and rinse mouth with water
- Testing for the source (if known)—after obtaining consent, take bloods for HBsAg, anti-HCV and HIV antibody etc
- Testing for injured healthcare worker—HBsAb, anti-HCV, HIV antibody and baseline LFT
- Tetanus toxoid booster if indicated (see Tetanus, p. 393)
- Counselling and follow-up arrangement for the injured healthcare worker

I.   HEPATITIS B

General principles

- If the status of the source and the healthcare worker is unknown or immunisation status cannot be obtained within 48 hours, give hep B immunoglobulin 400 IU IM and start the first dose of hep B vaccination
- If the source is HBsAg-negative and unlikely to be in the window period, no further testing is required for both the source and the healthcare worker
- If the healthcare worker has had HBV vaccination in the past, check hep B antibody titre and, if low, give hep B booster

- If the source is HBsAg-positive and the healthcare worker is HBsAb negative, the healthcare worker should receive hep B immunoglobulin 400 IU within 24 hours and receive the first hep B vaccination at the same time
- If the source is HBsAg-negative and the healthcare worker is HBsAb negative, the healthcare worker should receive a full course of HBV vaccination ASAP

2. HEPATITIS C

General principles

- If the source is anti-HCV negative and is unlikely to be in the window period, no further testing is required for both the source and the healthcare worker
- If the source is anti-HCV positive or negative but likely to be in the window period, the healthcare worker should have HCV RNA testing at 4–6 weeks, and anti-HCV and LFT at 4–6 months
- If seroconversion occurs, early therapy should be considered

There is no effective passive or active immunoprophylaxis for HCV infection

3. HUMAN IMMUNODEFICIENCY VIRUS (HIV)

Investigation

- If the source is HIV antibody negative and unlikely to be in the window period, no further testing is required for both the source and the healthcare worker
- In all other circumstances, the healthcare worker should have follow-up HIV antibody testing at 1, 3 and 6 months

Post-exposure prophylaxis

Post-exposure prophylaxis (PEP) can reduce the risk of HIV infection
PEP is indicated for non-occupational post-exposure:
If the source is known HIV-positive:

- All anal or vaginal intercourse, receptive or insertive
- Shared injection equipment

If the source's HIV status is unknown:

- Receptive anal intercourse between men who have sex with men (MSM) or with a heterosexual partner from a high-prevalence country (HPC)
- Shared injection equipment between MSM or with a person from a HPC

PEP may be considered for the following people:
If the source is known HIV-positive:

- Oral intercourse (with ejaculation), receptive with broken oral mucosa

If the source's HIV status is unknown:

- Insertive anal intercourse between MSM
- Receptive anal intercourse with a heterosexual IV drug user
- Receptive vaginal or insertive vagina/anal intercourse with a partner from a HPC
- Shared injection equipment between heterosexuals

PEP is not indicated for:

If the source is known HIV-positive:

- Oral intercourse (with ejaculation), receptive with intact oral mucosa
- Contamination of intact skin and mucosa with source body fluids

If the source's HIV status is unknown:

- Community-acquired needle-stick injury
- Heterosexual anal, vaginal or oral intercourse (not from a HPC)

PEP for post-occupational exposure:

- If the source is known HIV-positive—commence PEP ASAP within 72 hours of exposure (PEP may still be recommended after 72 hours post-exposure)
- Refer to or seek advice from an HIV practitioner, a sexual health centre or an S100 prescriber GP (check local guidelines or find your local centre for PEP at <www.getpep.info>)

PEP regimens for HIV

- Initiation of PEP should be the responsibility of an HIV practitioner or an S100 prescriber GP
- Two nucleoside or nucleotide reverse transcriptase inhibitors (to which the source has not been exposed) **plus** a third medicine if exposure is high risk

For low-risk exposure*

- Option 1: emtricitabine + tenofovir (Truvada) 200 + 300 mg PO daily for 4 weeks
- Option 2: lamivudine + zidovudine (Combivir) 150 + 300 mg PO q12h for 4 weeks

For high-risk exposure**

Either of the above regimens **plus** one of following:

- Option 1: lopinavir + ritonavir (Kaletra) 400 + 100 mg PO q12h for 4 weeks
- Option 2: raltegravir 400 mg PO q12h for 4 weeks

---

*Low-risk exposure: mucous membrane or intact skin exposure, superficial scratches, injuries involving solid needles, low HIV viral load in the source

**High-risk exposure: percutaneous injury with hollow blood-containing needle, deep injury, high viral load or late-stage disease of the source

4. Human T-cell lymphotropic virus type I

- Seek expert advice
- For high-risk exposures (e.g. percutaneous injury with a hollow blood-containing needle)
  - Lamivudine + zidovudine (Combivir) 150 + 300 mg PO q12h for 4 weeks

NEUTROPENIC SEPSIS

Other names: neutropenia, febrile neutropenia

Indication for antibiotic therapy

- Neutrophils $<0.5 \times 10^9$/L (usually occurs 7–10 days post chemotherapy)
- Neutrophils $<1 \times 10^9$/L with a predicted further decline
- Fever ≥38°C

Management

- Blood cultures (×2), FBC, CRP, EUC, LFT, Ca, Mg, Ph, BSL and CXR
- Collect urine, sputum, stool and swabs from any lesions for culture
- Consider removing intravascular devices

Antibiotic therapy

Commence ASAP after collection of the cultures

Empirical therapy

Use broad-spectrum antibiotics
  - Option 1: piperacillin/tazobactam 4 g (child: 100 mg/kg up to 4 g) IV q6h
  - Option 2: cefepime 2 g (child: 50 mg/kg up to 2 g) IV q8h
  - Option 3: ceftazidime 2 g (child: 50 mg/kg up to 2 g) IV q8h

For severe sepsis/septic shock with possible resistance to above antibiotics **add**

  - Gentamicin 4–7 mg/kg (child: 7.5 mg/kg up to 320 mg) IV for the 1st dose (further dosing, see p. 459)

For severe sepsis/septic shock and when vancomycin is indicated* **add**

  - Vancomycin 25–30 mg/kg IV for the 1st dose (further dosing, see p. 462)

---

*Indication of vancomycin for severe sepsis or septic shock:
- Pre-existing MRSA or MRSE infection or known MRSA colonisation
- Catheter-related infection with high risk of MRSA infection
- Prevalence of above organisms in the facility is high
- Fever persists after 48 hours of treatment and the culture results are not available

Duration of antibiotic therapy

For 24–48 hours, modify antibiotic as soon as pathogen is identified and the susceptibility is known; continue treatment until neutrophils $>1 \times 10^9$/L and patient has been afebrile for 24 hours

If fever persists >4 days of antibiotic therapy

Consider add antifungals

- Option 1: fluconazole 400 mg (child: 12 mg/kg up to 400 mg) IV daily
- Option 2: amphotericin B adult, child: 1 mg/kg IV daily
- Option 3: voriconazole adult, child: 4 mg/kg IV q12h

Seek expert advice

Low-risk neutropenic patients

May be treated at home with oral therapy

NOCARDIOSIS

NOCARDIAL BRAIN ABSCESS

Pathogens

- *Nocardia asteroids* and other spp

Clinical

- Usually seen in the immunocompromised
- Headache, lethargy, confusion, seizures, sudden onset of neurological deficit
- Nocardial meningitis—rare and difficult to diagnose

Diagnosis

- Modified Ziehl Neelsen stains—*Nocardiae* spp can be visualised
- Nocardia molecular sequencing—species identification
- Cultures (laboratory should be informed) and susceptibility testing
- CT brain scan—cerebral abscess

Treatment

- Surgical drainage of abscesses (potentially diagnostic)—the risks of a neurosurgical procedure should be balanced against the benefits of surgical drainage
- Antibiotic treatment—brain abscesses may respond to antibiotics without surgery (species identification and susceptibility testing provide a guide to treatment)

Empirical therapy

- Option 1: cotrimoxazole (IV **or** PO) **plus** imipenem (**or** meropenem*) (IV)

---

*Meropenem has a lower risk of seizures than imipenem

- Option 2: cotrimoxazole (IV **or** PO) **plus** amikacin (IV)
- Option 3: cotrimoxazole (IV **or** PO) **plus** imipenem (**or** meropenem*) (IV) **plus** amikacin (IV)

If susceptible to ceftriaxone

- Option 4: cotrimoxazole (IV **or** PO) **plus** ceftriaxone (IV)

Duration of initial therapy

- 3–6 weeks

Follow-up oral therapy (if susceptible to cotrimoxaole)
- Cotrimoxazole (PO) for up to 12 months

Alternative follow-up therapy (if susceptible)
- Amoxicillin/clavulanate, linezolid, moxifloxacin, or minocycline

Seek expert advice

Dosage of above antibiotics

- Cotrimoxazole 320/1600 mg (child >1 month: 8/40 mg/kg up to 320/1600 mg) IV **or** PO q12h
- Imipenem 500 mg (child: 15 mg/kg up to 500 mg) IV q6h
- Meropenem 2 g (child: 40 mg/kg up to 2 g) IV q8h
- Amikacin (adult and child): 15 mg/kg IV daily **or** 7.5 mg/kg IV q12h (monitor blood levels and adjust dose, see p. 459)
- Ceftriaxone 4 g (child: 100 mg/kg up to 4 g) IV daily **or** 2 g (child: 50 mg/kg up to 2 g) IV q12h

NOROVIRUS

Other names: Norwalk-like viruses, winter diarrhoea, winter vomiting disease

Norovirus is probably the commonest cause of gastroenteritis in adults and older children. Noroviruses are highly infectious and may cause outbreaks in schools, childcare centres, aged care facilities, cruise ships, restaurants and hospitals.

Pathogens

- Noroviruses—members of caliciviruses
- Noroviruses can survive on contaminated surfaces and are resistant to many common disinfectants
- Highly infectious (very few virus particles are needed to cause infection)

Transmission

- Ingestion of contaminated food or water (norovirus is in the vomit or faeces)
- Direct contact with an infected person or via contaminated surfaces
- Aerosol spread from vomitus has been suggested in some outbreaks
- Infectious for at least 3 days after symptoms have resolved; some may still be infectious up to 2 weeks after recovery
- Outbreaks typically occur in winter months

Incubation

- 1–2 days, but can appear as early as 12 hours after exposure

Clinical

- Sudden onset of profuse vomiting and/or watery diarrhoea, abdominal cramps, headache, low-grade fever, chills and muscle aches
- Symptoms usually last 1–3 days
- Immunity to norovirus may be strain-specific and lasts only a few months

Laboratory

- Norovirus RT-PCR (faeces, vomit samples or environmental swabs)
- Immune electron microscopy of faecal specimens
- Norovirus ELISA tests—low specificity, used in investigation of outbreaks

Treatment

- Symptomatic treatment
- Oral rehydration
- No vaccine available

Prevention

- Do not go to work until at least 2 days after symptoms have resolved
- Do not handle or prepare food for at least 2 days after symptoms have resolved
- Keep children home for at least 24 hours after symptoms have resolved
- Patients in hospitals and nursing homes should be nursed in their own rooms, with a private bathroom for at least 24 hours after symptoms have resolved
- Immediately remove and wash any clothes or bedding contaminated with vomit or diarrhoea (use hot water and soap)
- Thoroughly clean and disinfect contaminated surfaces immediately by using a bleach-based household cleaner
- Wash hands after using the bathroom or changing nappies

O

ORF

Other names: *Ecthyma contagiosum*, sheep pox
Orf is a viral disease that is widespread in sheep and goats and can be transmitted to humans by contact with an infected animal or contaminated fomites.

Pathogen

- Orf virus belongs to the Parapoxvirus genus

Transmission

- Humans acquire orf from contact with infected animals, carcasses or contaminated material
- Orf is very common among shepherds, veterinary surgeons and farmers who bottle-feed lambs, as well as butchers and meat porters from handling infected carcasses
- No person-to-person transmission

Incubation

- 1 week

Clinical

- The majority of orf infections go unreported
- Single or group of red weeping papules or nodules on dorsa of hands and fingers with an erythematous margin; may have mild fever and malaise
- Immunocompromised patients with orf may have progressive, destructive large fungating lesions

Laboratory

- Orf skin biopsy—histopathologically confirm the diagnosis
- PCR for orf virus—definitively identify orf virus
- Immune electron microscopy—negative staining of the crust or a small biopsy

Treatment

- Usually spontaneously resolves in 3–6 weeks without scaring
- Symptomatic treatment—moist dressings, local antiseptics and finger immobilisation
- Steroid injected into the pustular nodule can achieve a rapid healing
  - Corticosteroid with 1% lidocaine (lignocaine), intralesional injection
- Topic imiquimod may induce rapid regression
  - Imiquimod (e.g. Aldara) 5% cream top 3 times per week
- Secondary bacterial infection—treat with topical or systemic antibiotics

- Immunosuppressed patients with large fungating lesions require medical treatment such as antiviral therapy and surgical debridement
- Dissection of orf lesion from underlying dermis—for large exophytic lesions
- Curettage and electrodesiccation—if an orf lesion is persistent
- Shave excision
- Cryotherapy (liquid nitrogen)—speeds up the recovery process

OSTEOMYELITIS—EMPIRICAL THERAPY

Pathogens

- *Staphylococcus aureus*
- Group A Streptococcus spp
- *Enterobacter* spp
- Group B Streptococcus spp (newborns)
- *Haemophilus influenzae*
- *Kingella kingae* (gram-negative)

Clinical

- In children the long bones are usually affected
- In adults the vertebrae and the pelvis are most commonly affected

Diagnosis

- Blood culture—positive in 50% of patients with haematogenous osteomyelitis
- Bone biopsy—if blood cultures negative (open surgical biopsy is better than needle biopsy in vertebral osteomyelitis)
- Nucleic acid testing for *Kingella kingae*—particularly for infants and children
- X-ray—overlying soft-tissue oedema at 3–5 days after infection; periosteal elevation and cortical or medullary lucencies after 3–4 weeks
- MRI—for early detection and for surgical localisation of osteomyelitis
- Bone scan—the initial imaging modality of choice
- CT scan—most useful for spinal vertebral lesions
- Ultrasound scan and ultrasound-guided aspiration—soft-tissue abscess or fluid collection and periosteal elevation (particularly suitable for children)

Treatment

- Surgical intervention (chronic infections almost always require surgery)
- Hyperbaric oxygen therapy—a useful adjunct treatment for refractory cases
- Empirical antibiotic therapy

Long-bone osteomyelitis and child vertebral osteomyelitis

- Flucloxacillin (IV) (+ vancomycin [IV] if critically ill)

If non-immediate penicillin allergy
- Cefazolin (IV) (+ vancomycin [IV] if critically ill)

If immediate penicillin allergy or MRSA infection is likely
- Vancomycin (IV)

Adult vertebral osteomyelitis

- Ceftriaxone (IV) **plus** vancomycin (IV)

Modify therapy according to the results of cultures and susceptibility testing

Dosage of above antibiotics

- Flucloxacillin 2 g (child: 50 mg/kg up to 2 g) IV q6h **or** q4h for critically ill patients
- Cefazolin 2 g (child: 50 mg/kg up to 2 g) IV q8h **or** q6h for critically ill patients
- Vancomycin 25–30 mg/kg IV for the 1st dose (further dosing, see p. 462)
- Ceftriaxone 2 g IV daily

OSTEOMYELITIS—DIRECT THERAPY

1. Mssa (methicillin-susceptible *Staphylococcus aureus*)

Treatment

- Flucloxacillin (IV) **then** (PO)

If non-immediate penicillin allergy
- Cefazolin (IV), **then** cefalexin (PO)

If immediate penicillin allergy
- Clindamycin (**or** lincomycin) (IV), **then** clindamycin (PO)

If immediate penicillin allergy and MSSA is lincosamide resistant
- Vancomycin (IV), then seek expert advice on oral continuation therapy

Duration of treatment

See p. 258

Dosage of above antibiotics

- Flucloxacillin 2 g (child: 50 mg/kg up to 2 g) IV q6h **or** q4h for critically ill patients
  then flucloxacillin 1 g (child: 25 mg/kg up to 1 g) PO q6h
- Cefazolin 2 g (child: 50 mg/kg up to 2 g) IV q8h **or** q6h for critically ill patients
  then cefalexin 1 g (child: 25 mg/kg up to 1 g) PO q6h
- Clindamycin 600 mg (child: 15 mg/kg up to 600 mg) IV q8h
- Lincomycin 600 mg (child: 15 mg/kg up to 600 mg) IV q8h
- Clindamycin 450 mg (child: 10 mg/kg up to 450 mg) PO q8h
- Vancomycin 25–30 mg/kg iv for the 1st dose (further dosing, see p. 462)

2. MRSA (METHICILLIN-RESISTANT *STAPHYLOCOCCUS AUREUS*)

Treatment

* Vancomycin (IV)

Followed by (if bacteria are susceptible):

If MRSA is susceptible to clindamycin and patient is not critically ill
* Clindamycin (IV) **then** clindamycin (**or** doxycycline **or** cotrimoxazole) (PO)

If MRSA is resistant to all above oral drugs, but is susceptible to rifampicin and fusidate
* Rifampicin (PO) **plus** fusidate sodium (PO)

Duration of therapy

See p. 258

Dosage of above antibiotics

* Vancomycin 25–30 mg/kg IV for the 1st dose (further dosing, see p. 462)
* Clindamycin 600 mg (child: 15 mg/kg up to 600 mg) IV q8h, **then** 450 mg (child: 10 mg/kg up to 450 mg) PO q8h
* Doxycycline 100 mg (child >8 years: 2 mg/kg up to 100 mg) PO q12h
* Cotrimoxazole 320/1600 mg (child >1 month: 8/40 mg/kg up to 320/1600 mg) PO q12h
* Rifampicin 300 mg (child: 7.5 mg/kg up to 300 mg) PO q12h
* Fusidate sodium 500 mg (child: 12 mg/kg up to 250 mg) PO q12h

3. GRAM-NEGATIVE INFECTION

Pathogens

* Enterobacteriaceae (e.g. *E. coli* and *Klebsiella*) and *Pseudomonas* spp account for 20% of vertebral osteomyelitis
* *Haemophilus influenzae* type b (Hib) may be the cause in children <5 years who have not received Hib vaccination
* *Kingella kingae* may be a cause in infants and children with negative blood culture

Treatment

If *E. coli* or *Klebsiella* or Hib or *Kingella kingae* infection is suspected or confirmed
* Option 1: ceftriaxone (IV) (not for neonates and preterm infants)*
* Option 2: cefotaxime (IV)

---

*Ceftriaxone displaces bilirubin from albumin and may increase the risk of bilirubin encephalopathy in neonates

If immediate penicillin allergy, seek expert advice
- Ciprofloxacin (IV)

If *Pseudomonas* spp are confirmed
- Ceftazidime (IV)

Oral continuation therapy (guided by susceptibility testing), seek expert advice

- Ciprofloxacin (PO)

For other gram-negative infections, seek expert advice

- Antibiotic choice according to the culture and susceptibility

Duration of therapy

See below

Dosage of above antibiotics

- Ceftriaxone 2 g (child: 50 mg/kg up to 2 g) IV daily
- Cefotaxime 2 g (child: 50 mg/kg up to 2 g) IV q8h
- Ciprofloxacin 400 mg (child: 10 mg/kg up to 400 mg) IV q12h
- Ceftazidime 2 g (child: 50 mg/kg up to 2 g) IV q8h
- Ciprofloxacin 750 mg (child: 20 mg/kg up to 750 mg) PO q12h

Duration of therapy for osteomyelitis due to MSSA or MRSA

Acute osteomyelitis:

- Neonate—IV therapy for 4 weeks (all IV)
- Child—IV therapy for 3 days, followed by oral therapy for total of at least 3 weeks
- Adult—IV therapy for 4 weeks,* followed by oral therapy for total of at least 6 weeks

Chronic osteomyelitis:

- Child—oral therapy for at least 6 weeks
- Adult—IV therapy for 2 weeks,* followed by oral therapy for many months

Outpatient parenteral antimicrobial therapy

Once stable with inpatient IV therapy—may switch to outpatient IV therapy
- Flucloxacillin 8 g/day continuous infusion or intermittent bolus via programmable pump

For MRSA, MR-CNS or penicillin allergy
- Vancomycin** 24-hour continuous infusion or twice-daily intermittent infusions

---

*Once stable, outpatient parenteral antimicrobial therapy may be used
**Vancomycin dose is according to the plasma concentration monitoring (see p. 462)

OSTEOMYELITIS—INVOLVING PROSTHESES

Pathogens

- MSSA (methicillin-susceptible *Staphylococcus aureus*)
- MRSA (methicillin-resistant *Staphylococcus aureus*)
- MS-CNS (methicillin-sensitive, coagulase-negative staphylococci, e.g. *Staphylococcus epidermidis*)—late chronic infection
- MR-CNS (methicillin-resistant, coagulase-negative staphylococci, e.g. *Staphylococcus epidermidis*)—late chronic infection
- Beta-haemolytic streptococci—early postoperative and late haematogenous infection
- Aerobic gram-negative organisms—early postoperative and late haematogenous infection
- *Enterococcus* spp—late chronic infection
- *Propionibacterium* spp—late chronic infection
- Polymicrobial infections also occur

Classification of arthroplasty device infection

1. **Early postoperative infection** (within 1 month after original implantation)
2. **Late chronic infection** (>1 month after original implantation, insidious onset)
3. **Late acute haematogenous infection** (sudden onset in a previously well-functioning joint)

Specimen collection and culture

- At least 5 tissue biopsies and a specimen of synovial fluid during operation in the absence of antibiotics should be collected
- Treatment must be guided by the susceptibility of the organism isolated from aspiration or biopsies

1. EXCHANGE ARTHROPLASTY

Treatment

Two stage–exchange arthroplasty (85–95% success rate):

- Extensive debridement, removal of prosthesis, insertion of an antibiotic-impregnated spacer
- Followed by 6 weeks of IV antibiotic therapy (antibiotic treatment should be guided by susceptibility of organism isolated from aspiration or biopsies)

For empirical therapy while awaiting the results of cultures, or if cultures are negative

- Vancomycin (IV)
- Cease IV antibiotics at least 7–14 days prior to the second-stage operation
- A new prosthesis is inserted at the second-stage operation

- Intraoperative tissue cultures are taken at the second-stage operation; if positive, a further 6 weeks of IV antibiotics should be given

Dosage of above antibiotic

- Vancomycin IV daily (monitor blood levels and adjust dose, see p. 462)

One stage–exchange arthroplasty has similar success rate when performed in experienced centres

2. IMPLANT RETENTION

Debridement and implant retention (DAIR) may be used if the following criteria are met:

- Stable prosthesis with no periprosthetic lytic area on x-ray
- Good condition of surrounding skin and soft tissue
- Not immunocompromised
- No sepsis or septic shock
- Culture confirmation of a single organism that is susceptible to oral antibiotics suitable for treatment of bone infection

Treatment

- Extensive debridement, removal of exchangeable components; retain the prosthesis
- Followed by 6 weeks of IV antibiotic therapy with or without additional 6 weeks of oral antibiotic therapy (antibiotic choice, see Osteomyelitis—direct therapy)
- Alternative regimens: rifampicin-based regimens (1–2 weeks of IV beta-lactam antibiotic or vancomycin, followed by 3–6 months of oral rifampicin + fusidate or a quinolone)

If patient is not fit for surgery

- Long-term suppression therapy—a cure is unlikely, but suppression of infection with long-term antibiotics may be possible (seek expert advice)

OTITIS EXTERNA

1. ACUTE DIFFUSE OTITIS EXTERNA (SWIMMER'S EAR)

Pathogens

- Bacteria—*Pseudomonas aeruginosa*, *Staphylococcus aureus*, Corynebacteria, *Proteus* and *Klebsiella* spp
- Fungus—*Candida* and *Aspergillus* spp (frequently occur after prolonged topical steroid/antibiotic therapy)

Risk factors

- Maceration of the ear canals with water; skin damage of the ear canal (dermatitis)

Treatment

- Ear toilet—remove debris or exudate either by mechanical suction under direct vision or by dry mopping with small cottonwool ball; avoid syringing with water
- Send swabs for culture
- Antibiotic eardrops with or without corticosteroid

Treat bacterial infection

Options of eardrops

Treat bacterial infection
- Dexamethasone + framycetin + gramicidin eardrops (e.g. Sofradex, Otodex) 3 drops tds for 3–7 days

Treat bacterial and fungal infection
- Flumethasone + clioquinol eardrops (e.g. Locacorten-Vioform) 3 drops bid for 3–7 days
- Triamcinolone + neomycin + gramicidin + nystatin eardrops (e.g. Kenacomb Otic, Otocomb Otic) 3 drops tds for 3–7 days

If tympanic membrane perforation is present
- Ciprofloxacin eardrops (e.g. Ciloxan) 3 drops tds for 7 days

If no response or *P. aeruginosa* is isolated
- Ciprofloxacin + hydrocortisone eardrops (e.g. Ciproxin HC) 3 drops bid for 7 days

Treat bacterial infection without underlying dermatitis

Antibiotic-only eardrops may be used

- Framycetin eardrops (e.g. Soframycin Ear) 2–3 drops tds for 7 days

Note

- For children, preferred choice of eardrops is ciprofloxacin +/− hydrocortisone
- Do not use aminoglycoside-containing (framycetin, neomycin) eardrops for >7 days if tympanic membrane is perforated (to reduce the risk of ototoxicity)
- Secondary fungal infection usually occurs after prolonged topical steroid/antibiotic use
- If ear canal swelling, insert a gauze wick saturated with eardrops; review daily
- If severe infection fails to respond after 2–3 days, refer to ENT specialist
- If infection involves cartilage or perichondrium of canal, hospital admission

Prevention of swimmer's ear

See Recurrent otitis externa below

2. Recurrent otitis externa

Treatment

- Treat as Acute diffuse otitis externa
- Avoid aminoglycoside eardrops in children

Prevention

- Keep ear canals free of water—use either:

Earplugs during showering and swimming

- Disposable earplugs or petroleum jelly-coated cottonwool ball to cover the opening of the canals during swimming and showering

Eardrops to dry up (evaporate) ear canals after swimming or bathing

- Acetic acid/glycerol + isopropyl alcohol eardrops (e.g. Aquaear, Ear Clear for Swimmers Ear) 4–6 drops into each ear after shaking the water out

3. Necrotising otitis externa

Necrotising otitis externa (malignant otitis externa, MOE) occurs when infection spreads to the cartilage and bone of the external ear canal and skull base (skull base osteomyelitis).

Pathogen

- *Pseudomonas aeruginosa*

Risk factors

- Usually occurs in elderly, diabetic or immunocompromised patients

Clinical

- Severe pain, fever, visible granulation tissue and progressive cranial neuropathies

Treatment

- Swab for culture
- CT or bone scan if there is suspicion of skull base osteomyelitis
- Urgent referral to an ENT specialist or ID practitioner
- Antipseudomonal therapy (combination of systemic and topical treatment)
  - Option 1: ceftazidime (IV) **plus** gentamicin (IV)
  - Option 2: piperacillin/tazobactam (IV) **plus** gentamicin (IV)

If immediate penicillin allergy

- Ciprofloxacin (IV) **plus** gentamicin (IV)

Together with topical antipseudomonal therapy

- Ciprofloxacin eardrops (e.g. Ciloxan) 5 drops top q12h

Dosage of above antibiotics

- Ceftazidime 2 g (child: 50 mg/kg up to 2 g) IV q8h
- Gentamicin 4–7 mg/kg IV for the 1st dose (further dosing, see p. 459)

- Piperacillin/tazobactam 4 g (child: 100 mg/kg up to 4 g) IV q6h
- Ciprofloxacin 400 mg (child: 10 mg/kg up to 400 mg) IV q8h

4. ACUTE LOCALISED OTITIS EXTERNA

Pathogens

- A boil/furuncle involving ear canal or pinna—*Staphylococcus aureus*
- Erysipelas or cellulitis involving ear canal and pinna—*Streptococcus pyogenes*

Treatment

- Swabs for culture, if available
- Surgical drainage may be required
- Oral antibiotic treatment
  - Option 1: flucloxacillin (PO) for 5 days
  - Option 2: cefalexin (PO) for 5 days (if allergic to penicillin)
  - Option 3: clindamycin (PO) for 5 days (if immediate penicillin allergy)

Dosage of above antibiotics

  - Flucloxacillin 500 mg (child: 12.5 mg up to 500 mg) PO q6h
  - Cefalexin 500 mg (child: 12.5 mg/kg up to 500 mg) PO q6h
  - Clindamycin 300–450 mg (child: 7.5–10 mg/kg up to 450 mg) PO q8h

5. OTITIS EXTERNA—OTOMYCOSIS (FUNGAL EAR INFECTION, SINGAPORE EAR)

Pathogen

- *Candida albicans*, *Aspergillus niger* or *Aspergillus flavus*

Risk factors

- Prolonged use of topical antibiotics/steroids
- Diabetes
- Underlying dermatitis
- Warm, humid and/or wet environment
- Presence of cerumen

Clinical

- Presence of greyish-white thick debris

Diagnosis

- Swab for fungal culture

Treatment

- Thoroughly clean and dry the ear canal
Antifungal ear drops
  - Flumethasone/clioquinol ear drops (e.g. Locacorten-Vioform) 3 drops tds

- Triamcinolone/neomycin/gramicidin/nystatin ear drops (e.g. Kenacomb Otic, Otocomb Otic) 3 drops tds or insert gauze wick saturated with the drops

Antifungal cream
- Option 1: terbinafine 1% cream (e.g. Lamisil, SolvEasy) top daily
- Option 2: bifonazole1% cream (e.g. Mycospor) top daily
- Option 3: clotrimazole 1% cream (e.g. Canesten) top bid
- Option 4: econazole 1% cream (e.g. Dermazole, Pevaryl Topicals) top bid
- Option 5: ketoconazole 2% cream (e.g. Nizoral, DaktaGOLD) top bid
- Option 6: miconazole 2% cream (e.g. Daktarin) top bid

If no response

Referral to ENT specialist

OTITIS MEDIA

1. ACUTE OTITIS MEDIA

Pathogens

- Viral—frequently during a viral (e.g. respiratory syncytial virus) URTI
- Bacterial—*Streptococcus pneumoniae*, *Haemophilus influenzae*, *Moraxella catarrhalis* and *Streptococcus pyogenes*

Clinical

- Mild inflammation of the middle ear with reddening and fullness of the tympanic membrane

Treatment

Adult acute otitis media is treated in the same way as it is treated in children

Early antibiotic treatment is indicated for:

- All children with systemic features (i.e. vomiting and fever)
- All children aged <6 months (even without systemic features)
- All patients in remote Aboriginal and Torres Strait Islander communities (to prevent suppurative complications, e.g. mastoiditis)
- Immunocompromised patients with early acute otitis media

Delayed antibiotic therapy may be applied to:

- Children aged 6 months to 2 years with no systemic features—review after 24 hours, or provide a 'wait-and-see' antibiotic script; if condition worsens after 24 hours, start antibiotic
- Children aged ≥2 years with no systemic features—review in 2 days, or provide a 'wait-and-see' antibiotic script; if condition worsens after 2 days, start antibiotic

Antibiotic treatment

- Amoxicillin (PO) for 5 days

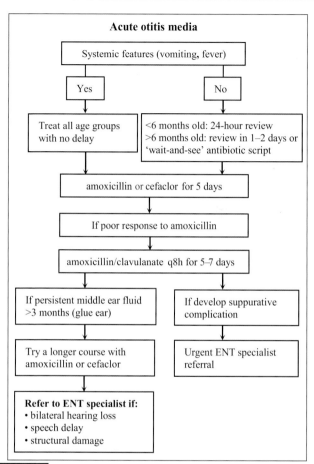

Management of otitis media in children

If poor response to amoxicillin (beta-lactamase–producing gram-negative bacteria)
- Amoxicillin/clavulanate (PO) q8h for 5–7 days

If non-immediate penicillin allergy
- Cefuroxime (PO) for 5 days

If immediate penicillin allergy
- Cotrimoxazole (PO) for 5 days

If still fails to respond, seek expert advice

For persistent middle ear fluid

- No antibiotic is indicated: 90% will spontaneously resolve in 3 months; 10% may develop into glue ear (see below)

If develops suppurative complication (e.g. mastoiditis or facial palsy)

- Urgent referral to ENT specialist

Dosage of above antibiotics

- Amoxicillin 500 mg (child: 15 mg/kg up to 500 mg) PO q8h **or** amoxicillin 1 g (child: 30 mg/kg up to 1 g) PO q12h
- Amoxicillin/clavulanate 875 mg (child: 22.5 mg/kg up to 500 mg) PO q12h
- Cefuroxime 500 mg (child 3 months–2 years: 10 mg/kg up to 125 mg; >2 years: 15 mg/kg up to 500 mg) PO q12h
- Cotrimoxazole 160/800 mg (child >1 month: 4/20 mg/kg up to 160/800 mg) PO q12h

2. RECURRENT BACTERIAL OTITIS MEDIA

- Defined as ≥3 distinct episodes in 6 months or ≥4 episodes in 12 months

Pathogens

- *Alloiococcus otitidis* (gram-positive cocci)—the most common pathogen of chronic otitis media in children
- *Corynebacterium*
- *Staphylococcus aureus*
- *Haemophilus influenzae*

Risk factors

- Exposure to smoke
- Allergic rhinitis
- Adenoid disease
- Structural anomalies (e.g. cleft palate, Down syndrome)
- Group childcare
- *Alloiococcus otitidis* infection is a major factor of chronicity (slow growth)

Laboratory

- Ear swab for culture and sensitivity
- PCR for *Alloiococcus otitidis*—fast and sensitive
- Ear swab for *Alloiococcus otitidis* culture—takes 7–14 days to grow

Treatment

- Remove risk factors
- Treat each episode as Acute otitis media (p. 264)
- *Alloiococcus otitidis* is resistant to beta-lactam antibiotics and erythromycin

- Antibiotic prophylaxis is not advised
- Frequent recurrence may need referral for grommet insertion

3. OTITIS MEDIA WITH EFFUSION (OME) (GLUE EAR)

Clinical

- Persistent middle ear effusion >3 months with dull earache, imbalance, conductive hearing loss, visible grey-white or blue fluid and immobile tympanic membrane with dilated blood vessels on pneumatoscopy, without signs of acute inflammation.
- Child may present with behavioural problems as a result of undetected hearing loss

Treatment

- **Hearing test**—for school-aged children with hearing loss, placement at the front of the class, hearing aids or amplification
- **ENT specialist referral for following conditions:**
    - Bilateral hearing loss on audiometry
    - Speech delay or educational disability
    - Tympanic membrane significant retraction
    - Cholesteatoma suspected or confirmed
- Try a longer course of antibiotic therapy
    - Amoxicillin (PO) for 10–30 days

If non-immediate penicillin allergy

- Cefuroxime (PO) for 10–30 days

If immediate penicillin allergy

- Cotrimoxazole (PO) for 10–30 days

Dosage of above antibiotics

- Amoxicillin 500 mg (child: 15 mg/kg up to 500 mg) PO q8h **or** Amoxicillin 1 g (child: 30 mg/kg up to 1 g) PO q12h
- Cefuroxime 500 mg (child 3 months–2 years: 10 mg/kg up to 125 mg; >2 years: 15 mg/kg up to 500 mg) PO q12h
- Cotrimoxazole 160/800 mg (child >1 month: 4/20 mg/kg up to 160/800 mg) PO q12h

4. CHRONIC SUPPURATIVE OTITIS MEDIA (CSOM)

Clinical

- Tympanic membrane perforation and ear discharge for at least 6 weeks
- It can cause conductive hearing loss, intracranial infections and mastoiditis (occasionally)

Treatment

Ear toilet prior to topical treatment—dry mopping with rolled tissue spears 4 times daily, or suction under direct vision until the ear canal is dry
If tympanic membrane perforation <6 weeks—oral antibiotic + eardrops

- If ear discharge has persisted >6 weeks—eardrops alone
- If persistent discharge >3 months—refer to ENT specialist

Oral antibiotics

- Amoxicillin (**or** amoxicillin/clavulanate) (PO) for 7 days

If non-immediate penicillin allergy

- Cefuroxime (PO) for 7 days

If immediate penicillin allergy

- Cotrimoxazole (PO) for 7 days

Eardrops

- Ciprofloxacin eardrops (e.g. Ciloxan) 5 drops q12h

If secondary fungal infection occurs

- Flumethasone/clioquinol ear drops (e.g. Locacorten-Vioform) 3 drops tds

For persistent aural discharge

- Refer to ENT specialist for assessment of possible cholesteatoma or chronic osteitis

Dosage of above antibiotics

- Amoxicillin 500 mg (child: 15 mg/kg up to 500 mg) PO Q8h **or** amoxicillin 1 g (child: 30 mg/kg up to 1 g) PO q12h
- Cefuroxime 500 mg (child 3 months–2 years: 10 mg/kg up to 125 mg; >2 years: 15 mg/kg up to 500 mg) PO q12h
- Cotrimoxazole 160/800 mg (child >1 month: 4/20 mg/kg up to 160/800 mg) PO q12h

Vaccination

- Vaccines against a wide range of pneumococcal serotypes and *Haemophilus influenzae* serotypes including non-typeable *Haemophilus influenzae* (NTHi) (e.g. Synflorix) provide protection against otitis media

PANCREATITIS—ACUTE NECROTISING

About 30% of people with acute necrotising pancreatitis (ANP) develop infection of the damaged pancreatic tissue.

Pathogens

- *Escherichia coli*
- *Klebsiella pneumoniae*
- *Enterococcus faecalis*
- *Staphylococcus aureus*
- *Pseudomonas aeruginosa*
- *Proteus mirabilis*
- *Streptococcus* spp

Diagnosis

- Elevated WBCs with a left shift—suggests infected necrosis or pancreatic abscess
- Blood cultures—if positive, suggest infected necrosis or pancreatic abscess
- Pancrease needle aspiration under CT or ultrasound guidance for Gram stain and culture
- Abdominal x-ray—presence of air in a pseudocyst is specific for infection
- Abdominal CT with IV contrast—lack of uptake of contrast may reveal ischaemic pancreatic tissue
- Endoscopic or transabdominal ultrasound
- MRI (with gadolinium)—decreased contrast on MRI

Treatment

- Supportive—pay attention to blood pressure and volume status
- Percutaneous or surgical drainage and/or debridement of infected necrosis and abscess
- CT-guided drainage for the patient who is intolerant of open drainage
- Endoscopic ultrasound (EUS) with transgastric drainage is another option
- Prophylactic antibiotics are not recommended

Antibiotic treatment

Antibiotic treatment is indicated for:

- Newly developed sepsis
- Evidence of systemic inflammatory response syndrome (SIRS)
- Newly developed multiorgan failure

Empirical treatment
  - Piperacillin/tazobactam (IV)

If non-immediate penicillin allergy
  - Ceftriaxone (**or** cefotaxime) (IV) **plus** metronidazole (IV)

If immediate penicillin allergy seek expert advice

If a pancreatic abscess develops, treat as Peritonitis—post viscus perforation (p. 278)

Dosage of above antibiotics

- Piperacillin/tazobactam 4 g (child: 100 mg/kg up to 4 g) IV q6h
- Ceftriaxone 1 g (child: 50 mg/kg up to 1 g) IV daily
- Cefotaxime 1 g (child: 50 mg/kg up to 1 g) IV q8h
- Metronidazole 500 mg (child: 12.5 mg/kg up to 500 mg) IV q12h

PARONYCHIA AND WHITLOW—ACUTE

Acute paronychia—an infection of the tissue at the side or base of the nail

Whitlow—an infection of the pulp of the distal finger

Felon—abscess of the pulp of the distal finger

Eponychia—an infection that extends into the eponychium

Pathogens

- *Staphylococcus aureus*
- Anaerobes (contracted through nail biting or finger sucking)

Clinical

- Red and swollen around the nail. Pus may collect under the skin of the lateral fold (paronychia)
- If untreated, the infection can extend into the eponychium (eponychia)
- Further extension of the infection can involve both lateral folds as it tracks under the nail sulcus (run-around infection)
- The infection may produce a concomitant abscess of the pulp of the distal finger (felon)
- The infection of the nail bed may lift the nail off the nail bed

Treatment

- Rule out herpetic whitlow (p. 165)
- Warm water soaks of the affected finger three times a day until symptoms resolve
- Drainage if abscess forms, wound/pus swab for culture
- Oral antibiotics
  - Option 1: flucloxacillin (PO) for 5–7 days
  - Option 2 (to cover anaerobes): amoxicillin/clavulanate (PO) for 5–7 days

If penicillin allergy
  - Option 1: cefalexin 500 mg (PO) for 5–7 days
  - Option 2 (to cover anaerobes): clindamycin (PO) for 5–7 days

Dosage of above antibiotics

- Flucloxacillin 500 mg (child: 25 mg/kg up to 500 mg) PO q6h
- Amoxicillin/clavulanate 500–875 mg (child: 22.5 mg/kg) PO q12h
- Cefalexin 500 mg (child: 12.5 mg/kg up to 500 mg) PO q6h
- Clindamycin 300–450 mg (child: 10 mg/kg up to 450 mg) PO q8h

PARONYCHIA—CHRONIC

Chronic paronychia is a slow progressive nail infection with painless nail dystrophy.

Pathogens

- *Candida* spp
- Gram-negative bacilli
- *Staphylococcus aureus*
- Medication-induced chronic paronychia—toxicity from medications such as retinoids and protease inhibitors (e.g. the antiretroviral drug indinavir may cause chronic paronychia in HIV patients)

Clinical

- Swollen, red and tender nail folds without fluctuance
- Eventually, the nail plates become thickened and discoloured, with pronounced transverse ridges; the cuticles and nail folds may separate from the nail plate, forming a space for the invasion of various microorganisms

Treatment

- Keep hands dry and warm—avoid exposure to moisture or skin irritants
- Avoid manipulation of the nails (such as manicuring and finger sucking)
- Medication-induced chronic paronychia usually resolves after the medication has been discontinued
- Antibiotic/antifungal + topical steroid

For staphylococcal infection
- Antibiotics as Acute paronychia (p. 270)

For *Candida* infection
- Miconazole 2% tincture (e.g. Daktarin) top bid for 5–7 days

Topical steroid ointment
- Potent corticosteroid oint (e.g. Diproson OV) top daily for 14–21 days

More severe cases
- Fluconazole 150–300 mg PO weekly for 3–12 months

When there is persistent exudate—to dry out the area
- Thymol 4% in alcohol 70%, apply to the base of the nail*

---

*Require extemporaneous preparation

If the area is dry—to waterproof the area
* White soft paraffin top 5–10 times daily

Refer unresponsive patients to a dermatologist

PAROTITIS

Other names: acute suppurative parotitis, salivary gland infection
Parotitis is inflammation of one or both parotid glands.

Pathogen

* *Staphylococcus aureus*, occasionally polymicrobial

Causes and risk factors

* Blockage of main parotid duct or one of its branches by a salivary stone, a mucus plug or a benign tumour
* More common in older people, who often take medications that cause dry mouth (xerostomia) or who are dehydrated or debilitated by chronic disease; when saliva flow is reduced, bacteria may cause the parotid gland infection

Clinical

* Swelling and pain in parotid gland with tender and inflamed skin

Diagnosis

Parotid gland stones may be detected by:

* Ultrasonography of the parotid gland
* X-ray (sialography)
* CT scan of the parotid gland

Treatment

* Remove the salivary stones by manipulation, lithotripsy or surgery
* Early surgical drainage may be required
* Gram stain, culture and sensitivity testing for the drained pus
* Antibiotic therapy
  * Flucloxacillin (IV **then** PO) for a total of 10 days
If penicillin allergy
  * Clindamycin (IV **then** PO) for a total of 10 days

Adjust antibiotics according to culture and sensitivity report

Dosage of above antibiotics

* Flucloxacillin 1–2 g (child: 25–50 mg/kg up to 2 g) IV q6h
* Flucloxacillin 250–500 mg (child: 12.5–25 mg up to 500 mg) PO q6h
* Clindamycin 450 mg (child: 10 mg/kg up to 450 mg) IV q8h
* Clindamycin 300–450 mg (child: 5–10 mg/kg up to 450 mg) PO q8h

PELVIC INFLAMMATORY DISEASE

Pelvic inflammatory disease (PID) includes endometritis, chorioamnionitis, salpingitis, tubo-ovarian abscess, pelvic cellulitis and pelvic peritonitis.

1. SEXUALLY ACQUIRED PID

Pathogens

- *Chlamydia trachomatis*
- *Neisseria gonorrhoeae*
- *Mycoplasma genitalium* (10–20%)
- Endogenous vaginal flora may subsequently be involved

Clinical

- Pelvic or lower abdominal pain, dysuria, dyspareunia, vaginal discharge/bleeding
- Fever, pelvic tenderness, cervical motion tenderness/adnexal tenderness, adnexal mass

Laboratory

- Self-collected vaginal swab or endocervical swab—PCR testing for *C. trachomatis*, *N. gonorrhoea* and *M. genitalium*
- Endocervical swab—for microscopy, Gram stain and culture of *N. gonorrhoea* for susceptibility testing (required on any isolated gonococci)
- APTIMA® assay for *Chlamydia* and gonorrhoea (urine/vaginal or endocervical swab)—more sensitive and specific than PCR testing (requires green-topped urine container and APTIMA® swab collection kit)

Treatment

Mild to moderate infection

- Ceftriaxone (IM or IV) **plus** azithromycin (**or** doxycycline) (PO) **plus** metronidazole (PO) for 2 weeks

If immediate penicillin allergy seek expert advice

Severe infection (treat in hospital)

- Ceftriaxone (**or** cefotaxime) (IV) **plus** azithromycin (IV) **plus** metronidazole (IV)

If immediate penicillin allergy

- Gentamicin (IV) **plus** azithromycin (IV) **plus** clindamycin (IV)

Continue IV therapy until clinical improvement then change to oral

- Metronidazole (PO) **plus** doxycycline (PO)

Duration of treatment

- Total (IV + oral) for at least 2 weeks

If *M. genitalium* PCR test is positive and above treatment fails
- Moxifloxacin 400 mg PO daily for 10 days

Sexual contacts should be examined, investigated and treated

Dosage of above antibiotics

Mild to moderate infection
- Ceftriaxone 500 mg in 2 mL 1% lidocaine (lignocaine) IM or 500 mg IV st
- Azithromycin 1 g PO st, a 2nd dose 1 week later
- Doxycycline 100 mg PO q12h
- Metronidazole 400 mg PO q12h

Severe infection
- Ceftriaxone 2 g IV daily
- Cefotaxime 2 g IV q8h
- Azithromycin 500 mg IV daily
- Metronidazole 500 mg IV q12h
- Gentamicin 4–7 mg/kg IV for the 1st dose (further dosing, see p. 459)
- Clindamycin 600 mg IV q8h
- Doxycycline 100 mg PO q12h
- Metronidazole 400 mg PO q12h

2.   NON-SEXUALLY ACQUIRED PID

Pathogens

Mixed organisms from vaginal flora, including:
- Anaerobes
- Facultative gram-negative bacteria
- *Mycoplasma hominis*

Risk factors

- Post-termination of pregnancy
- After delivery
- Pelvic surgery
- Following insertion of an intrauterine contraceptive device (IUCD)

Clinical

- Pelvic or lower abdominal pain, dysuria, dyspareunia, vaginal discharge/bleeding
- Fever, pelvic tenderness, cervical motion tenderness/adnexal tenderness, adnexal mass

Treatment

- Removal of retained products of conception
- Removal of IUCD if infection is severe and response to treatment is poor

Mild to moderate infection

* Amoxicillin/clavulanate (PO) **plus** doxycycline (PO) for 14 days

If penicillin allergy

* Ciprofloxacin **plus** metronidazole (PO) for 14 days

Severe infection (treat in hospital)

* Ampi(amoxi)cillin (IV) **plus** gentamicin (IV) **plus** metronidazole (IV)

If penicillin allergy or if gentamicin is contraindicated

* Ceftriaxone (**or** cefotaxime) (IV) **plus** azithromycin (IV) **plus** metronidazole (IV)

If immediate penicillin allergy seek expert advice

* Clindamycin (IV) **plus** gentamicin (IV)

Continue IV therapy until clinical improvement then change to oral

* Option 1: amoxicillin/clavulanate (PO) **plus** doxycycline (PO)
* Option 2: ciprofloxacin (PO) **plus** metronidazole (PO) (if penicillin allergy)

Duration of treatment

* Total (IV + oral) for at least 2 weeks

Dosage of above antibiotics

* Amoxicillin/clavulanate 875 mg PO q12h
* Doxycycline 100 mg PO q12h
* Ciprofloxacin 500 mg PO q12h
* Metronidazole 400 mg PO q12h
* Ampi(amoxi)cillin 2 g IV q6h
* Gentamicin 4–7 mg/kg IV for the 1st dose (further dosing, see p. 459)
* Metronidazole 500 mg IV q12h
* Ceftriaxone 1 g IV daily
* Cefotaxime 2 g IV q8h
* Azithromycin 500 mg IV daily
* Clindamycin 600 mg IV q8h

3. PELVIC ACTINOMYCOSIS

* A rare cause of PID, often associated with IUCD use (see Actinomycosis, p. 3)

PERIANAL INFECTION

1. PERIANAL CELLULITIS

Pathogen

* *Streptococcus pyogenes*

Laboratory

* Anal swab for culture

Treatment

- Option 1: penicillin V 500 mg PO q6h for 7 days
- Option 2: amoxicillin 500 mg PO q8h for 7 days

2. PERIANAL ABSCESS

Other names: anorectal abscess, perirectal abscess

Treatment

- Surgery—incision and drainage of the abscess
- Antibiotics—to cover rectal flora (not the skin flora)
- An anorectal abscess that is untreated or not fully drained can worsen and cause a severe local or systemic infection, which can be life-threatening (e.g. Fournier's gangrene, p. 123 or sepsis)

Mild perianal abscess

- Option 1: amoxicillin/clavulanate 875 mg PO q12h for 5–10 days
- Option 2: cefalexin 500 mg PO q6h **plus** metronidazole 400 mg PO q12h for 5–10 days (if non-immediate penicillin allergy)
- Option 3: cotrimoxazole 160/800 mg PO q12h **plus** metronidazole 400 mg PO q12h for 5–10 days (if immediate penicillin allergy)

Severe perianal abscess

- Option 1: ampi(amoxi)cillin 2 g IV q6h **plus** gentamicin 4–7 mg/kg IV daily **plus** metronidazole 500 mg IV q12h
- Option 2: piperacillin/tazobactam 4 g IV q8h
- Option 3: ticarcillin/clavulanate 3 g IV q6h
- Option 4: ceftriaxone 1 g IV daily (**or** cefotaxime 1 g IV q8h) **plus** metronidazole 500 mg IV q12h (if non-immediate penicillin allergy)
- Option 5: vancomycin 1 g IV q12h **plus** gentamicin 4–7 mg/kg IV daily **plus** metronidazole 500 mg IV q12h (if immediate penicillin allergy)

Change to oral after improvement: see Mild perianal abscess (above)

PERIORBITAL AND ORBITAL CELLULITIS

Both periorbital and orbital cellulitis are potentially life-threatening.

1. PERIORBITAL (PRE-SEPTAL) CELLULITIS

- Caused by local trauma or local infection, e.g. stye, dacrycystitis, impetigo or boil

Pathogens

- Children <5 years—*Streptococcus pneumoniae*, *Streptococcus anginosus*/*milleri* group or *Haemophilus influenzae* type b (Hib)
- Adults and children >5 years—*Staphylococcus aureus*

Treatment

Child <5 years

Mild infection (afebrile)
- Option 1: cefalexin (PO) for 7 days (does not cover Hib)
- Option 2: amoxicillin/clavulanate (PO) for 7 days (covers Hib)
- Option 3: cefuroxime (PO) for 7 days (covers Hib)
- Option 4: clindamycin (PO) for 7 days (if immediate penicillin allergy)

Severe infection (regardless of Hib immunisation)
- Option 1: cefotaxime (IV)
- Option 2: ceftriaxone (IV) **plus** flucloxacillin (IV)

After improvement, change to oral amoxicillin/clavulanate to complete 7-day course

Adult or child >5 years

Mild infection
- Option 1: flucloxacillin (PO) for 7 days
- Option 2: cefalexin (PO) for 7 days
- Option 3: clindamycin (PO) for 7 days (if immediate penicillin allergy)

Severe infection
- Option 1: cefotaxime (IV)
- Option 2: ceftriaxone (IV) **plus** flucloxacillin (IV)

After improvement, change to oral amoxicillin/clavulanate to complete 7-day course

Refer to an ophthalmologist
If MRSA is suspected, seek expert advice

Dosage of above antibiotics

Child <5 years
- Cefalexin 12.5 mg/kg PO q6h
- Amoxicillin/clavulanate 22.5 mg/kg PO q12h
- Cefuroxime (child 3 months–2 years: 10 mg/kg up to 125 mg; >2 years: 15 mg/kg up to 500 mg) PO q12h
- Clindamycin 10 mg/kg PO q8h
- Cefotaxime 50 mg/kg IV q8h
- Ceftriaxone 50 mg/kg IV daily
- Flucloxacillin 25–50 mg/kg IV q6h

Adult or child >5 years
- Flucloxacillin 500 mg PO q6h
- Cefalexin 500 mg PO q6h
- Clindamycin 450 mg PO q8h
- Cefotaxime 2 g IV q8h
- Ceftriaxone 2 g IV daily
- Flucloxacillin 2 g IV q6h

2. ORBITAL (POST-SEPTAL) CELLULITES

- Caused by spreading of paranasal sinus infection or orbital trauma

Pathogens

- *Haemophilus influenzae*
- *Streptococcus pneumoniae*, *Streptococcus anginosus*/*milleri* group
- *Staphylococcus aureus*
- Aerobic gram-negative bacteria
- Anaerobes

Clinical

- Painful and limited eye movement, reduced vision or proptosis
- Blood culture
- CT scan of sinuses

Treatment

- Urgent ophthalmologist referral for drainage of sinuses or abscess (to prevent loss of vision)
- Antibiotic therapy
  - Option 1: cefotaxime (IV) for 3–14 days
  - Option 2: ceftriaxone (IV) **plus** flucloxacillin (IV) for 3–14 days

If immediate penicillin allergy
  - Clindamycin (**or** vancomycin) (IV) for 3–14 days

After improvement, change to oral
  - Amoxicillin/clavulanate (PO) for a further 10 days

Dosage of above antibiotics

  - Cefotaxime 2 g (child: 50 mg/kg up to 2 g) IV q8h
  - Ceftriaxone 2 g (child: 50 mg/kg up to 2 g) IV daily
  - Flucloxacillin 2 g (child: 50 mg/kg up to 2 g) IV q6h
  - Clindamycin 600 mg (child: 15 mg/kg up to 600 mg) IV q8h
  - Vancomycin 25–30 mg/kg IV for the 1st dose (further dosing, see p. 462)
  - Amoxicillin/clavulanate 850 mg (child: 22.5 mg/kg up to 850 mg) PO q12h

PERITONITIS—POST VISCUS PERFORATION

Pathogens

Mixed infection with aerobic and anaerobic bowel flora, including:

- Gram-negative bacilli (e.g. *Escherichia coli*)
- Anaerobic bacteria (e.g. *Bacteroides fragilis*)

Treatment

- Surgical intervention is usually required
- Antibiotic therapy

Triple therapy

- Ampicillin (IV) **plus** gentamicin (IV) **plus** metronidazole (IV)

After 3 days of gentamicin or if gentamicin is contraindicated

- Option 1: piperacillin/tazobactam (IV)
- Option 2: ticarcillin/clavulanate (IV)

If non-immediate penicillin allergy

- Ceftriaxone (**or** cefotaxime) (IV) **plus** metronidazole (IV)

If immediate penicillin allergy

- Gentamicin (IV) **plus** clindamycin (IV)

After clinical improvement, switch to oral

- Option 1: amoxicillin/clavulanate (PO)
- Option 2: cotrimoxazole (PO) **plus** metronidazole (PO)

Duration of therapy

- Total of 7 days

Dosage of above antibiotics

- Ampicillin 2 g (child: 50 mg/kg up to 2 g) IV q6h
- Gentamicin 4–7 mg/kg (child: 7.5 mg/kg up to 320 mg) IV for the 1st dose (further dosing, see p. 459)
- Metronidazole 500 mg (child: 12.5 mg/kg up to 500 mg) IV q12h
- Piperacillin/tazobactam 4 g (child: 100 mg/kg up to 4 g) IV q8h
- Ticarcillin/clavulanate 3 g (child: 50 mg/kg up to 3 g) IV q6h
- Ceftriaxone 1 g (child: 50 mg/kg up to 1 g) IV daily
- Cefotaxime 1 g (child: 50 mg/kg up to 1 g) IV q8h
- Clindamycin 600 mg (child: 15 mg/kg up to 600 mg) IV q8h
- Amoxicillin/clavulanate 875/125 mg (child: 22.5/3.2 mg/kg up to 875/125 mg) PO q12h
- Cotrimoxazole 160/800 mg (child >1 month: 4/20 mg/kg up to 160/800 mg) PO q12h
- Metronidazole 400 mg (child: 10 mg/kg up to 400 mg) PO q12h

PERITONITIS—PERITONEAL DIALYSIS

Peritonitis is the most common complication of continuous ambulatory peritoneal dialysis.

Source of infection

- Bacteria may gain access to the peritoneal cavity through the subcutaneous tunnel around a catheter or via the catheter during bag exchange

Pathogens

- Gram-positive skin organisms e.g. *Staphylococcus epidermidis*, *S. aureus*
- Enteric gram-negative bacilli (less frequent)
- *Streptococcus* and *Enterococcus* spp
- Fungi, such as *Candida* spp (uncommon but difficult to eradicate)

Clinical

- Suspect peritonitis—dialysate becomes cloudy

Treatment

- Gram stain and culture of dialysate fluid (10 mL in blood culture bottles or centrifugation of several hundred mL of dialysate fluid before culture)
- Antibiotics can be given intraperitoneally and/or IV if the patient is severely ill
- Indication for catheter removal:
    - Failure to respond to antibiotics within 5 days
    - Exit-site and tunnel infections fail to respond to antibiotic treatment
    - Relapsing peritonitis
    - Fungal peritonitis
    - Mycobacteria peritonitis fails to respond to treatment
    - Polymicrobial infection with enteric pathogens fails to respond to treatment

If gram-positive bacteria in dialysate fluid
- Cefazolin (IP)

If gram-negative bacteria in dialysate fluid
- Option 1: gentamicin (IP)
- Option 2: cefepime (IP) (if non-anuric or gentamicin is contraindicated)

If Gram stain does not help—to cover both gram-positive and gram-negative bacteria
- Cefazolin (IP) **plus** gentamicin (**or** ceftazidime) (IP)

If MRSA is colonised or if immediate penicillin allergy
- Vancomycin (IP) **plus** gentamicin (**or** ceftazidime) (IP)

If diverticular disease or if bowel perforation is suspected **add**
- Metronidazole 500 mg IV q12h **or** 400 mg PO q12h

Modify antibiotic according to the culture and susceptibility results

Duration of treatment

- If gram-positive infection—for at least 14 days or 7 days after dialysate clears
- If gram-negative or *S. aureus* or *Enterococcus* infection—for at least 21 days

Dosage of above antibiotics

- Cefazolin (adult and child) 15 mg/kg added to 1 bag per day (intermittent administration)
  or cefazolin (adult and child) added to the 1st bag of dialysate to get concentration of 500 mg/L, then to get 125 mg/L in each subsequent bag of dialysate (continuous administration)

- Gentamicin (adult and child) 0.6 mg/kg up to 50 mg, added to 1 bag per day (intermittent administration)
  or gentamicin (adult and child) added to the 1st bag of dialysate to get concentration of 8 mg/L, then to get 4 mg/L in each subsequent bag of dialysate, up to a maximum of 40 mg/day (continuous administration)
- Cefepime 1 g (child: 15 mg/kg up to 1 g) added to 1 bag of dialysate per day (intermittent administration)
  or cefepime (adult and child) added to the 1st bag of dialysate to get concentration of 500 mg/L, then to get 125 mg/L in each subsequent bag of dialysate (continuous administration)
- Vancomycin 2 g (child: 50 mg/kg up to 2 g) added to 1 bag of dialysate every 5–7 days (intermittent administration)
  or vancomycin (adult) added to the 1st bag of dialysate to get concentration of 1 g/L, then to get 25 mg/L (child: 30 mg/L) in each subsequent bag of dialysate (continuous administration)

PERITONITIS—SPONTANEOUS BACTERIAL PERITONITIS

Other names: primary peritonitis, SBP

Pathogens

- Gram-negative bacilli—e.g. *Escherichia coli* (the most common) and *Klebsiella* spp
- Gram-positive organisms—e.g. *Streptococcus pneumoniae*, other streptococci and enterococci—more common in patients receiving prophylaxis with cotrimoxazole or norfloxacin
- Anaerobic bacteria—uncommon
- In children—*S. pneumoniae* (the most common cause)

Clinical

- Usually occurs in patients with chronic liver disease and ascites
- SBP should be considered in any patient with ascites whose clinical state deteriorates

Laboratory

Should exclude an intra-abdominal source of infection

- Ascitic tap—ascetic fluid culture (add 10 mL of peritoneal fluid into blood culture bottle)
- Ascitic fluid microscopy—WBC count (>500/mm^3) or neutrophil count (>250/mm^3)
- Ascites lactate level (elevated)
- Blood and urine cultures
- Chest and abdominal x-rays to exclude viscus perforation (free air)

Antibiotic treatment

If indicated, should be initiated ASAP

- Option 1: ceftriaxone 2 g (child >1 month: 50 mg/kg up to 2 g) IV daily
- Option 2: cefotaxime 2 g (child: 50 mg/kg up to 2 g) IV q8h

If streptococcal or enterococcal infection is suspected (common in patients receiving prophylaxis)

- Piperacillin/tazobactam 4 g (child: 100 mg/kg up to 4 g) IV q8h

If immediate penicillin allergy see expert advice

- Option 1: ciprofloxacin 400 mg (child: 10 mg/kg up to 400 mg) IV q12h
- Option 2: aztreonam 2 g (child: 50 mg/kg up to 2 g) IV q6–8h

Duration of treatment

- Modify antibiotics according to culture results and continue until the infection resolves (usually 5–10 days)

Prophylaxis

SBP has a high rate of recurrence
Indication for prophylaxis:

- Patients with previous SBP
- Patients with low ascitic protein levels (<10 g/L)

Children with ascites—prophylaxis is not routinely recommended

Long-term prophylaxis*

Cotrimoxazole 160/800 mg PO daily
If above regimen is contraindicated or has failed

- Norfloxacin 400 mg PO daily

PERTUSSIS

Other names: whooping cough

Pathogen

- *Bordetella pertussis*, a gram-negative pleomorphic bacillus

Transmission

- By droplets
- Highly infectious
- Becomes non-infectious 3 weeks after onset of cough or 5 days after antibiotic treatment

Incubation

4–21 days (average 7–10 days)

---

*Long-term antibiotic prophylaxis has been shown to increase the risk of severe staphylococcal or quinolone-resistant gram-negative bacterial infections

Clinical

- **Infants <6 months and preterm babies**—may become cyanotic or apnoeic during coughing attacks; high morbidity and mortality in non-immunised infants
- **Children**
  - Paroxysmal coughing bouts (may last up to 12 weeks)
  - Inspiratory whoop (a deep gasp after coughing bouts)
  - Post-tussive vomiting
  - Nil or mild fever
- **Adults** (90% of cases are adults)—prolonged cough with post-tussive vomiting, usually no whoop; infections in adults are less severe, but adults are the main source of disease spread to children

Complications

- Pneumonia, hypoxic encephalopathy and bronchiectasis (later)

Clinical diagnosis

- Acute cough lasting ≥14 days with post-tussive vomiting, apnoea or whoop
- Acute cough with history of contacting a laboratory-confirmed case

Laboratory confirmation of diagnosis

Should be notified to public health authority

- Pertussis PCR—nasopharyngeal swab or aspirate (good sensitivity and specificity, early diagnosis)
- Pertussis serology (IgA)—test 2–12 weeks following cough onset (sensitivity is low and negative cannot exclude pertussis)

Antibiotic treatment

- In catarrhal and early paroxysmal stages treatment may ameliorate the disease
- After early stage but within 3 weeks of onset, treatment may eliminate the bacteria (after 5 days of treatment) and reduce the infectious period, but may not reduce the duration and severity of cough
- After 3 weeks from onset, antibiotic treatment is not necessary
- Infants <6 months or with other conditions such as asthma may require hospital admission
  - Option 1: azithromycin (PO) for 5 days
  - Option 2: cotrimoxazole (PO) for 7 days
  - Option 3: clarithromycin (PO) for 7 days
- If allergic to macrolides
  - Option 4: cotrimoxazole (PO) for 7 days

Dosage of above antibiotics

- Azithromycin 500 mg (child >6 months: 10 mg/kg up to 500 mg) PO on day 1, then 250 mg (child >6 months: 5 mg/kg up to 250 mg)

PO daily for further 4 days (neonate and child <6 months: 10 mg/kg PO daily for 5 days)
- Cotrimoxazole 160/800 mg (child >1 month: 4/20 mg/kg up to 160/800 mg) PO q12h
- Clarithromycin 500 mg (child: 7.5 mg/kg up to 500 mg) PO q12h

Antibiotic prophylaxis

To prevent the spread of the infection—recommended for the following close contacts:

- Women in the last month of pregnancy (regardless of vaccination status)
- Children <2 years who have not received 3 doses of pertussis (DTPa) vaccine (all household members should also receive antibiotic prophylaxis)
- If an infectious case attended childcare and there are at-risk children (<6 months old or who have not received 3 doses of pertussis vaccine)—all at-risk children and staff who have not had a pertussis-containing vaccine in last 10 years should receive antibiotic prophylaxis
- If an infectious healthcare worker or child in a maternity ward or newborn nursery—all exposed babies and healthcare workers in the ward and nursery should receive antibiotic prophylaxis

Prophylaxis antibiotic choice

Same as the treatment (above), should be given ASAP within 3 weeks after contacting the index case

Vaccination

Pertussis vaccination is recommended for all children

Primary schedule
- DTPa 0.5 mL IM, 3 doses at 6 weeks, 4 months and 6 months

Boosters
- DTPa 0.5 mL IM, at age of 18 months and 4 years
- DTpa (e.g. Boostrix) 0.5 mL IM, at age of 12–17 years (school), then every 10 years

A single pertussis booster is recommended (if no previous DTPa booster) to prevent transmission of pertussis to children in the following groups:

- Women planning a pregnancy (pre-conceptive vaccination)
- Pregnant women in the third trimester (if no pre-conception vaccination)
- Women postpartum vaccination (ASAP after baby is born) (if not received before or during pregnancy)
- Other household members
- Adults working with or caring for young children (e.g. childcare and healthcare workers)

- Any adult who wants to have a booster and to avoid getting whooping cough
- All adults aged 50 years (the routine tetanus and diphtheria booster (e.g. ADT) can be replaced by DTpa (e.g. Boostrix) to protect against pertussis as well

School exclusion

- Infected children should be excluded from school until antibiotics have been taken for 5 days, or until 21 days have passed after the onset of cough
- Uninfected children <1 year should be kept out of school unless they have had previous pertussis infection or have received ≥2 DTPa vaccinations more than 4 weeks apart
- Uninfected children >1 year may attend school even if they have had no pertussis infection in the past or have not been vaccinated

PILONIDAL SINUS INFECTION

A pilonidal sinus (PNS) occurs in the cleavage between the buttocks, which often contains hair and skin debris.

Pathogens and causes

- Anaerobic bacteria—*Bacteroides* and *Enterococci* (predominately)
- Aerobic bacteria—*Staphylococci* and *Streptococcus pyogenes*
- Pilonidal sinus infection may be caused by obstruction of natal cleft hair follicles and ingrowing hairs

Clinical

- More common in males (M:F = 10:1)
- Pilonidal sinus infection can cause discomfort, embarrassment and absence from work for thousands of young people (mostly men) annually
- It may cause secondary tracks, which open laterally and may develop into pilonidal abscesses

Treatment

- Surgical—incision and drainage of the abscess and excision of the sinus tract
- Antibiotics—empirical antibiotic therapy should cover both anaerobic and aerobic bacteria, then be guided by cultures
  - Flucloxacillin (PO or IV) **plus** metronidazole (PO or IV)
If non-immediate penicillin allergy
  - Cefalexin (PO) (**or** cefazolin [IV]) **plus** metronidazole (PO or IV)
If immediate penicillin allergy
  - Clindamycin (PO or IV)

IV therapy is for more severe cases

Duration of treatment

- At least 2 weeks

Dosage of above antibiotics

- Flucloxacillin 250–500 mg (child: 12.5–25 mg up to 500 mg) PO q6h
- Flucloxacillin 1–2 g (child: 25–50 mg/kg up to 2 g) IV q6h
- Metronidazole 200–400 mg (child: 7.5 mg/kg up to 400 mg) PO q8h
- Metronidazole 500 mg (child: 10 mg/kg up to 500 mg) IV q12h
- Cefalexin 250–500 mg (child: 6.25-12.5 mg/kg up to 500 mg) PO q6h
- Cefazolin 1 g (child: 25 mg/kg up to 1 g) IV q6h
- Clindamycin 150–300 mg (child: 5–7.5 mg/kg up to 300 mg) PO q8h
- Clindamycin 450 mg (child: 10 mg/kg up to 450 mg) IV q8h

PITYRIASIS VERSICOLOR

Other names: tinea versicolor

Pathogens

- *Malassezia globosa* (the most common)
- *Malassezia furfur* (previously called *Pityrosporum orbiculare*) (less common)

These yeasts are normally found on the human skin and become troublesome under certain circumstances, such as a warm and humid environment

Clinical

- Commonly seen in teenagers and young adults who sweat excessively
- Macular rash (brown or red on pale skin or pale on tanned skin) with fine scales
- The rash is often found on covered areas, particularly the upper trunk, shoulders and neck
- The maculas may coalesce and become slightly itchy

Laboratory

- Skin scraping—yeast cells and hyphae ('spaghetti with meatballs')
- Wood's light—lesions may show up as pale yellow to orange fluorescence

Treatment

Permanent cure is difficult

Localised disease

Any of the following azole antifungal creams for 1–2 weeks

- Bifonazole cream (e.g. Canesten once daily, Mycospor) top daily
- Clotrimazole cream (e.g. Clonea) top bid
- Econazole cream (e.g. Dermazole, Pevaryl Topicals) top bid
- Ketoconazole cream (e.g. DaktaGOLD, Nizoral) top daily
- Miconazole cream (e.g. Daktarin) top daily

Extensive disease

Any of the following solutions or shampoos

- Econazole 1% solution (e.g. Pevaryl Topicals) 1 sachet to wet skin, leave on overnight, for 3 nights
- Ketoconazole 2% shampoo (e.g. Nizoral, Sebizole) top for 5–10 min then wash off, daily for 5–7 days
- Miconazole 2% shampoo (e.g. HairScience for Dandruff Shampoo) top for 5–10 min then wash off, daily for 10 days
- Selenium sulfide 2.5% shampoo (e.g. Selsun) top for 15–30 min then wash off, daily for 2 weeks

Unresponsive or severe disease

Oral antifungals

- Itraconazole (e.g. Sporanox) 200 mg PO daily for 5–7 days

Prevention of recurrence

One of the following regimens

- Any above effective topic preparation, apply once every 2–4 weeks
- Itraconazole (e.g. Sporanox) 400 mg PO monthly

PLAGUE

Plague can be a very severe disease with a fatality rate of 30–60% if left untreated.
Pneumonic plague may be used as a biological warfare agent.

Pathogen

- *Yersinia pestis*, a zoonotic disease

Transmission

- By the bite of infected fleas
- Direct contact
- Inhalation
- Ingestion of infective materials (rare)

Incubation

- 2–7 days

Clinical

Three forms of plague

- **Bubonic plague**—the most common form of plague, results from flea bites; presents with very painful swollen lymph nodes, called bubo
- **Septicaemic plague**—results from flea bites and direct contact with infective materials through cracks in the skin
- **Pneumonic plague**—primary pneumonic plague results from inhalation of aerosolised infective droplets; secondary pneumonic plague is due to the spread of advanced infection of an initial bubonic plague

Laboratory

- Rapid dipstick tests—quickly screen for *Y. pestis* antigen
- *Y. pestis* culture—lymph node (bubo) aspirates, blood and sputum samples

Treatment

- Isolate pneumonic plague patients
- Antibiotic treatment
  - Option 1: gentamicin (IV)
  - Option 2: doxycycline (IV)*
  - Option 3: ciprofloxacin (IV)

After improvement, switch to oral

  - Option 1: doxycycline (PO) for total of 14 days
  - Option 2: ciprofloxacin (PO) for total of 14 days

Dosage of above antibiotics

  - Gentamicin 4–7 mg/kg (child: 7.5 mg/kg up to 320 mg) IV for the 1st dose (further dosing, see p. 459)
  - Doxycycline 200 mg (child >8 years: 5 mg/kg up to 200 mg) IV for 1 dose, then 100 mg (child >8 years: 2.5 mg/kg up to 100 mg) IV q12h
  - Ciprofloxacin 400 mg (child: 15 mg/kg up to 400 mg) IV q12h
  - Doxycycline 100 mg (child >8 years: 2.5 mg/kg up to 100 mg) PO q12h
  - Ciprofloxacin 500 mg (child: 15 mg/kg up to 500 mg) PO q12h

Post-exposure prophylaxis

  - Option 1: doxycycline 100 mg (child >8 years: 2.5 mg/kg up to 100 mg) PO q12h for 7 days

---

*IV doxycycline is available via Special Access Scheme <www.tga.gov.au/hp/access-sas.htm>

- Option 2: ciprofloxacin 500 mg (child: 15 mg/kg up to 500 mg) PO q12h for 7 days

Prevention

- Be aware of the areas where zoonotic plague is active, take precautions against flea bites and when handling carcasses while in plague-endemic areas
- Avoid direct contact with infective tissues or from being exposed to patients with pneumonic plague

Vaccination

- Only recommended for high-risk groups (e.g. laboratory personnel who are constantly exposed to the risk of contamination)

PLEURAL EMPYEMA

Pathogens

Pleural empyema complicating community-acquired pneumonia

- *Streptococus pneumoniae*
- *Streptococus milleri* group (e.g. *S. anginosus*, *S. intermedius*, *S. constellatus*)
- *Staphylococcus* spp (<10% of cases)

Pleural empyema complicating hospital-acquired pneumonia

- Methicillin-resistant *Staphylococcus aureus* (MRSA)
- Enteric gram-negative bacteria (e.g. *Enterobacter* spp, *Klebsiella pneumoniae*, *Escherichia coli*, *Serratia marcescens*, *Proteus* spp, *Acinetobacter* spp. and *Stenotrophomonas maltophilia*)
- *Pseudomonas aeruginosa*

Clinical

- Up to 50% of cases of pneumonia can develop pleural effusion (parapneumonic effusion); if pleural effusion is not drained appropriately, it can develop into pleural empyema
- Fever, shivers, chest pain and SOB
- Pleural effusion is confirmed by chest x-ray
- Pleural empyema is confirmed by aspiration/drainage + microscopy and culture

Laboratory

- Pleural aspiration/drainage—for M/C/S (pleural empyema are often culture-negative due to antibiotic use for pneumonia)
- Blood cultures, FBC and CRP (monitor response to treatment)

Treatment

- Pleural empyema requires adequate drainage

Pleural empyema complicating community-acquired pneumonia

- Option 1: amoxicillin/clavulanate (PO)
- Option 2: clindamycin (PO) (if gram-negative pathogens are not suspected)

For severe case or if oral therapy is not tolerated

- Option 1: piperacillin/tazobactam (IV)
- Option 2: ticarcillin/clavulanate (IV)
- Option 3: moxifloxacin (IV) (if penicillin allergy)

Pleural empyema complicating hospital-acquired pneumonia

- Treat as hospital-acquired pneumonia (see p. 308)

Pleural empyema complicating atypical pneumonia

- Treat as *Mycoplasma*, *Chlamydia* pneumonia (p. 304) or *Legionella* (p. 198)

Dosage of above antibiotics

- Amoxicillin/clavulanate 875/125 mg (child: 22.5/3.2 mg/kg up to 875/125 mg) PO q12h
- Clindamycin 450 mg (child: 10 mg/kg up to 450 mg) PO q8h
- Piperacillin/tazobactam 4 g (child: 100 mg/kg up to 4 g) IV q8h
- Ticarcillin/clavulanate 3 g IV q6h
- Moxifloxacin 400 mg (child: 10 mg/kg up to 400 mg) IV daily

PNEUMOCOCCAL DISEASE

Other names: invasive pneumococcal disease (IPD)
Pneumococcal disease is a leading cause of serious illness and death among Australian children under 5 years of age. The infection rate is highest in Indigenous children, especially in central Australia.

Pathogens

- *Streptococcus pneumoniae* (pneumococcus) with 90 different strains

Transmission

- Most people carry pneumococcus in their nose and throat
- Via droplets or contact—sneezing, coughing, sharing toys or kissing

Incubation

- 1–3 days

Clinical

IPD includes:

- Pneumococcal pneumonia (more common in adults)
- Pneumococcal meningitis (the most common bacterial cause of meningitis)
- Pneumococcal bacteraemia and septicaemia (more common in children)

Other infections caused by pneumococcus:

- Otitis media
- Sinusitis
- Osteomyelitis and septic arthritis

High-risk groups

Asplenia (functional or anatomical), multiple myeloma, hypogammaglobulinaemia, lymphoid malignancies, HIV/AIDS, corticosteroid therapy, complement (C1–C4) defect, CSF leakage after cranial trauma or surgery, diabetes, chronic renal and liver disease, frequent otitis media, alcoholism, smoking and malnutrition

Laboratory

- Pneumococcal urinary antigen test (UAT)—aids early diagnosis of pneumococcal disease (less helpful in children)
- Bacterial culture and MIC testing—blood, sputum and CSF

All isolated *Streptococcus pneumoniae* cases should undergo MIC testing

Antibiotic treatment

- Pneumococcal pneumonia—see Pneumococcal pneumonia (p. 300)
- Pneumococcal meningitis—see Pneumococcal meningitis (p. 226)
- Pneumococcal sepsis—see Pneumococcal sepsis (p. 371)

Pneumococcal vaccines (see Appendix 3)

- 10vPCV (Synflorix)—for children from 6 weeks of age up to 5 years
- 13vPCV (Prevenar 13®)—for children from 6 weeks of age
- 23vPPV (Pneumovax 23®)—for children aged ≥2 years and adults

PNEUMONIA—ASPIRATION AND LUNG ABSCESS

Pathogens

- Gram-positive aerobes—e.g. *S. anginosus/milleri* group
- Gram-negative bacilli—e.g. *H. influenzae*, *K. pneumoniae*
- Anaerobes—e.g. *Bacteroides*

Risk factors

- Altered conscious state (e.g. anaesthesia, alcohol intoxication, postictal)
- Swallowing abnormality
- Periodontal and gingival disease

Diagnosis

- Sputum culture (aerobes and anaerobes)
- Bronchoalveolar lavage (BAL) or fine-needle aspiration—to obtain culture specimens
- Chest x-ray or CT

Treatment

- Mild aspiration does not require antibiotic therapy

Not systemically unwell

- Option 1: amoxicillin/clavulanate (PO)
- Option 2: clindamycin (PO)

Systemically unwell

- Option 1: benzylpenicillin (IV) **plus** metronidazole (IV or PO) then amoxicillin/clavulanate (PO)
- Option 2: clindamycin (IV or PO)

Severely unwell or if gram-negative infection is suspected

- Option 1: ceftriaxone (**or** cefotaxime) (IV) **plus** metronidazole (IV) then cefuroxime (PO) **plus** metronidazole (PO)
- Option 2: piperacillin/tazobactam (IV) (also for hospital-acquired)
- Option 3: ticarcillin/clavulanate IV q6h

If immediate penicillin allergy see expert advice

If staphylococcal infection is suspected or confirmed

- Option 1: flucloxacillin (IV)
- Option 2: cefalotin (**or** ephazolin) (IV) (if non-immediate penicillin allergy)
- Option 3: vancomycin (IV) (If MRSA or severely ill or immediate penicillin allergy)

For vancomycin-intermediate *S. aureus* (VISA) pneumonia

- Linezolid (PO) (seek expert advice)

After significant improvement switch to oral (as above)

Duration of treatment*

- Total (IV + oral) 3–4 weeks

Dosage of above antibiotics

Not systemically unwell

- Amoxicillin/clavulanate 875/125 mg (child: 22.5/3.2 mg/kg up to 875/125 mg) PO q12h
- Clindamycin 450 mg (child: 10 mg/kg up to 450 mg) PO q8h

Systemically unwell

- Benzylpenicillin 1.2 g (child: 50 mg/kg up to 1.2 g) IV q6h

---

*Serum C-reactive protein (CRP) is useful for monitoring the response to therapy

- Metronidazole 500 mg (child: 12.5 mg/kg up to 500 mg) IV q12h **or** metronidazole 400 mg (child: 10 mg/kg up to 400 mg) PO q12h
- Amoxicillin/clavulanate 875/125 mg (child: 22.5/3.2 mg/kg up to 875/125 mg) PO q12h
- Clindamycin 450 mg (child: 10 mg/kg up to 450 mg) IV or PO q8h

Severely unwell or gram-negative infection is suspected

- Ceftriaxone 1 g (child: 50 mg/kg up to 1 g) IV daily
- Metronidazole 500 mg (child: 12.5 mg/kg up to 500 mg) IV q12h
- Cefuroxime 500 mg (child <2 years: 10 mg/kg up to 125 mg; >2 years: 15 mg/kg up to 500 mg) PO q12h
- Metronidazole 400 mg (child: 10 mg/kg up to 400 mg) PO q8h
- Cefotaxime 1 g (child: 50 mg/kg up to 1 g) IV q8h
- Piperacillin/tazobactam 4 g (child: 100 mg/kg up to 4 g) IV q6h
- Ticarcillin + clavulanate 3 g (child: 50 mg/kg up to 3 g) IV q8h

If staphylococcal infection is suspected or confirmed

- Flucloxacillin 2 g (child: 50 mg/kg up to 2 g) IV q4–6h, then 1 g (child: 25 mg/kg up to 1 g) PO q6h
- Cefalotin 2 g (child: 50 mg/kg up to 2 g) IV q4h
- Cefazolin 2 g (child: 50 mg/kg up to 2 g) IV q8h
- Vancomycin 25–30 mg/kg IV for the 1st dose (further dosing, see p. 462)
- Linezolid 600 mg (child: 10 mg/kg up to 600 mg) PO q12h

PNEUMONIA—COMMUNITY-ACQUIRED (ADULT)

Community-acquired pneumonia (CAP) affects individuals who are not hospitalised or who have been in hospital for less than 48 hours and who are not significantly immunocompromised.

Pathogens

Often a single organism

- *Streptococcus pneumoniae* (the most common)
- *Haemophilus influenzae* (often the cause of bronchial pneumonia in COPD)
- *Mycoplasma pneumoniae* (atypical pneumonia)
- *Chlamydia pneumoniae* (atypical pneumonia)
- *Legionella* spp (atypical pneumonia)
- Gram-negative bacilli e.g. *Klebsiella pneumoniae*, *Pseudomonas aeruginosa* (uncommon)
- *Staphylococcus aureus* (uncommon)
- *Burkholderia pseudomallei* and *Acinetobacter baumannii* (in tropical Australia)

Clinical features

The following features plus consolidation on chest x-ray:

- New-onset cough
- Change in sputum colour
- SOB
- Fever and rigors
- Pleuritic chest pain
- Crackles in lungs

Laboratory

- Blood cultures (10–20 mL in an adult, 3–5 mL in a child)
- Mycoplasma/*Chlamydia*/*Legionella* serology (2nd test at >3 weeks after onset of disease)
- Sputum Gram stain/culture; sputum *Legionella* culture and PCR
- Urine *Legionella* (LP1) antigen test; urine pneumococcal antigen test
- Nose/throat swab for influenza PCR (during May to November)
- Pleural fluid aspiration for microscopy, biochemistry and culture

Assess pneumonia severity using pneumonia comorbidity and severity indicators (PCSIs) (see Box 16.1)

BOX 16.1

ASSESSING SEVERITY USING PCSIS

MILD CAP

- Comorbidity indicators: **no**
- Severity indicators: **no**

  Outpatient treatment or social admission

MODERATE CAP

- Comorbidity indicators: **yes**
- Severity indicators: **no**

  Hospital admission is indicated

SEVERE CAP

- Comorbidity indicators: **yes/no**
- Severity indicators: **any 1 or more**

  ICU admission is indicated

Comorbidity indicators

- Age ≥70
- Malignant disease
- Chronic lung disease
- Chronic liver disease
- Chronic renal disease
- Heart failure
- Uncontrolled diabetes
- Immunocompromised

Severity indicators

- Acute onset confusion
- Temperature <35°C or ≥40°C
- Respiratory rate >30/min
- Systolic BP <90 mmHg
- O_2 sat <92% or PaO_2 <60 mmHg
- Acidosis: arterial pH <7.35 or venous pH <7.31

Empirical antibiotic therapy for adult CAP

- Early commencement of empirical antibiotic therapy (within 4–8 hours of presentation) significantly reduces morbidity and the length of hospital stay
- The more severe the CAP, the wider the spectrum the antibiotic should cover
- Empirical therapy should be carefully reviewed and substituted with directed (targeted) therapy once the pathogen has been isolated

Sputum Gram stain—for early judgement of possible pathogens

- Gram-positive diplococci—suggests *S. pneumoniae*
- Small gram-negative rods—suggests *H. influenzae*
- Gram-positive cocci in clusters—suggests *S. aureus*

1. Mild CAP

- Outpatient treatment with oral antibiotic therapy; closely reviewed by GP
- Consider hospital admission for IV therapy if oral treatment fails
- May need hospital admission for social or other reasons (e.g. social isolation, inability to take oral antibiotics, alcoholism or illicit drug use)
    - Amoxicillin (PO) for 5–7 days
    - Doxycycline (**or** clarithromycin) (PO) for 5–7 days (if atypical pathogens suspected)

If gram-negative organism identified by sputum Gram stain
    - Amoxicillin/clavulanate (PO) for 5–7 days

If non-immediate penicillin allergy
    - Cefuroxime (PO) for 5–7 days

If immediate penicillin allergy
    - Doxycycline (**or** clarithromycin) (PO) for 5–7 days

If no improvement by 48 hours, dual therapy
    - Amoxicillin (**or** cefuroxime) (PO) **plus** doxycycline (PO) (**or** clarithromycin) (PO) for 5–7 days

Dosage of above antibiotics

- Amoxicillin 1 g PO q8h for 5–7 days
- Doxycycline 100 mg PO q12h for 5–7 days
- Clarithromycin 500 mg PO q12h for 5–7 days
- Cefuroxime 500 mg PO q12h for 5–7 days

2.   Moderate CAP

- Hospital admission and IV antibiotic therapy
- May use hospital-in-the-home care for less severe patients
- Always consider influenza as a potential cause
  - Benzylpenicillin (IV) then amoxicillin (PO) **plus** doxycycline (**or** clarithromycin) (PO) for total 7 days*

In rural and remote areas, where hospitalisation is difficult
  - Procaine penicillin (IM) then amoxicillin (PO), **plus** doxycycline (**or** clarithromycin) (PO) for total 7 days*

If gram-negative bacilli infection is suspected or identified in sputum or blood
  - Option 1: ceftriaxone[1] (**or** cefotaxime) (IV) then cefuroxime (PO), **plus** doxycycline (**or** clarithromycin) (PO) for total 7 days*
  - Option 2: benzylpenicillin (IV) **plus** gentamicin (IV) then amoxicillin (PO) **plus** doxycycline (**or** clarithromycin) (PO) for total 7 days

If non-immediate penicillin allergy
  - Above Option 1

If immediate penicillin allergy
  - Moxifloxacin (PO) for total 7 days

In tropical Australia, if there are risk factors for *B. pseudomallei* and *A. baumannii* (i.e. diabetes, alcoholism, chronic renal failure or chronic lung disease)
  - Ceftriaxone[2] (IV) **plus** gentamicin (IV) st **plus** doxycycline (**or** clarithromycin) (PO)

Dosage of above antibiotics

- Benzylpenicillin 1.2 g IV q6h until significant improvement
- Amoxicillin 1 g PO q8h
- Doxycycline 100 mg PO q12h
- Clarithromycin 500 mg PO q12h
- Procaine penicillin 1.5 g IM daily until significant improvement
- Ceftriaxone[1] 1 g IV daily until significant improvement
- Cefotaxime 1 g IV q8h until significant improvement
- Cefuroxime 500 mg PO q12h
- Gentamicin 4–7 mg/kg IV for the 1st dose (further dosing, see p. 459)
- Moxifloxacin 400 mg IV daily until significant improvement, then 400 mg PO daily
- Ceftriaxone[2] 2 g IV daily

3.   Severe CAP

- Hospital ICU admission and IV antibiotic therapy
- Broad-spectrum antibiotic cover
- Treat possible influenza
  - Option 1: ceftriaxone (**or** cefotaxime) (IV) **plus** azithromycin (IV)
  - Option 2: benzylpenicillin (IV) **plus** gentamicin (IV) **plus** azithromycin (IV)

---

*Oral antibiotics alone may be sufficient for some cases

After significant improvement switch to oral

- Amoxicillin/clavulanate (PO) **plus** azithromycin (PO) for total 7–14 days

If non-immediate penicillin allergy

- Ceftriaxone (**or** cefotaxime) (IV) **plus** azithromycin (IV)

After significant improvement switch to oral

- Cefuroxime (PO) **plus** azithromycin (PO) for total 7–14 days

If immediate penicillin allergy

- Moxifloxacin (IV)

After significant improvement switch to oral

- Moxifloxacin (PO) for total 7–14 days

In tropical regions, if risk factors for *B. pseudomallei* and *A. baumannii* (i.e. diabetes, alcoholism, chronic renal failure or chronic lung disease), as initial therapy use

- Option 1: meropenem (IV) **plus** azithromycin (IV) (wet season)
- Option 2: piperacillin/tazobactam (IV) **plus** azithromycin (IV) (dry season)

When pathogen is isolated, adjust antibiotic regimen accordingly

Dosage of above antibiotics

- Ceftriaxone 1 g IV daily
- Cefotaxime 1 g IV q8h
- Azithromycin 500 mg IV daily
- Benzylpenicillin 1.2 g IV q4h
- Gentamicin 4–7 mg/kg IV for the 1st dose (further dosing, see p. 459); if IV therapy is still required after 3 doses, change to ceftriaxone or cefotaxime regimen
- Amoxicillin/clavulanate 875 mg PO q12h
- Azithromycin 500 mg PO daily
- Cefuroxime 500 mg PO q12h
- Moxifloxacin 400 mg IV daily
- Moxifloxacin 400 mg PO daily
- Meropenem 1 g IV q8h
- Piperacillin/tazobactam 4 g IV q8h

PNEUMONIA—COMMUNITY-ACQUIRED (CHILD)

BIRTH TO 1 MONTH

Pathogens

The pneumonia is usually acquired from maternal perineal flora

- Group B streptococcus (*S. agalactiae*)
- *E. coli*
- Herpes simplex virus (HSV)

Empirical therapy

- Benzylpenicillin (IV) **plus** gentamicin (IV) for 7 days

If *Chlamydia* or pertussis pneumonia are suspected **add**
- Azithromycin (IV) for 7 days

For HSV pneumonitis see expert advice

Dosage of above antibiotics
- Benzylpenicillin 50 mg/kg IV (neonate 0–7 days: q12h; >7 days: q6h)
- Gentamicin IV for 7 days (dosage, see p. 459)
- Azithromycin 10 mg/kg IV daily

1 MONTH TO 3 MONTHS

Pathogens

- *S. pneumoniae* (most common)
- *C. trachomatis* and *B. pertussis*

Empirical therapy

If acute bronchiolitis is not present

If baby is afebrile and only mildly ill
- Option 1: azithromycin (PO) for 5 days
- Option 2: clarithromycin (PO) for 7 days

If baby is febrile and unwell
- Benzylpenicillin (IV) **then** amoxicillin (PO) for total 7 days

If baby is severely ill (systemic toxicity, rapidly progressive pneumonia)
- Cefotaxime* (**or** ceftriaxone) (IV) **plus** flucloxacillin (IV) **then** amoxicillin (PO) for total 7 days

If MRSA is suspected or is prevalent in the region
- Vancomycin (IV)

Dosage of above antibiotics
- Azithromycin 10 mg/kg PO daily
- Clarithromycin 7.5 mg/kg PO q12h
- Benzylpenicillin 50 mg/kg IV q6h
- Amoxicillin 25 mg/kg PO q8h
- Cefotaxime 50 mg/kg IV q8h
- Ceftriaxone 50 mg/kg IV daily
- Flucloxacillin 50 mg/kg IV q6h
- Vancomycin 15 mg/kg IV q12h for 2 doses (further dosing, see p. 462)

3 MONTHS TO 5 YEARS

Pathogens

- Viral (most common)
- *S. pneumoniae*
- *S. aureus* (systemic toxicity, empyema, pneumatoceles on chest x-ray)

---

*Do not use ceftriaxone in neonates and preterm infants (displaces bilirubin from albumin and increases risk of bilirubin encephalopathy)

Empirical therapy

- If bacterial infection is suspected (e.g. elevated WBC count and neutrophils and chest x-ray suggests bacterial pneumonia), antibiotic therapy should be commenced

Mild pneumonia
- Amoxicillin (PO) for 5 days (review after 48 hours if no response)

Moderate pneumonia or if oral therapy is not tolerated
- Benzylpenicillin (IV) for 5 days

In rural and remote regions, where hospitalisation may be difficult
- Procaine penicillin (IM) for 5 days

Severe pneumonia (systemic toxicity, hypoxia)
- Cefotaxime (**or** ceftriaxone) (IV) **plus** flucloxacillin (IV)

If staphylococcal pneumonia is suspected (systemic toxicity, large pleural effusion, pneumatoceles)
- Vancomycin (IV)

Dosage of above antibiotics

- Amoxicillin 25 mg/kg PO q8h
- Benzylpenicillin 50 mg/kg IV q6h
- Procaine penicillin child 3–6 kg: 250 mg; 6–10 kg: 375 mg; 10–15 kg: 500 mg; 15–20 kg: 750 mg IM daily
- Cefotaxime 50 mg/kg IV q8h
- Ceftriaxone 50 mg/kg IV daily
- Flucloxacillin 50 mg/kg IV q6h
- Vancomycin IV (dosing, see p. 462)

5 YEARS OR OLDER

Pathogens

- *S. pneumoniae* (the most common)
- *M. pneumoniae* (more common in this age group)
- *C. pneumoniae*
- *B. pseudomallei*—may cause CAP in tropical Australia in children with chronic diseases such as diabetes, cystic fibrosis and congenital/ rheumatic heart disease

Empirical therapy

Mild pneumonia

- Amoxicillin (PO) **plus** doxycycline (**or** azithromycin **or** clarithromycin) (PO) for 5 days

Severe pneumonia

- Cefotaxime (**or** ceftriaxone) (IV) **plus** flucloxacillin (IV) **plus** azithromycin (IV)

If allergic to penicillin
- Vancomycin (IV) **plus** azithromycin (IV)

After significant improvement switch to oral (see above) for total of 7 days

If staphylococcal pneumonia is suspected
- Treat as staphylococcal pneumonia (p. 301)

In tropical Australia, to cover *B. pseudomallei* (melioidosis) in children with chronic diseases
- Meropenem (**or** piperacillin/tazobactam) (IV) **plus** vancomycin (IV) **plus** azithromycin (IV)

After significant improvement switch to oral (see above Mild pneumonia)

Dosage of above antibiotics

Mild pneumonia
- Amoxicillin 25 mg/kg up to 1 g PO q8h
- Doxycycline (child >8 years) 2 mg/kg up to 100 mg PO q12h
- Azithromycin 10 mg/kg up to 500 mg PO daily
- Clarithromycin 7.5 mg/kg up to 500 mg PO q12h

Severe pneumonia
- Cefotaxime 50 mg/kg up to 1 g IV q8h
- Ceftriaxone 50 mg/kg up to 1 g IV daily
- Flucloxacillin 50 mg/kg up to 2 g IV q6h
- Azithromycin 10 mg/kg up to 500 mg IV daily
- Vancomycin IV (dosing, see p. 462)
- Meropenem 25 mg/kg up to 1 g IV q8h (wet season)
- Piperacillin/tazobactam 100 mg/kg up to 4 g IV q8h (dry season)

PNEUMONIA—DIRECT THERAPY

1. PNEUMOCOCCAL PNEUMONIA

Pathogen

- *Streptococcus pneumoniae* (pneumococcus)

Laboratory

- Pneumococcal urinary antigen test (UAT)—aids early diagnosis of pneumococcal disease (less useful in children)

Prevention

- Pneumococcal vaccination—for patients at risk of recurrence

Treatment

Antibiotic choice should be based on susceptibility

- Option 1: benzylpenicillin* (IV), then amoxicillin (PO) for total 7 days
- Option 2: amoxicillin (PO) for 7 days (some mild cases)

---

*Penicillin-resistant strains are a rare cause of pneumonia in Australia

If non-immediate penicillin allergy
  - Option 1: ceftriaxone (**or** cefotaxime) (IV), then cefuroxime (PO) for total 7 days
  - Option 2: cefuroxime (PO) for 7 days (some mild cases)

If immediate penicillin allergy (adult)
  - Option 1: moxifloxacin (PO or IV) for 7 days
  - Option 2: doxycycline (PO) for 7 days (some mild cases)
  - Option 3: vancomycin (IV), then oral for total 7 days

For child with immediate penicillin allergy—seek expert advice

For penicillin-resistant (MIC ≥2 mg/L) strain*
  - Vancomycin (IV), then oral for total 7 days

Seek expert advice

Dosage of above antibiotics

  - Benzylpenicillin 1.2 g (child: 50 mg/kg up to 1.2 g) IV q6h
  - Amoxicillin 1 g (child: 25 mg/kg up to 1 g) PO q8h
  - Ceftriaxone 1 g (child: 50 mg/kg up to 1 g) IV daily
  - Cefotaxime 1 g (child: 50 mg/kg up to 1 g) IV q8h
  - Cefuroxime 500 mg (child 3 months–2 years: 10 mg/kg up to 125 mg; >2 years: 15 mg/kg up to 500 mg) PO q12h
  - Moxifloxacin 400 mg PO or IV daily
  - Doxycycline 100 mg PO q12h
  - Vancomycin 25–30 mg/kg IV for the 1st dose (further dosing, see p. 462)

2. STAPHYLOCOCCAL PNEUMONIA

Pathogens

- *Staphylococcus aureus*, including methicillin-susceptible *S. aureus* (MSSA) and methicillin-resistant *S. aureus* (MRSA)

Causes

- Primary infection
- Secondary to aspiration, right-sided endocarditis or influenza
- Pneumonia cases caused by community-associated MRSA (CA-MRSA) are increasing, especially among IV drug users, Indigenous Australians and Pacific Islanders (these strains may be clinically more aggressive, but may be susceptible to some routine antibiotics such as clindamycin and cotrimoxazole)

Laboratory

- Sputum Gram stain—gram-positive cocci in clusters
- Sputum culture—*S. aureus* in sputum culture may represent colonisation
- Susceptibility testing for all *S. aureus* isolates is crucial for antibiotic choice

*Penicillin-resistant strains are a rare cause of pneumonia in Australia

Treatment

MSSA pneumonia
- Option 1: flucloxacillin (IV)
- Option 2: cefalotin (**or** cefazolin) (IV) (if non-immediate penicillin allergy)
- Option 3: vancomycin (IV) (if immediate penicillin allergy)

For MRSA pneumonia or severe illness before susceptibility available
- Vancomycin (IV)

If CA-MRSA confirmed step-down with
- Clindamycin (**or** cotrimazole) (PO)

Seek expert advice on timing and type of step-down oral therapy

For vancomycin-intermediate *S. aureus* (VISA) pneumonia
- Linezolid (PO) (seek expert advice)

Duration of treatment
- Uncomplicated case—7–14 days
- More severe cases (e.g. cavitatory)—longer therapy

Dosage of above antibiotics
- Flucloxacillin 2 g (child: 50 mg/kg up to 2 g) IV q4–6h, then 1 g (child: 25 mg/kg up to 1 g) PO q6h
- Cefalotin 2 g (child: 50 mg/kg up to 2 g) IV q4h
- Cefazolin 2 g (child: 50 mg/kg up to 2 g) IV q8h
- Vancomycin 25–30 mg/kg IV for the 1st dose (further dosing, see p. 462)
- Clindamycin 600 mg (child: 10 mg/kg up to 600 mg) IV q6h
- Cotrimoxazole 160/800 mg PO q12h
- Linezolid 600 mg (child: 10 mg/kg up to 600 mg) PO q12h

3. *HAEMOPHILUS* PNEUMONIA

Pathogens

- *Haemophilus influenzae*—a small pleomorphic, gram-negative coccobacillus
- The most virulent strain is *H. influenzae* type b (Hib)

Transmission

- Direct contact or inhalation of droplets

Clinical

- Hib pneumonia is clinically indistinguishable from other bacterial pneumonias
- Patients with Hib pneumonia tend to have more pleural and pericardial involvement (50% patients) than those with other bacterial pneumonias
- Hib infection is more common in patients with asplenia, splenectomy, sickle cell disease, malignancies and congenital or acquired immunodeficiencies

Laboratory

- Gram stain—sputum or pleural effusion
- Bacterial culture—blood, sputum or pleural effusion
- Detection of the polysaccharide capsule in serum, urine and pleural fluid
- Chest x-ray—alveolar infiltrates in patchy or lobar distributions (none specific)

Treatment

- Antibiotic therapy
- Hib vaccine has led to a dramatic decline in incidence of the infection

Mild infection—oral regimen

- Amoxicillin (PO)

For beta-lactamase productive strains

- Amoxicillin/clavulanate (PO)

If non-immediate penicillin allergy

- Cefuroxime (PO)

If immediate penicillin allergy (if susceptible)

- Option 1: doxycycline (PO)
- Option 2: ciprofloxacin (PO)

More severe infection—IV regimen

- Benzylpenicillin (IV)

For beta-lactamase productive strains

- Option 1: ceftriaxone (**or** cefotaxime) (IV)
- Option 2: ciprofloxacin (IV) (if immediate penicillin allergy)

Duration of therapy

- 7–14 days

Dosage of above antibiotics

- Amoxicillin 1 g (child: 25 mg/kg up to 1 g) PO q8h
- Amoxicillin/clavulanate 875 mg (child: 22.5 mg up to 875 mg) PO q12h
- Cefuroxime 500 mg (child 3 months–2 years: 10 mg/kg up to 125 mg; >2 years: 15 mg/kg up to 500 mg) PO q12h
- Doxycycline 100 mg (child >8 years: 2 mg/kg up to 100 mg) PO q12h
- Ciprofloxacin 500 mg (child: 12.5 mg/kg up to 500 mg) PO q12h
- Benzylpenicillin 1.2 g (child: 50 mg/kg up to 1.2 g) IV q6h
- Ceftriaxone 1 g (child: 50 mg/kg up to 1 g) IV daily
- Cefotaxime 1 g (child: 50 mg/kg up to 1 g) IV q8h
- Ciprofloxacin 400 mg (child: 10 mg/kg up to 400 mg) IV q12h

4. MYCOPLASMA PNEUMONIA

Mycoplasma pneumonia is an atypical pneumonia.

Pathogen

- *Mycoplasma pneumoniae*

Transmission

- Respiratory droplets

Incubation

- 2–3 weeks

Clinical

- Gradual and insidious onset of several days to weeks
- Persistent progressive dry cough; usually not critically ill; may have fever, chills, malaise, headache, scratchy sore throat and sore chest

Complications

- Haemolytic anaemia
- Otitis media
- Respiratory failure
- Pericarditis
- Gullain-Barré syndrome
- Encephalitis and meningitis

Diagnosis

- *Mycoplasma* antigen PCR—from pharyngeal swab, bronchoalveolar lavage, sputum or biopsy tissue
- *Mycoplasma* serology—positive after 4–6 weeks of infection
- Chest x-ray—bilateral bronchopneumonia, reticulonodular or interstitial infiltrates; pleural effusions in <20% of patients

Treatment

- Option 1: doxycycline (PO) for 7–10 days
- Option 2: azithromycin (IV or PO) for 3–5 days
- Option 3: clarithromycin (PO) for 7–10 days

Dosage of above antibiotics

- Doxycycline 100 mg (child >8 years: 2 mg/kg up to 100 mg) PO q12h
- Azithromycin 500 mg (child: 10 mg/kg up to 500 mg) PO or IV daily
- Clarithromycin 500 mg (child: 7.5 mg/kg up to 500 mg) PO q12h

5.   *CHLAMYDIA* PNEUMONIA

Chlamydia pneumonia is an atypical pneumonia.

Pathogens

Small, gram-negative, obligate intracellular organisms

- *Chlamydophila pneumoniae*—causes mild pneumonia or bronchitis in adolescents and young adults; older adults may have more severe pneumonia

- *Chlamydophila psittaci*—causes psittacosis (ornithosis, parrot fever) after exposure to infected birds; patients with ornithosis most commonly present with pneumonia or fever of unknown origin (see Psittacosis, p. 340)
- *Chlamydophila trachomatis*—an important cause of sexually transmitted infections, it can also cause pneumonia, primarily in infants and young children and in immunocompromised adults

Transmission

- Respiratory droplets

Complications

- Meningoencephalitis, arthritis, myocarditis and Guillain-Barré syndrome
- It has also been associated with Alzheimer's disease, fibromyalgia, chronic fatigue syndrome and prostatitis

Diagnosis

- *Chlamydia* serology—IgM positive (after 4–6 weeks of infection)
- *Chlamydia* antigen PCR—from pharyngeal swab, bronchoalveolar lavage, sputum or tissue); PCR can distinguish different *Chlamydia* species
- Chest x-rays—a single subsegmental infiltrate in lower lobes; *C. trachomatis* pneumonia may show bilateral interstitial infiltrates with hyperinflation

Treatment

- Option 1: doxycycline (PO) for 7–10 days
- Option 2: azithromycin (IV or PO) for 3–5 days
- Option 3: clarithromycin (PO) for 7–10 days

Dosage of above antibiotics

- Doxycycline 100 mg (child >8 years: 2 mg/kg up to 100 mg) PO q12h
- Azithromycin 500 mg (child: 10 mg/kg up to 500 mg) PO or IV daily
- Clarithromycin 500 mg (child: 7.5 mg/kg up to 500 mg) PO q12h

6. *KLEBSIELLA* PNEUMONIA

Pathogen

- *Klebsiella pneumoniae*—an aerobic gram-negative bacillus

Clinical

- *K. pneumoniae* usually causes bronchopneumonia or bronchitis
- *Klebsiella* lobar pneumonia—a necrotising pneumonia associated with abscess formation, cavitations, empyema and pleural adhesions—has a rapid onset and often-fatal outcome despite early and appropriate antibiotic treatment

- Typically abundant, thick, tenacious and blood-tinged sputum
- Usually exhibits unilateral chest signs, predominantly in the upper lobes

Diagnosis

- Sputum for Gram stain and culture
- Blood, pleural fluid or bronchoalveolar lavage for culture
- Chest x-ray: typically affects one of the upper lobes, which appears swollen with a bulging fissure sign and cavitation; pleural effusion, empyema and pleural adhesions are more common

Treatment

- Option 1: ceftriaxone (**or** cefotaxime) (IV)
- Option 2: piperacillin/tazobactam (IV or IVI)
- Option 3: ciprofloxacin (IV or PO) (**or** cotrimoxazole (PO))
- Option 4: meropenem (IV or IVI)

Duration of treatment

- 8–14 days (adjust according to susceptibility)

Dosage of above antibiotics

- Ceftriaxone 1 g (child: 50 mg/kg up to 1 g) IV daily or q12h
- Cefotaxime 1–2 g (child: 50–100 mg/kg up to 1–2 g) IV q8h
- Piperacillin/tazobactam 4 g (child: 100 mg/kg up to 4 g) IV q8h or continuous infusion
- Ciprofloxacin 400 mg (child: 10 mg/kg up to 400 mg) IV q12h
- Ciprofloxacin 500 mg (child 12.5 mg/kg up to 500 mg) PO q12h
- Cotrimoxazole 160/800 mg (child >1 month: 4/20 mg/kg up to 160/800 mg) PO q12h
- Meropenem 0.5–1 g (child: 12.5 mg/kg up to 500 mg) IV q8h or continuous infusion

7. *PSEUDOMONAS* PNEUMONIA

Pathogen

- *Pseudomonas aeruginosa*, a gram-negative rod
- It is a frequent cause of hospital-acquired pneumonia and bacteraemia

Risk factors

- Patients with immunosuppression and chronic lung disease
- Patients in ICU, particularly on positive-pressure ventilation
- Chemotherapy-induced neutropenic patients (bacteraemic spread to the lungs)

Diagnosis

- Sputum and tracheal secretions culture—isolation of *Pseudomonas* may indicate airways colonisation

- Protected bronchoalveolar lavage and specimen brushings for quantitative cultures—confirms diagnosis
- Chest x-ray—often reveals bilateral bronchopneumonia consisting of nodular infiltrates with or without pleural effusion; lobar pneumonia is uncommon

Treatment

- Most experts recommend starting with two anti-pseudomonal antibiotics and then de-escalating to monotherapy based on organism culture sensitivity
- Except in cystic fibrosis, the role of an aerosolised aminoglycoside or ceftazidime is controversial
  - Option 1: ceftazidime (IV) **plus** gentamicin (IV) (**or** ciprofloxacin [IV or PO])
  - Option 2: piperacillin/tazobactam) (IV) **plus** gentamicin (IV) (**or** ciprofloxacin [IV or PO])
  - Option 3: meropenem (IV) **plus** gentamicin (IV) (**or** ciprofloxacin [IV or PO])

Duration of therapy

- 14–21 days (individualised)
- Adjust treatment according to susceptibility

Dosage of above antibiotics

- Ceftazidime 2 g (child: 50 mg/kg up to 2 g) IV q8h
- Gentamicin 4–7 mg/kg IV for the 1st dose (further dosing, see p. 459)
- Ciprofloxacin 400 mg (child: 10 mg/kg up to 400 mg) IV q8h
- Ciprofloxacin 750 mg (child 20 mg/kg up to 750 mg) PO q12h
- Piperacillin/tazobactam 4 g (child: 100 mg/kg up to 4 g) IV q6h
- Meropenem 0.5–1 g (child: 12.5–25 mg/kg up to 500 mg–1 g) IV q8h

8. *ENTEROBACTER, SERRATIA, MORGANELLA* AND *ACINETOBACTER* PNEUMONIA

Pathogens

- *Enterobacter* spp, *Serratia* spp, *Morganella* spp, *Acinetobacter baumannii*—aerobic gram-negative bacilli

Treatment

Choose antibiotic according to antimicrobial susceptibility testing

- Option 1: cefepime (IV)
- Option 2: piperacillin/tazobactam (IV)
- Option 3: cotrimoxazole (PO)
- Option 4: ciprofloxacin (IV or PO)
- Option 5: meropenem (IV) (if susceptibilities are unknown initially)

Duration of therapy

- 14–21 days
- Adjust treatment according to susceptibility

Dosage of above antibiotics

- Cefepime 2 g (child: 50 mg/kg up to 2 g) IV q8h
- Piperacillin/tazobactam 4 g (child: 100 mg/kg up to 4 g) IV q6h
- Cotrimoxazole 160/800 mg (child >1 month: 4/20 mg/kg up to 160/800 mg) PO q12h
- Ciprofloxacin 400 mg (child: 10 mg/kg up to 400 mg) IV q8–12h
- Ciprofloxacin 500 mg (child 12.5 mg/kg up to 500 mg) PO q12h
- Meropenem 0.5–1 g (child: 12.5–25 mg/kg up to 500 mg–1 g) IV q8h

PNEUMONIA—HOSPITAL-ACQUIRED

Hospital-acquired pneumonia (HAP) is also known as nosocomial pneumonia.

Definition

- Pneumonia developed at least 48 hours after hospital admission (not nursing home)
- HAP includes
  - Ventilator-associated pneumonia (VAP)
  - Post-operative pneumonia
  - Healthcare-associated pneumonia (HCAP)

Pathogens

Pathogens and antibiotic resistance patterns vary among hospitals

- Aerobic gram-negative bacilli (oropharynx colonisation)
- Methicillin-resistant *Staphylococcus aureus* (MRSA)
- Enteric gram-negative bacteria (e.g. *Enterobacter* spp, *Klebsiella pneumoniae*, *Escherichia coli*, *Serratia marcescens*, *Proteus* spp, *Acinetobacter* spp and *Stenotrophomonas maltophilia*)
- *Pseudomonas aeruginosa* (the most important pathogen)
- *Acinetobacter* spp
- *Legionella*, *Aspergillus* spp
- Respiratory viruses (e.g. influenza/parainfluenza virus, respiratory syncytia virus and adenovirus)

Causes and risk factors

- Microaspiration of bacteria that colonise the oropharynx and upper airways
- Macroaspiration of oesophageal or gastric material
- Endotracheal intubation with mechanical ventilation
- Inhalation of aerosols containing *Legionella* or *Aspergillus* spp

- Previous antibiotic treatment greatly increases the risk of polymicrobial infection and infections from resistant organisms, particularly MRSA and *Pseudomonas*
- Coexisting cardiac, pulmonary, hepatic or renal insufficiency
- High gastric pH (from stress ulcer prophylaxis or therapy)
- High-dose corticosteroids increase the risk of *Legionella* and *Pseudomonas* infections
- Abdominal or thoracic surgery

Diagnosis

- Newly developed respiratory symptoms and fever at least 2 days after admission
- Chest x-ray—new infiltration (exclude atelectasis)
- Sputum or endotracheal aspirate cultures (in the presence of pneumonia) may identify colonised pathogen(s), which may be responsible for the infection
- Bronchoscopy for diagnosis of ventilator-associated pneumonia
- Blood culture

Treatment

- Antibiotics should cover both resistant gram-negative and gram-positive organisms
- The initial antibiotic regimen may need to be modified to cover local pathogens

1. PATIENT IN LOW-RISK WARD

In low-risk ward for any duration or in ICU, high-dependency unit or any ward with known multiple antibiotic resistance (MDR) for <5 days

Pathogen

- Most likely *S. pneumoniae* (non-multiple antibiotic resistance) infection

Antibiotic therapy

Mild pneumonia

- Amoxicillin/clavulanate (PO) for 8 days

If penicillin allergy

- Cefuroxime (PO) for 8 days

If immediate penicillin allergy (adult)

- Moxifloxacin (PO or IV) for 8 days

For child with immediate penicillin allergy—seek expert advice

Moderate and severe pneumonia

- Ceftriaxone (**or** cefotaxime) (IV) for 8 days

If immediate penicillin allergy (adult)

- Moxifloxacin (PO or IV) for 8 days

For child with immediate penicillin allergy—seek expert advice

Dosage of above antibiotics

- Amoxicillin/clavulanate 875 mg (child: 22.5 mg/kg up to 875 mg) PO q12h
- Cefuroxime 500 mg (child 3 months–2 years: 10 mg/kg up to 125 mg; >2 years: 15 mg/kg up to 500 mg) PO q12h
- Moxifloxacin 400 mg PO or IV daily
- Ceftriaxone 1 g (child: 50 mg/kg up to 1 g) IV daily
- Cefotaxime 1 g (child: 50 mg/kg up to 1 g) IV q8h

2. PATIENT IN HIGH-RISK WARD

In ICU, high-dependency unit or any ward with known MDR for >5 days

Pathogens

- More likely MDR infection

Antibiotic therapy

- Option 1: piperacillin/tazobactam (**or** ticarcillin/clavulanate) (IV)
- Option 2: cefepime (IV) (if allergic to penicillin)
- Option 3: meropenem (IV) (if no response to above medications)

If immediate penicillin allergy seek expert advice

- Vancomycin (IV) **plus** gentamicin (**or** ciprofloxacin **or** aztreonam) (IV)

If MRSA pneumonia is suspected **add**

- Vancomycin (IV)

Discontinue if cultures are negative and patient is improving after 48 hours

If *P. aeruginosa* or other gram-negative pathogens are suspected **add**

- Option 1: gentamicin (IV)
- Option 2: ciprofloxacin (IV)

Discontinue if cultures are negative and patient is improving after 48 hours

Duration of treatment

- Continue until causative pathogen is identified, then adjust antibiotic regimen; treatment for 8 days is recommended

Dosage of above antibiotics

- Piperacillin/tazobactam 4 g (child: 100 mg/kg up to 4 g) IV q6h
- Ticarcillin/clavulanate 3 g (child: 50 mg/kg up to 3 g) IV q6h
- Cefepime 2 g (child: 50 mg/kg up to 2 g) IV q8h
- Meropenem 2 g (child: 40 mg/kg up to 2 g) IV q8h
- Vancomycin 25–30 mg/kg IV for the 1st dose (further dosing, see p. 462)
- Gentamicin 4–7 mg/kg (child: 7.5 mg/kg up to 320 mg) IV for the 1st dose (further dosing, see p. 459)

- Ciprofloxacin 400 mg (child: 10 mg/kg up to 400 mg) IV q8h
- Aztreonam 2 g (child: 50 mg/kg up to 2 g) IV q6–8h

PNEUMONIA IN COPD

Pathogens

Frequently due to overgrowth of colonised organisms in patient's lower airways

- *Haemophilus influenzae*
- *Streptococcus pneumoniae*
- *Moraxella catarrhalis*

Clinical

- Increase in sputum purulence
- Increase in coughing
- Increase in SOB
- Increase in sputum volume
- Fever
- Pleuritic chest pain
- Leucocytosis

Diagnosis

- Chest x-ray usually shows bronchopneumonia
- Sputum culture frequently isolates the colonised bacteria and may indicate the causative pathogen(s)

Antibiotic treatment

- Need hospital admission
- Treat as moderate to severe CAP
- Amoxicillin/ampicillin may not be suitable for the treatment, as the causative bacteria may have developed resistance to the frequently used antibiotics
  - Ceftriaxone (**or** cefotaxime) (IV) then cefuroxime (PO) **plus** azithromycin (**or** doxycycline **or** clarithromycin) (PO) for total of 7–14 days

If immediate penicillin allergy

  - Moxifloxacin (PO) **plus** azithromycin (**or** doxycycline **or** clarithromycin) (PO) for total of 7–14 days

Dosage of above antibiotics

- Ceftriaxone 1 g IV daily
- Cefotaxime 1 g IV q8h
- Cefuroxime 500 mg PO q12h
- Azithromycin 500 mg PO daily
- Doxycycline 100 mg PO q12h
- Clarithromycin 500 mg PO q12h
- Moxifloxacin 400 mg PO daily

PNEUMONIA IN THE IMMUNOCOMPROMISED

Pathogens

1. **T-cell immunodeficiency** (e.g. AIDS, immunosuppressive therapy, severe combined immunodeficiency)
- *Pneumocystis jirovecii*—see *Pneumocystis jirovecii* pneumonia (p. 173)
- *Streptococcus pneumoniae*—see Pneumococcal pneumonia (p. 300)
- *Legionella* spp—see Legionella (p. 198)
- Mycobacterium tuberculosis (see Tuberculosis, p. 405)
- Mycobacterium avium complex (MAC) (see p. 240)
- *Nocardia* spp—treat as brain abscess in Nocardiosis (see p. 251)
- *Cryptococcus neoformans*—see *Cryptococcus* pneumonia (p. 171)
- Cytomegalovirus (see p. 73)
- Varicella zoster—see Herpes zoster (p. 162)
- *Strongyloides stercoralis*
- Respiratory syncytial virus (RSV)
2. **B-cell immunodeficiency** (e.g. AIDS, chronic lymphocytic leukaemia, common variable immunodeficiency, immunosuppressive therapy, myeloma, nephrotic syndrome, X-linked agammaglobulinaemia)
- *Streptococcus pneumoniae*
- *Haemophilus influenzae*
- *Neisseria meningitides*
3. **Neutrophil deficiency** (e.g. neutropenia, chronic granulomatous disease)
- Gram-negative bacilli including *Pseudomonas* spp
- *Staphylococcus aureus*
- Viridans streptococci (if bacteraemia)
- *Aspergillus* spp (see p. 11)
- *Candida* spp—treatment as *Candida* sepsis (see p. 36)

Note

- Patients presenting with recurrent pneumonias, especially those involving unusual organisms, should arouse suspicion of an underlying immunodeficiency disorder
- If examination of sputum or tracheal aspirates is unhelpful, induced sputum, bronchoscopy, fine-needle aspiration or open lung biopsy may be necessary to establish a specific diagnosis
- Consultation with a clinical microbiologist or an ID specialist should be sought

POLIOMYELITIS

Other names: polio, infantile paralysis

Pathogens

- Poliovirus type 1, 2 or 3

Transmission

- Faecal–oral (virus is excreted in faeces)

Incubation

- 7–21 days

Infectious period

- 7–10 days before and 7–10 days after onset of symptoms (virus may be shed in faeces for 6 weeks)

Clinical

- Asymptomatic infection (95% of infected cases)
- Abortive poliomyelitis (4–5% of cases)—fever, sore throat and myalgia only
- Non-paralytic poliomyelitis—symptoms of abortive poliomyelitis plus meningeal irritation; recovery is complete
- Paralytic poliomyelitis (1% of cases)—muscle pain, asymmetrical paralysis
- Bulbar poliomyelitis—cranial nerve damage, respiratory muscle paralysis

Complications

- Aspiration pneumonia
- Myocarditis
- Paralytic ileus

Laboratory

Consult pathologist

- Poliovirus culture (faeces, CSF)
- Poliovirus PCR testing (faeces, CSF)—detection of wild-type poliovirus
- Poliovirus serology

Treatment

- Supportive, occupational therapy, physiotherapy and surgery

Vaccination

Primary vaccination for children

- IPV (inactivated poliomyelitis vaccine) combination vaccine (e.g. Infanrix Hexa): 0.5 mL IM, 3 doses at age 2, 4 and 6 months

Booster at 4 years of age

- DTPa-IPV (e.g. Infanrix IPV) 0.5 mL IM st

Primary vaccination for adults

No adult should remain unvaccinated

- IPV (e.g. IPOL®) **or** DTPa-IPV (e.g. Boostrix-IPV, Adacel® Polio) 0.5 mL IM, 3 doses at 4 weeks apart

Indication for adult booster

- Travel to affected countries (see www.polioeradication.org)—single IPV (e.g. IPOL)
- Healthcare workers in contact with poliomyelitis cases—single IPV (e.g. IPOL)
- Exposure to a continuing risk of infection—single IPV (e.g. IPOL) every 10 years

Vaccination of the immunocompromised and their household contacts

- Immunocompromised persons should receive a 4th dose of IPV 12 months after the 3rd dose
- HIV-positive individuals and their household contacts must receive IPV

PROCTITIS

Proctitis is an infection of the anus and rectum.

Transmission

- During anal sex in men who have sex with men (MSM) or women practising anal sex
- Shared enema usage may facilitate the spread of *Chlamydia* proctitis

Pathogens and clinical features

- *Neisseria gonorrhoeae* (gonococcal proctitis)—the most common cause; anorectal itching, bloody or mucopurulent discharge, diarrhoea
- *Chlamydia trachomatis*—*Chlamydia proctitis*—25% of cases; may have no symptoms or mild anorectal pain, discharge and cramping; severe cases may have bloody rectal discharge, severe pain and diarrhoea; some may develop rectal strictures
- Herpes simplex virus 1 and 2—herpes proctitis—multiple vesicles/ulcers, tenesmus, rectal pain, discharge and haematochezia; may be recurrent, more prolonged and severe in patients with immunodeficiency
- *Treponema pallidum*—syphilitic proctitis—primary stage: a painless sore with raised borders at the site of sexual contact, and enlarged firm and rubbery groin lymph nodes; secondary stage: a contagious diffuse rash over the body, particularly on hands and feet; third stage: affects mostly the heart and nervous system
- *Chlamydia trachomatis* L1–3—lymphogranuloma venereum (LGV) proctitis—cases have been reported in Australia; most cases are HIV-positive MSM with proctitis; transient painless genital ulcer followed by inguinal lymphadenopathy; may be complicated with perirectal/perianal strictures and fistulae

Laboratory

- HIV and syphilis serology
- Proctoscopy or sigmoidoscopy +/– biopsy
- Rectal swab—for *C. trachomatis* and *N. gonorrhoeae* PCR

- Rectal swab—for culture of *N. gonorrhoeae*
- Swabs from sores or ulcers—for syphilis PCR
- Swabs from de-roofed vesicles and ulcers—for herpes simplex virus PCR
- Swabs from sores or ulcers—for LGV PCR
- Serovar-specific LGV testing—if rectal swab is positive for *C. trachomatis* PCR
- Stool culture (if diarrhoea)
- Colonoscopy or barium enema—to exclude Crohn's disease or ulcerative colitis

Treatment

- Ceftriaxone (IM or IV) st **plus** doxycycline (PO) for 10 days

Proctitis with painful vesicles/ulceration **add**

- Valaciclovir 500 mg PO q12h for 5–10 days

In severe cases, longer treatment may be required

For lymphogranuloma venereum proctitis
- Option 1: doxycycline 100 mg PO q12h for 21 days
- Option 2: azithromycin 1 g PO weekly for 3 weeks

Dosage of above antibiotics

- Ceftriaxone 500 mg in 2 mL 1% lidocaine (lignocaine) IM **or** 500 mg IV as a single dose
- Doxycycline 100 mg PO q12h

PROPHYLAXIS—ABDOMINAL SURGERY
Indication for antibiotic prophylaxis

- Prophylaxis is appropriate in all patients undergoing abdominal surgery

Pathogens

- Aerobic gram-negative bacilli (e.g. *Escherichia coli*, *Klebsiella* spp)—the most common contaminating organisms
- Anaerobic gram-negative organisms (e.g. *Bacteroides* spp)—may be involved, depending on the site and risk factors

Antibiotic prophylaxis

- If operation ≤3 hours, a single dose of antibiotics is sufficient
- If operation >3 hours, a second dose should be given if a short-acting antibiotic is used
- The spectrum covered by the antibiotic must be relevant for the site
- If major peritoneal soiling occurs, a full course of antibiotic therapy should be given (see Peritonitis—post viscus perforation, p. 278)

Gastroduodenal and oesophageal surgery

Prophylaxis is recommended for:

- Procedures that enter the GI tract lumen
- GI tract perforation, bleeding or malignancy

- Significant obesity or immunocompromised
- Gastric outlet obstruction
- Reduced gastric acidity or motility

Prophylactic antibiotics
  - Cefazolin 2 g (child: 30 mg/kg up to 2 g) IV, 15–60 min before incision

Biliary surgery, including laparoscopic surgery

Prophylaxis is recommended for:

- Patients older than 70 years
- Obstructive jaundice, common bile duct stones
- With acute cholecystitis or a non-functional gall bladder
- Open cholecystectomy
- Patients with diabetes

Prophylaxis is **not** required for low-risk uncomplicated elective biliary procedures, including laparoscopic surgery

Prophylactic antibiotics
  - Cefazolin 2 g (child: 30 mg/kg up to 2 g) IV, 15–60 min before incision

Small bowel surgery

Prophylaxis is recommended for:

- All small bowel surgeries, except endoscopic procedures

Prophylactic antibiotics
  - Cefazolin (IV)

If bowel obstruction is present
  - Option 1: cefazolin (IV) **plus** metronidazole (IV)
  - Option 2: cefoxitin (IV) as a single drug

Dosage of above antibiotics

  - Cefazolin 2 g (child: 30 mg/kg up to 2 g) IV, 15–60 min before incision
  - Metronidazole 500 mg (child: 12.5 mg/kg up to 500 mg) IV, 15–60 min before incision
  - Cefoxitin 2 g (child: 40 mg/kg up to 2 g) IV, 15–60 min before incision

Colorectal surgery and appendicectomy

Prophylactic antibiotic
  - Option 1: cefazolin (IV) **plus** metronidazole (IV)
  - Option 2: gentamicin (IV) **plus** metronidazole (IV)
  - Option 3: cefoxitin (IV) as a single drug

Dosage of above antibiotics

  - Cefazolin 2 g (child: 30 mg/kg up to 2 g) IV, 15–60 min before incision
  - Metronidazole 500 mg (child: 12.5 mg/kg up to 500 mg) IV, 15–60 min before incision

- Gentamicin (adult and child) 2 mg/kg IV, 15–60 min before incision
- Cefoxitin 2 g (child: 40 mg/kg up to 2 g) IV, 15–60 min before incision

Hernia repair

Prophylaxis is recommended only if prosthetic material (mesh) is used **plus** the following conditions:

- Advanced age
- Immunocompromised
- Prolonged duration of operation
- Reoperation
- Use of surgical drains

Prophylactic antibiotics
  - Cefazolin 2 g (child: 30 mg/kg up to 2 g) IV, 15–60 min before incision

Endoscopic procedures

Prophylaxis is not required for routine upper or lower gastrointestinal endoscopy

ENDOSCOPIC RETROGRADE CHOLANGIOPANCREATOGRAPHY (ERCP)

Indication for antibiotic prophylaxis:

- ERCP with biliary tract obstruction if biliary drainage may not be achieved
- ERCP in patients with communicating pancreatitic cysts or pseudocysts and before transpapillary or transmural drainage of pseudocysts

Prophylactic antibiotics
  - Option 1: cefazolin 2 g (child: 30 mg/kg up to 2 g) IV, 15–60 min before incision
  - Option 2: gentamicin (adult and child) 2 mg/kg IV, 15–60 min before incision

ENDOSCOPIC ULTRASOUND-GUIDED FINE-NEEDLE ASPIRATION (EUS-FNA)

Indication for antibiotic prophylaxis:

- EUS-FNA of cystic lesions adjacent to GI tract
- May be considered for solid lesions adjacent to low GI tract

Prophylactic antibiotics
  - Option 1: cefazolin (IV) **plus** metronidazole (IV)
  - Option 2: gentamicin (IV) **plus** metronidazole (IV)
  - Option 3: cefoxitin (IV) as a single drug

Dosage of above antibiotics

  - Cefazolin 2 g (child: 30 mg/kg up to 2 g) IV, 15–60 min before incision
  - Metronidazole 500 mg (child: 12.5 mg/kg up to 500 mg) IV, 15–60 min before incision

- Gentamicin (adult and child) 2 mg/kg IV, 15–60 min before incision
- Cefoxitin 2 g (child: 40 mg/kg up to 2 g) IV, 15–60 min before incision

GASTROSTOMY OR JEJUNOSTOMY TUBE INSERTION

Indication for antibiotic prophylaxis:

- Percutaneous gastrostomy, endoscopically or radiologically
- Percutaneous jejunostomy tube insertion, endoscopically or radiologically

Prophylactic antibiotics

- Cefazolin 2 g (child: 30 mg/kg up to 2 g) IV, 15–60 min before incision

If at risk of MRSA colonisation/infection **add**

- Vancomycin (child and adult) 15 mg/kg IVI (10 mg/min), start 30–120 min before incision

PROPHYLAXIS—ASPLENIA

Pathogens

Encapsulated bacteria

- *Streptococcus pneumoniae*
- *Neisseria meningitides*
- *Haemophilus influenzae* type b (Hib)
- Bacteria acquired from animal bites
- Some parasites (including malaria)

High-risk patients

- Splenectomy
- Sickle cell disease or other congenital haemoglobinopathy with hyposplenia
- Asplenic and hyposplenic patients age <16 years or >50 years
- Previous invasive pneumococcal disease
- Severe underlying immunosuppression

Prophylactic antibiotics

- Amoxicillin (PO) **or** penicillin V (PO)
- Erythromycin (PO) (if allergic to penicillin)

Duration of prophylaxis

- Up to 5 years for asplenic children or hyposplenic children due to sickle cell anaemia or other congenital haemoglobinopathy
- At least 3 years for any patient post splenectomy
- At least 6 months for any asplenic patient post an episode of severe sepsis
- Lifelong for severely immunosuppressed patients or those with severe sepsis after splenectomy

Dosage of above antibiotics

- Amoxicillin 250 mg (child: 20 mg/kg up to 250 mg) PO daily
- Penicillin V 250 mg (child <1 years: 62.5 mg; 1–5 years: 125 mg) PO q12h
- Erythromycin 250 mg (child >1 month: 10 mg/kg up to 250 mg) PO daily

  or erythromycin (ethyl succinate) 400 mg (child >1 month: 10 mg/kg up to 400 mg) PO daily

Vaccination

Pneumococcal vaccination

- Child 6–9 years: 13vPCV (Prevenar 13®) 0.5 mL IM, 2 doses, 2 months apart, then 1 dose of 23vPPV (Pneumovax 23®) 0.5 mL IM®, at least 2 months later, followed by 1 dose every 5 years
- Adult, child ≥10 years: 13vPCV (Prevenar 13®) 0.5 mL IM single dose, then 1 dose of 23vPPV (Pneumovax 23®) 0.5 mL IM, at least 2 months later or 2 weeks before splenectomy or shortly after recovery from surgery, followed by 1 dose every 5 years

Meningococcal vaccination

- MenCCV (Meningitec, Menjugate) 0.5 mL IM (6 weeks–5 months: 2 doses, 2 months apart; 6–11 months: 1 dose) **then** 4vMenCV (Menactra, Menveo) 0.5 mL IM at 12 months, booster 5 yearly
- MenBV (Bexsero) 0.5 mL IM

  2–5 months of age: 3 doses, ≥1 month apart + booster at 12 months

  6–11 months of age: 2 doses, ≥2 months apart + booster at 12 months

  1–10 years of age: 2 doses, ≥2 months apart

  11–50 years of age: 2 doses, ≥1 month apart

Hib vaccination

Any age if unvaccinated or if vaccination has not completed, give a single dose of Hib vaccine 2 weeks before splenectomy

Influenza vaccination

2 weeks before splenectomy, then annually

PROPHYLAXIS—BREAST SURGERY

Indication for antibiotic prophylaxis

- Breast cancer surgery
- Reduction mammoplasty
- Prosthetic implantation or wire localisation
- Reoperation

Prophylactic antibiotics

- Cefazolin 2 g (child: 30 mg/kg up to 2 g) IV, 15–60 min before incision

If at risk of MRSA colonisation/infection **add**

- Vancomycin (child and adult) 15 mg/kg IVI (10 mg/min), start 30–120 min before incision

PROPHYLAXIS—BURNS AND EXTENSIVE SKIN LOSS

Pathogens

- *Staphylococcus aureus*
- *Streptococcus pyogenes*
- *Pseudomonas aeruginosa*
- Aerobic gram-negative bacilli

Prophylaxis

For dressing change

Regular use of a topical agent at each dressing change

- Silver sulfadiazine 1% + chlorhexidine 0.2% cream (e.g. Flamazine) topically, at each dressing change

For surgical debridement

Antibiotic choice according to culture results

- A single dose of an antibiotic (IV) before surgical debridement

If the procedure is >3 hours, repeat the dose or give as a continuous infusion

PROPHYLAXIS—CARDIAC SURGERY

Pathogens

- Gram-positive organisms—*Staphylococcus aureus* and coagulase-negative staphylococci
- Aerobic gram-negative organisms

Indication for antibiotic prophylaxis

- Valve replacement
- Coronary artery bypass surgery
- Cardiac transplantation
- Transcatheter aortic valve implantation
- Insertion of ventricular assist device

Preoperative screening and eradication of MRSA (p. 24) for all patients undergoing cardiac surgery

Prophylactic antibiotics

- Cefazolin (IV)

If at risk of MRSA colonisation/infection

- Cefazolin (IV) **plus** vancomycin (IVI)

If immediate penicillin allergy

- Vancomycin (IVI) **plus** gentamicin (IV)

Dosage of above antibiotics

- Cefazolin 2 g (child: 30 mg/kg up to 2 g) IV, 15–60 min before incision, then q8h up to 2 further doses
- Vancomycin (adult and child) 15 mg/kg IVI (10 mg/min), start 30–120 min before incision, may repeat the dose after 12 hours
- Gentamicin (adult and child) 5 mg/kg IV, 15–60 min before incision

IMPLANTABLE CARDIAC DEVICE INSERTION

Indication for antibiotic prophylaxis:

- Permanent pacemaker device
- Cardioverter-defibrillator
- Cardiac resynchronisation device

Prophylactic antibiotics

- Cefazolin (IV)

If at risk of MRSA colonisation/infection

- Cefazolin (IV) **plus** vancomycin (IVI)

Dosage of above antibiotics

- Cefazolin 2 g (child: 30 mg/kg up to 2 g) IV, 15–60 min before incision
- Vancomycin (adult and child) 15 mg/kg IVI (10 mg/min), start 30–120 min before incision
- Gentamicin (adult and child) 2 mg/kg IV, 15–60 min before incision

PROPHYLAXIS—CIRRHOSIS WITH GIT BLEEDING

Indication for prophylaxis

- Patient with cirrhosis who has active GI tract bleeding

Aim of prophylaxis

- To reduce the risk of subsequent bacterial infections, e.g. bacteraemia, pneumonia, spontaneous bacterial peritonitis (SBP) and urinary tract infections

Short-term prophylaxis

To reduce quinolone resistance

- Norfloxacin (PO) for 2 days

If oral therapy is not feasible

- Option 1: ceftriaxone (IV) for 2 days
- Option 2: ciprofloxacin (IV) for 2 days

Dosage of above antibiotics

- Norfloxacin 400 mg (child: 10 mg/kg up to 400 mg) PO q12h
- Ceftriaxone 1 g (child >1 month: 50 mg/kg up to 1 g) IV daily
- Ciprofloxacin 400 mg (child: 10 mg/kg up to 400 mg) IV q12h

PROPHYLAXIS—ENDOCARDITIS

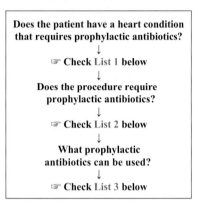

Does the patient have a heart condition that requires prophylactic antibiotics?
↓
☞ **Check List 1 below**
↓
Does the procedure require prophylactic antibiotics?
↓
☞ **Check List 2 below**
↓
What prophylactic antibiotics can be used?
↓
☞ **Check List 3 below**

FIGURE 16.1

Step guide for endocarditis prophylaxis

List 1: Heart conditions requiring prophylactic antibiotics

- Previous infective endocarditis
- Prosthetic cardiac valve or prosthetic material used for cardiac valve repair
- Congenital heart disease—unrepaired cyanotic defects (including palliative shunts and conduits)
- Congenital heart disease—completely repaired defects with prosthetic material or devices, during the first 6 months after the repair
- Congenital heart disease—repaired defects with residual defects at or adjacent to the site of a prosthetic patch or device
- Rheumatic heart disease in high-risk patients

List 2: Procedures requiring prophylactic antibiotics

Dental procedures requiring prophylaxis

- Extraction
- Periodontal procedures including surgery, subgingival scaling and root planing
- Replanting avulsed teeth
- Others: implant placement, apicoectomy

Dental procedures that may require prophylaxis

- Full periodontal probing for patients with periodontitis
- Intraligmentary and intraosseous local anaesthetic injection
- Supragingival calculus removal/cleaning
- Rubber dam placement with clamps (where there is a risk of damaging gingiva)
- Restorative matrix band/strip placement
- Endodontics beyond the apical foramen

- Placement of orthodontic bands
- Placement of interdental wedges
- Subgingival placement of retraction cords, antibiotic fibres or strips

Respiratory tract procedures requiring prophylaxis

- Invasive ear/nose/throat or respiratory tract procedure to treat an infection
- Tonsillectomy/adenoidectomy
- Laryngectomy, pharyngectomy, complex septorhinoplasty

Genitourinary and gastrointestinal tract procedures requiring prophylaxis

- Suspected or confirmed genitourinary tract or intra-abdominal infection
- Genitourinary or gastrointestinal tract procedure where antibiotic prophylaxis is routinely indicated
- Caesarean section
- Prevention of group B streptococcal disease in pre-term pre-labour rupture of membranes
- Third- or fourth-degree perineal tear

List 3: Prophylactic antibiotics

For dental and respiratory tract procedures

- Option 1: amoxicillin (PO) (**or** ampi(amoxi)cillin [IV or IM])
- Option 2: cefalexin (PO) (**or** cefazolin [IV or IM])

If immediate penicillin allergy or taken beta-lactam recently

- Clindamycin (PO or IV) (**or** lincomycin [IV])

For genitourinary and gastrointestinal tract procedures

- Ampi(amoxi)cillin (IV or IM)

If immediate penicillin allergy

- Vancomycin (IVI) (**or** teicoplanin [IV])

Dosage of above antibiotics

For dental and respiratory tract procedures

- Amoxicillin 2 g (child: 50 mg/kg up to 2 g) PO 1 hour before procedure
- Ampi(amoxi)cillin 2 g (child: 50 mg/kg up to 2 g) IV 15–60 min before procedure
- Ampi(amoxi)cillin 2 g (child: 50 mg/kg up to 2 g) IM 30 min before procedure
- Cefalexin 2 g (child: 50 mg/kg up to 2 g) PO 1 hour before procedure
- Cefazolin 2 g (child: 30 mg/kg up to 2 g) IV 15–60 min before procedure
- Cefazolin 2 g (child: 30 mg/kg up to 2 g) IM, 30 min before procedure
- Clindamycin 600 mg (child: 20 mg/kg up to 600 mg) PO 1 hour before procedure
- Clindamycin 600 mg (child: 20 mg/kg max 600 mg) IV over 20 min, 15–60 min before procedure

For genitourinary and GI procedures
- Ampi(amoxi)cillin 2 g (child: 50 mg/kg up to 2 g) IV 15–60 min before procedure
- Ampi(amoxi)cillin 2 g (child: 50 mg/kg up to 2 g) IM 30 min before procedure
- Vancomycin (adult and child) 15 mg/kg IVI at 10 mg/min 30–120 min before procedure
- Teicoplanin 400 mg (child: 10 mg/kg up to 400 mg) IV just before procedure

PROPHYLAXIS—EYE SURGERY

Prevention of endophthalmitis

- Preoperative screening and treatment of active conjunctivitis, dacryocystitis or blepharitis
- Antisepsis of periocular area and ocular surface
- Good intraoperative techniques
- Intracameral (anterior chamber) injection of antibiotics at the end of cataract surgery
  - Cefazolin 1–2.5 mg intracamerally, at the end of surgery
- Postoperative topical antibiotic use lacks evidence; if considered use
  - Chloramphenicol 0.5% eye drops, 1–2 drops qid for 7 days

If allergic to chloramphenicol
  - Tobramycin eye drops, 1–2 drops qid for 7 days

PROPHYLAXIS—HEAD, NECK AND THORACIC SURGERY

Indication for antibiotic prophylaxis

- Procedures that involve incision through oral, nasal, pharyngeal or oesophageal mucosa
- Stapedectomy or similar operations
- Insertion of prosthetic material
- Head and neck cancer operation

Prophylactic antibiotics

  - Cefazolin (IV)

If incisions through mucosal surfaces
  - Cefazolin (IV) **plus** metronidazole (IV)

If immediate penicillin allergy
  - Clindamycin (IV)

Dosage of above antibiotics

  - Cefazolin 2 g (child: 30 mg/kg up to 2 g) IV 15–60 min before incision
  - Metronidazole 500 mg (child: 12.5 mg/kg up to 500 mg) IV 15–60 min before incision
  - Clindamycin 600 mg (child: 15 mg/kg up to 600 mg) IV 15–60 min before incision

PROPHYLAXIS—LOWER LIMB AMPUTATION

Pathogens and risk factors

- Aerobic skin bacteria
- Anaerobic bacteria, e.g. *Clostridia* spp
- Ischaemic leg is particularly at risk of infection

Prophylactic antibiotics

- Cefazolin (IV)

If at risk of MRSA colonisation/infection

- Cefazolin (IV) **plus** vancomycin (IVI)

If immediate penicillin allergy

- Vancomycin (IVI) **plus** gentamicin (IV)

For amputation of an ischaemic limb **add**

- Metronidazole (IV)

Dosage of above antibiotics

- Cefazolin 2 g (child: 30 mg/kg up to 2 g) IV 15–60 min before incision, then q8h up to 2 further doses
- Vancomycin (adult and child) 15 mg/kg IVI (10 mg/min), start 30–120 min before incision, may repeat the dose after 12 hours
- Gentamicin (adult and child) 5 mg/kg IV, 15–60 min before incision
- Metronidazole 500 mg (child: 12.5 mg/kg up to 500 mg) IV 15–60 min before incision, may repeat the dose after 12 hours

PROPHYLAXIS—MENINGITIS

Pathogens

- *Neisseria meningitidis* (meningococcus)
    - Serogroup B—the most common in most areas of Australia
    - Serogroup C—the most common in Victoria and Tasmania
    - Serotype A, Y and W135—nationally, for <5% of cases
- *Haemophilus influenzae* type b (Hib) (less common)

Aim of chemoprophylaxis

To eradicate asymptomatic carriage in close contacts so that susceptible members of the group do not acquire the organism

Prophylactic antibiotics

N. meningitidis (meningococcus)

- Option 1: ciprofloxacin (PO) (preferred option for women on OCP)
- Option 2: ceftriaxone (IM) (preferred option for pregnant women)
- Option 3: rifampicin (PO) (preferred option for children)

H. influenzae type b (Hib)

- Option 1: rifampicin (PO)
- Option 2: ceftriaxone (IM)—if rifampicin is unsuitable

Dosage of above antibiotics

N. meningitidis (meningococcus)
- Ciprofloxacin 500 mg (child <5 years: 30 mg/kg up to 125 mg; 5–12 years: 250 mg) PO st
- Ceftriaxone 250 mg (child >1 month: 125 mg) IM* st
- Rifampicin 600 mg (neonate: 5 mg/kg; child: 10 mg/kg up to 600 mg) PO q12h for 2 days

H. influenzae type b (Hib)
- Rifampicin 600 mg (neonate: 10 mg/kg; child: 20 mg/kg up to 600 mg) PO daily for 4 days
- Ceftriaxone 1 g (child >1 month: 50 mg/kg up to 1 g) IM* or IV daily for 2 days

Meningococcal vaccines

1. Conjugate vaccines (MenCCV) against serogroup C
2. Quadrivalent conjugate vaccines (4vMenCV) against serogroups A, C, Y and W135
3. Polysaccharide vaccines (4vMenPV) against serogroups A, C, Y and W135
4. Multicomponent B vaccine (4CMenB) against serogroup B

Meningococcal C

- Children at age of 12 months—1 dose of MenCCV
- Age <6 months with high risk—additional 2 doses (8 weeks apart) before 12 months
- Age 6–11 months with high risk—additional 1 dose before 12 months

Meningococcal A, W135 or Y

- Age 17–18 who have not been vaccinated previously—1 dose of 4vMenCV

Meningococcal B

- Age 2–5 months—3 doses of 4CMenB (>1 month apart), booster after 12 months
- Age 6–11 months—2 doses of 4CMenB (>2 months apart), booster after 12 months
- Age 1–10 years—2 doses of 4CMenB (>2 months apart)
- Age 11–50 years—2 doses of 4CMenB (>1 month apart)

Vaccination for close contacts of meningococcal C

Only indicated for household and household-like contacts who were unvaccinated before
- Infant 2–5 months—2 doses of MenCCV 0.5 mL IM, at least 8 weeks apart, followed by a booster dose at 12 months
- Infant 6–12 months—1 dose of MenCCV 0.5 mL IM, followed by a booster dose at 12 months or 8 weeks after the 1st dose, whichever is later

---

*IM injection of ceftriaxone needs to be reconstituted with 1% lidocaine (lignocaine)

- Child >12 months and adult who is unvaccinated—1 dose of MenCCV 0.5 mL IM

Control of outbreaks caused by serogroup C

- Unvaccinated high-risk people—as close contacts (above)
- Patient with meningococcal C disease who is a child, an adolescent or a young adult—1 dose of MenCCV 0.5 mL IM (vaccine may be administered on discharge from hospital, or when the patient recovers from the infection)

Travellers to group A, W135 or Y epidemic areas

- 1 dose of 4vMenPV 0.5 mL SC

A current list of these countries is available at http://who.int/ith/en

Control of outbreaks of serogroup A, W135 or Y

- 4vMenCV **or** 4vMenPV 0.5 mL IM st

High-risk persons of A, W135 or Y infection

Such as those living in epidemic areas and with immunodeficiency (if last vaccination was 3–5 years ago)
- 4vMenCV **or** 4vMenPV 0.5 mL IM st

Laboratory personnel who frequently handle *N. meningitides*

- MenCCV 0.5 mL IM **and** 4vMenCV **or** 4vMenPV 0.5 mL IM*

Persons with inherited defects of properdin or complement, or asplenia

- MenCCV 0.5 mL IM (≥6 weeks of age) **and** 4vMenPV 0.5 mL IM (≥2 years of age)**, revaccination 5 yearly

Hib vaccination

- Index case <2 years of age—commence a full course of Hib vaccination as soon as possible after recovery from meningitis, regardless of any previous Hib immunisation
- Unvaccinated contacts <5 years of age—full course of immunisation as soon as possible

PROPHYLAXIS—NEUROSURGERY

Pathogens

- *Staphylococcus aureus*
- Coagulase-negative staphylococci
- Diphtheroids

Indication for antibiotic prophylaxis

- Craniotomy in prolonged procedures
- Re-explorations and microsurgery
- Insertion of prosthetic material (e.g. acrylic plates)

---

*If MenCCV is given first, ≥2 weeks should lapse before 4vMenPV is given
**If 4vMenPV is given first, 6 months should lapse before MenCCV is given

Not indicated for antibiotic prophylaxis

- CSF leakage following trauma
- Insertion of shunts, ventricular drains or pressure monitors (benefit unproven)

Prophylactic antibiotics

- Cefazolin (IV)

If at risk of MRSA colonisation/infection
- Cefazolin (IV) **plus** vancomycin (IVI)

If immediate penicillin allergy
- Vancomycin (IVI) **plus** gentamicin (IV)

Dosage of above antibiotics

- Cefazolin 2 g (child: 30 mg/kg up to 2 g) IV, 15–60 min before incision
- Vancomycin (adult and child) 15 mg/kg IVI (10 mg/min), start 30–120 min before incision
- Gentamicin (adult and child) 5 mg/kg IV, 15–60 min before incision

PROPHYLAXIS—OBSTETRIC AND GYNAECOLOGICAL SURGERY

Not indicated for antibiotic prophylaxis

- Insertion of intrauterine device
- Laparoscopy
- Medical termination of pregnancy

Indication for antibiotic prophylaxis

1. Surgical termination of pregnancy

- Screening and treatment of BV prior to vaginal termination can reduce the risk of post-procedure infection (see Bacterial vaginosis, p. 432)
- Screen and treat *Chlamydia* infection prior to the procedure (see *Chlamydia*, p. 53)

Prophylactic antibiotics

- Doxycycline 100 mg PO 60 min before procedure, then 200 mg PO 90 min after procedure

2. Caesarean section

Antibiotic prophylaxis is indicated for all caesarean sections to reduce wound sepsis and endometritis

Prophylactic antibiotics

- Cefazolin 2 g IV, 15–60 min before incision

If immediate penicillin allergy

- Clindamycin 600 mg IV over 20–30 min, 15–60 min before incision

3. Hysterectomy

Preoperative screening and treatment of BV can reduce the risk of postoperative infection (see Bacterial vaginosis, p. 432)

Prophylactic antibiotics

For vaginal hysterectomy
  * Cefazolin (IV) **plus** metronidazle (IV)

For abdominal hysterectomy
  * Cefazolin (IV)

If immediate penicillin allergy
  * Clindamycin (IV)

Dosage of above antibiotics
  * Cefazolin 2 g IV 15–60 min before incision
  * Metronidazole 500 mg IV 15–60 min before incision
  * Clindamycin 600 mg IV over 20–30 min, 15–60 min before incision

4. Pre-term pre-labour rupture of membranes (PPROM)

PPROM is membrane rupture before 37 weeks' gestation and before the onset of uterine contractions—antibiotic prophylaxis is associated with prolonged pregnancy and reduction in maternal and neonatal infections

Antibiotic prophylaxis and therapy

For PPROM without chorioamnionitis
  * Ampi(amoxi)cillin (IV) then amoxicillin (PO) **plus** erythromycin (PO)

If allergic to penicillin
  * Erythromycin (PO) as a single drug

For PPROM with chorioamnionitis
  * Ampi(amoxi)cillin (IV) **plus** gentamicin (IV) **plus** metronidazole (IV)

If immediate penicillin allergy seek expert advice

Dosage of above antibiotics
For PPROM without chorioamnionitis
  * Ampi(amoxi)cillin 2 g IV q6h for 2 days, then amoxicillin 250 mg PO q8h for 5 days
  * Erythromycin 250 mg PO q6h for 7 days

For PPROM with chorioamnionitis
  * Ampi(amoxi)cillin 2 g IV q6h
  * Gentamicin 5 mg/kg IV daily (monitor blood level and adjust dose, see p. 459)
  * Metronidazole 500 mg IV q12h

5. Third- or fourth-degree perineal tear

Antibiotic prophylaxis and therapy

Preoperative prophylaxis

- Option 1: cefazolin (IV) **plus** metronidazole (IV) as early as possible before repair

- Option 2: cefoxitin (IV) as early as possible before repair

Postoperative therapy (following anal sphincter repair)

- Amoxicillin/clavulanate (PO) for 7 days
If penicillin allergy
- Cefalexin (PO) **plus** metronidazole (PO) for 7 days
If immediate penicillin allergy
- Cotrimoxazole (PO) **plus** metronidazole (PO) for 7 days

Dosage of above antibiotics

- Cefazolin 2 g IV as early as possible before repair
- Metronidazole 500 mg IV as early as possible before repair
- Cefoxitin 2 g IV as early as possible before repair
- Amoxicillin/clavulanate 875 mg PO q12h
- Cefalexin 500 mg PO q6h
- Metronidazole 400 mg PO q12h
- Cotrimoxazole 160/800 mg PO q12h

PROPHYLAXIS—ORTHOPAEDIC SURGERY

Pathogens

- *Staphylococcus aureus*
- Coagulase-negative staphylococci
- Aerobic gram-negative bacilli (less common)
- Anaerobes (less common)

Indication for antibiotic prophylaxis

- Prosthetic large joint replacement
- Procedure involving insertion of prosthetic or transplant material
- Internal fixation of fracture of large bones
- Spinal surgery
- Open fracture

Preoperative treatment

- Treat chronic or recurrent skin infections, genitourinary tract infections, dental infections or other infections before the elective surgery

Prophylactic antibiotics

- Cefazolin (IV)
If at risk of MRSA colonisation/infection
- Cefazolin (IV) **plus** vancomycin (IVI)

If immediate penicillin allergy
- Vancomycin (IVI)

Dosage of above antibiotics

- Cefazolin 2 g (child: 30 mg/kg up to 2 g) IV 15–60 min before incision
- Vancomycin (adult and child) 15 mg/kg IVI (10 mg/min), start 30–120 min before incision

PROPHYLAXIS—PLASTIC SURGERY

Indication for antibiotic prophylaxis

- Implantation of prosthetic material
- Prior skin irradiation
- Clean-contaminated procedures (operative wounds enter respiratory, alimentary, genital or urinary tracts without unusual contamination)

Prophylactic antibiotics

- Cefazolin (IV)

If at risk of MRSA colonisation/infection
- Cefazolin (IV) **plus** vancomycin (IVI)

If immediate penicillin allergy
- Vancomycin (IVI)

Dosage of above antibiotics

- Cefazolin 2 g (child: 30 mg/kg up to 2 g) IV 15–60 min before incision
- Vancomycin (adult and child) 15 mg/kg IVI (10 mg/min), start 30–120 min before incision

PROPHYLAXIS—POST-SEXUAL ASSAULT

Management

- Discuss with a sexual assault service and referral
- Full range of tests for STIs before treatment (if given) and on follow-up
- Pregnancy test for a female victim
- Forensic specimens should be collected by an experienced professional and follow protocols

1. For STI

Indication for antibiotic prophylaxis:

- If the offender is known to have an STI or is at high risk of having an STI

Prophylactic antibiotics

- If it is likely that the victim will not return for follow-up
  - Ceftriaxone (IM or IV) **plus** azithromycin (PO) **plus** metronidazole (**or** tinidazole) (PO)

Dosage of above antibiotics

- Ceftriaxone 500 mg (child: 250 mg) in 2 mL of 1% lidocaine (lignocaine) IM or IV st
- Azithromycin 1 g (child: 20 mg/kg up to 1 g) PO st
- Metronidazole 2 g (child: 30 mg/kg up to 2 g) PO st
- Tinidazole 2 g (child: 50 mg/kg up to 2 g) PO st

2. For hepatitis B virus (HBV)

- If the victim is immune to HBV (HBsAb positive)—no action required
- If the victim is not immune to HBV (HBsAb negative)
  - If the source is HBsAg negative and unlikely in window period: start hep B vaccination
  - If the source is HBsAg positive or status unknown: 1) test the victim for HBsAg at baseline, 3 months and 6 months after exposure; 2) give HBIg within 72 hours of exposure; 3) start hep B vaccination ASAP
  - Hep B immunoglobulin (HBIg) 100–400 U IM ASAP (within 72 hours)
  - Hep B vaccine (e.g. Engerix B, H-B-VAX II or Twinrix 720/20) 1 mL IM, 3 doses at 0, 1 and 6 months, commence ASAP (1st dose given preferably within 24 hours of exposure)

3. For hepatitis C virus (HCV)

- If the source is HCV antibody negative and unlikely in window period—no action
- If the source is HCV antibody negative but is likely in window period—test the victim for HCV serology in 3 months
- If the source is HCV antibody positive—test the victim's HCV serology + HCV PCR in 3 months
- If the victim's HCV antibody and HCV PCR become positive at 3 months' follow-up testing—refer for early antiviral therapy

4. For HIV

- If the source is HIV antibody/antigen negative and unlikely in window period—no action
- If the source is known or suspected to be infected with HIV
  - Refer the victim to an experienced HIV practitioner—initiation of prophylaxis should be the responsibility of an HIV practitioner
  - General principles and medication choices, see Needle-stick injuries and blood exposure (p. 247)

PROPHYLAXIS—SBP IN ASCITIC PATIENT

SBP has a high rate of recurrence.

Indication for prophylaxis

- After first episode of SBP (secondary antibiotic prophylaxis)
- Patients with low ascitic protein level (<15 g/L) + liver failure and/or renal impairment (primary antibiotic prophylaxis)

Prophylactic antibiotics

- Cotrimoxazole 160/800 mg (child >1 month: 4/20 mg/kg up to 160/800 mg) PO daily

If cotrimoxazole is contraindicated or has previously failed

- Norfloxacin 400 mg (child: 10 mg/kg up to 400 mg) PO daily

PROPHYLAXIS—SURGICAL (GENERAL PRINCIPLES)

Indications

- If there is a significant risk of postoperative infection (e.g. colonic resection)
- If postoperative infection would cause severe consequences (e.g. a prosthetic implant)

Limitations

Antibiotic prophylaxis cannot be relied upon to overcome:

- Inadequate medical management (e.g. diabetes)
- Excessive soiling
- Tissue damage
- Inadequate debridement and poor surgical technique

Causative organisms

- Most postsurgical infections are due to the patient's own flora
- In hospitalised patients, postoperative infection may be due to multi-resistant organisms

Antibiotic choice

- Take into account the organisms causing infection within the institution, their patterns of susceptibility and the selection pressure of antibiotic use
- Avoid third-generation cefalosporins (e.g. cefotaxime and ceftriaxone)
- Do not use vancomycin for routine prophylaxis, in order to prevent selection pressure for vancomycin-resistant enterococci (VRE) and vancomycin-intermediate MRSA (VISA)
- Vancomycin is only indicated in the following situations
    - Preoperative patients infected or colonised with an MRSA strain (hospital-acquired or community-associated) currently or in the past
    - Patients having major surgery who are at high risk of MRSA colonisation (e.g. >5 days in a healthcare facility where MRSA is endemic)
    - Patients undergoing prosthetic cardiac valve, joint or vascular surgery where the procedure is a re-operation (return to theatre or revision)
    - Patients allergic to penicillin and/or cefalosporin

If vancomycin is used, intraoperative and postoperative doses are not required except in cardiac and vascular surgery

Preoperative MRSA screening and decolonisation

- Preoperative MRSA screening and decolonisation for targeted patients undergoing high-risk surgery can reduce the incidence of MRSA infection (see Fig. 16.2)

Route of administration of prophylactic antibiotics

- Parental, either IV or IM—usual way
- Rectal or oral—in certain instances

Timing of administration of prophylactic antibiotics

- Vancomycin—slow infusion (<10 mg/min), start 30–120 min before surgical incision, can be completed after surgical incision
- Other IV antibiotics—within 60 min before surgical incision; IV infusion should be finished before surgical incision
- IM antibiotics—at the time of premedication for surgery
- Rectal metronidazole—should be given 2–4 hours before surgery
- Oral tinidazole—should be given 6–12 hours prior to surgery

Dose of prophylactic antibiotics

- In general, a single dose of parenteral drug is sufficient
- A second dose may be necessary under the following conditions:
    - A significant delay in starting the operation
    - If cefazolin or flucloxacillin is used and the operation is prolonged, give a second dose after 3 hours
    - Excessive blood loss during the procedure
    - Postoperative prophylactic doses up to 24 hours are only required for some cardiac and vascular surgeries, and low limb amputation

Continuing prophylactic antibiotics until surgical drains have been removed is of unproven benefit and should be avoided

PROPHYLAXIS—THORACIC SURGERY

Prophylactic antibiotics

- Cefazolin (IV)

If at risk of MRSA colonisation/infection

- Cefazolin (IV) **plus** vancomycin (IVI)

If immediate penicillin allergy

- Vancomycin (IVI)

Dosage of above antibiotics

- Cefazolin 2 g (child: 30 mg/kg up to 2 g) IV 15–60 min before incision
- Vancomycin (adult and child) 15 mg/kg IVI (10 mg/min), start 30–120 min before incision

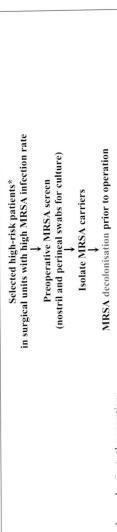

Selected high-risk patients*
in surgical units with high MRSA infection rate

↓

Preoperative MRSA screen
(nostril and perineal swabs for culture)

↓

Isolate MRSA carriers

↓

MRSA decolonisation prior to operation

In the week prior to the operation:

➤ Option 1: mupirocin 2% nasal oint (e.g. Bactroban) intranasal bid for 5 days

➤ Option 2: chlorhexidine 0.3% nasal cream (e.g. Nasalate) intranasal tds for 5 days

PLUS wash whole body daily for 5 days with either of following:

➤ Option 1: chlorhexidine 2% solution (e.g. Microshield 2)

➤ Option 2: triclosan 1% solution (e.g. pHisoHex) or soap (e.g. Sapoderm, Solyptol)

Pay particular attention to hair-bearing areas

↓

Vancomycin prophylaxis just prior to induction of anaesthesia

Alternatively, routine decolonisation for all high-risk patients prior to operation + vancomycin prophylaxis

* High-risk patients are those undergoing prosthetic cardiac valve, joint or vascular surgery who have been in the hospital for more than 5 days.

FIGURE 16.2
Preoperative MRSA screening and decolonisation

PROPHYLAXIS—UROLOGICAL SURGERY

General considerations

- Sterile urine should be confirmed before urological surgery
- Asymptomatic bacteriuria should be treated preoperatively
- Antibiotic choice should be guided by urine culture and susceptibility results
- Using antibiotics to cover the period of catheterisation is not recommended

Perioperative treatment of bacteriuria

- Choose antibiotic according to urine culture and susceptibility result

If no urine culture result

- Gentamicin (adult and child) 3 mg/kg IV, as a single preoperative dose

1.   Endoscopic procedures

Indication for antibiotic prophylaxis:

- Endoscopic intrarenal and ureteric stone procedures (e.g. percutaneous nephrolithotomy, pyeloscopy for renal stones or ureteroscopy for ureteric stones)
- Endoscopic resection of large or necrotic tumours
- Risk of bleeding
- Bladder outlet obstruction (incomplete bladder emptying)
- Lithotripsy in patients with an internal stent, nephrostomy tube or indwelling catheter

Prophylactic antibiotics

- Cefazolin (IV)

If at risk of MRSA colonisation/infection

- Cefazolin (IV) **plus** vancomycin (IVI)

If immediate penicillin allergy

- Gentamicin (IV)

Dosage of above antibiotics

- Cefazolin 2 g (child: 30 mg/kg up to 2 g) IV 15–60 min before procedure
- Vancomycin (adult and child) 15 mg/kg IVI (10 mg/min), start 30–120 min before procedure
- Gentamicin (adult and child) 2 mg/kg IV 15–60 min before procedure

2.   Transurethral resection of prostate (TURP)

Prophylactic antibiotics

- Option 1: gentamicin 2 mg/kg IV, 15–60 min before procedure
- Option 2: cefazolin 2 g IV, 15–60 min before procedure
- Option 3: trimethoprim 300 mg PO, 60 min before procedure

If MRSA urinary tract colonisation/infection **add**
* Vancomycin 15 mg/kg IVI (10 mg/min), start 30–120 min before procedure

3. Transrectal prostatic biopsy
Prophylactic antibiotics

* Prebiopsy screen for ciprofloxacin-resistant Enterobacteriaceae (faecal sample or rectal swabs) should be done for at-risk patients (e.g. quinolone treatment within past 3 months or travel to Asia or southern Europe within past 3–6 months)
  * Ciprofloxacin 500 mg PO 60–120 min before procedure

4. Transperineal prostatic biopsy
* Lower rates of postoperative infection than transrectal prostatic biopsy

Prophylactic antibiotics

* Cefazolin 2 g IV 15–60 min before procedure

5. Open or laparoscopic urological procedures
Indication for antibiotic prophylaxis:

* Urinary tract obstruction or abnormality
* Implantation of prosthetic devices (e.g. penile prosthesis, artificial urinary sphincter, mesh)
* Immediate operation and bacteriuria cannot be excluded
* All urological procedures where urinary tract is entered

Antibiotic prophylaxis is not indicated for:

* Vasectomy
* Scrotal surgery
* Varicocele ligation

Prophylactic antibiotics

* Cefazolin (IV)

For implantation of prosthetic devices or for radical prostatectomy
* Option 1: cefazolin (IV) **plus** gentamicin (IV)
* Option 2: cefazolin (IV) **plus** trimethoprim (PO)

If MRSA urinary tract colonisation/infection **add**
* Vancomycin (IVI)

If urinary tract is entered and immediate penicillin allergy
* Vancomycin (IVI) **plus** gentamicin (IV)

If at risk of entry into bowel lumen **add**
* Metronidazole (IV)

Dosage of above antibiotics
* Cefazolin 2 g (child: 30 mg/kg up to 2 g) IV 15–60 min before incision
* Gentamicin (adult and child) 2 mg/kg IV 15–60 min before incision

- Trimethoprim 300 mg PO 60 min before incision
- Vancomycin (adult and child) 15 mg/kg IVI (10 mg/min), start 30–120 min before incision
- Metronidazole 500 mg (child: 12.5 mg/kg up to 500 mg) IV, 15–60 min before incision

PROPHYLAXIS—VASCULAR SURGERY

Antibiotic prophylaxis is indicated for:

- Abdominal aorta reconstructive surgery with implantation of foreign material
- Lower limb arterial reconstructive surgery with a groin incision or with implantation of foreign material
- Arteriovenous fistula formation (single preoperative dose)

Antibiotic prophylaxis is not indicated for:

- Operations on brachial and carotid arteries, not involving prosthetic materials
- Operation on varicose veins

Prophylactic antibiotics

- Cefazolin (IV)

If at risk of MRSA colonisation/infection

- Cefazolin (IV) **plus** vancomycin (IVI)

If immediate penicillin allergy

- Vancomycin (IVI) **plus** gentamicin (IV)

Dosage of above antibiotics

- Cefazolin 2 g (child: 30 mg/kg up to 2 g) IV 15–60 min before incision, then q8h for up to 2 further doses
- Vancomycin (adult and child) 15 mg/kg IVI (10 mg/min), start 30–120 min before incision, may repeat the dose after 12 hours
- Gentamicin (adult and child) 5 mg/kg IV, 15–60 min before incision

PROSTATITIS

1.   ACUTE BACTERIAL PROSTATITIS

Pathogens

- Urinary tract pathogens—*Escherichia coli*, *Proteus*, *Klebsiella*, enterococci and group B streptococci
- Sexually transmitted pathogens (occasionally)—*Chlamydia* and gonorrhoea

Clinical

- Fever, perineal pain with extreme tenderness of prostate on rectal examination, urinary frequency, urgency, dysuria, weak stream and urethral discharge
- Can be complicated by the development of abscess or bacteraemia

Laboratory

- Urine and/or prostatic fluid microscopy and cultures

Treatment

- Urine and blood for culture and sensitivity test—sent before starting treatment
- Repeat urine cultures 1–2 weeks after treatment is completed

Mild to moderate infection

- Option 1: trimethoprim 300 mg PO daily for 2–4 weeks
- Option 2: cefalexin 500 mg PO q12h for 2–4 weeks
- Option 3: amoxicillin/clavulanate 500 mg PO q12h for 2–4 weeks

If resistant to above agents

- Option 1: ciprofloxacin 500 mg PO q12h for 2–4 weeks
- Option 2: norfloxacin 400 mg PO q12h for 2–4 weeks

Severe infection

- Ampi(amoxi)cillin (IV) **plus** gentamicin (IV)

If penicillin allergy

- Gentamicin (IV) alone

If aminoglycoside is contraindicated

- Ceftriaxone (**or** cefotaxime)* (IV)

If multidrug-resistant gram-negative organism is suspected

- Meropenem 500–1000 mg IV q8h

Modify therapy based on result of cultures and susceptibility testing

Duration of therapy and follow-up

- Continue IV antibiotics until afebrile for 24–48 hours, switch to oral antibiotic (above) for a total of 2 weeks (4 weeks for severe disease or bacteraemia)

Dosage of above antibiotics

Severe infection

- Ampi(amoxi)cillin 2 g IV q6h
- Gentamicin 4–7 mg/kg IV for the 1st dose (further dosing, see p. 459)
- Ceftriaxone 1 g IV daily
- Cefotaxime 1 g IV q8h

2. CHRONIC BACTERIAL PROSTATITIS

Pathogens

- *Escherichia coli*
- *Proteus* spp
- *Klebsiella* spp
- *Chlamydia trachomatis* (sexually transmitted)

---

*Ceftriaxone/cefotaxime does not cover enterococci or *Pseudomonas aeruginosa*

- *Mycoplasma genitalium* (sexually transmitted)
- *Ureaplasma urealyticum* (sexually transmitted)

Suspect chronic prostatitis

- Recurrent lower UTIs with the same organism
- Persistent symptoms after treatment of sexually acquired urethritis

Clinical

- Chronic prostate pain, intermittent dysuria and/or obstructive urinary tract symptoms

Laboratory

- Microscopy and culture—terminal urine and post-massage secretions
- *Chlamydia trachomatis* PCR—first-void urine (if bacterial culture negative)
- *Mycoplasma genitalium* PCR—first-void urine (if bacterial culture negative)
- *Ureaplasma urealyticum* PCR—prostate secretions (if bacterial culture negative)

Treatment

Treatment is difficult as few antibiotics penetrate into the non-inflamed prostate

Antibiotics are effective in curing only about one-third of cases

For conventional bacterial infection
  - Option 1: ciprofloxacin 500 mg PO q12h for 4 weeks
  - Option 2: norfloxacin 400 mg PO q12h for 4 weeks
  - Option 3: trimethoprim 300 mg PO daily for 4 weeks
If *Chlamydia* or *Mycoplasma* or *Ureaplasma* is identified
  - Doxycycline 100 mg PO q12h for 2–4 weeks

Treat sexual partners at the same time

PSITTACOSIS

Other names: ornithosis, parrot fever

Pathogens

- *Chlamydia psittaci*
- Principally carried by birds of the parrot family, including budgerigars, lovebirds and parakeets
- Other birds that may harbour the germ include canaries, poultry and pigeons

Transmission

- Inhaling *Chlamydia* from shed feathers, secretions and droppings
  (*C. psittaci* can live for several months in shed feathers and droppings)
- Person-to-person transmission is extremely rare

Incubation

- 1 week to 1 month

People at risk

- People who have birds as pets or who work in aviaries or pet shops;
  poultry workers
- Even casual contact with an infected bird can result in infection
- Some people develop psittacosis with no recognised history of bird
  contact

Clinical

- Some people may have no symptoms
- Symptoms: fever, headache, malaise, muscle aches, dry cough and
  SOB

Complications

- Encephalitis
- Myocarditis

Diagnosis

- *C. psittaci* PCR
- *C. psittaci* serology (≥ four-fold titre rise at least 2 weeks apart)
- *C. psittaci* culture (can be hazardous to laboratory personnel)

Antibiotic treatment

- Option 1: doxycycline (PO) for 10–14 days
- Option 2: clarithromycin (PO) for 10–14 days
- Option 3: roxithromycin (PO) for 10–14 days (for children)

For severe infection

- Azithromycin (IV then PO) for 7–10 days

Dosage of above antibiotics

- Doxycycline 200 mg (child >8 years: 5 mg/kg up to 200 mg) PO for
  the first dose, then 100 mg (child >8 years: 2.5 mg/kg up to
  100 mg) PO daily
- Clarithromycin 250–500 mg (child: 7.5–15 mg/kg up to 500 mg) PO
  q12h

- Roxithromycin child: 4 mg/kg up to 150 mg PO q12h
- Azithromycin 500 mg IV daily for at least 2 days, then 500 mg PO daily to complete a 7–10-day course (child: 10 mg/kg PO on 1st day, then 5 mg/kg PO daily)

Prevention

- Avoid inhalation of dust from dried bird droppings, feathers or cage dust by wearing mask and gloves when cleaning cages; wash hands after contacting birds
- Isolate sick birds and treat infected birds with antibiotics for at least 1 month

Q FEVER

Other name: query fever

Pathogen

- *Coxiella burnetii*, a rickettsia-like organism

Transmission

- Air-borne through aerosols from animal birth products and contaminated dust
- Unpasteurised milk is another source of infection
- Cases may occur without direct animal exposure

Incubation

- 7–14 days

Risk factors

- Animal-related industries

Clinical features

Q fever should be considered in any undiagnosed febrile illness

- Flu-like symptoms, fever, cholestatic hepatitis, some may develop atypical pneumonia, endocarditis, encephalitis, epididymo-orchitis, iritis or osteomyelitis

Laboratory

- *Coxiella burnetii* PCR testing
- Q fever serology (four-fold rise in antibody titre over 10–14 days)

Treatment

- Most cases resolve readily within 2 weeks without antibiotic treatment
- All patients with pre-existing heart valve disease require careful exclusion of endocarditis
- Antibiotic therapy is indicated for more severe or prolonged infections

For adult and child >8 years

- Doxycycline (PO) for 2 weeks

For child 2 months to 8 years

- Doxycycline (PO) for 5 days only
- If still has fever, continue with cotrimoxazole (PO) **plus** folic acid (PO) for 2 weeks

For pregnant women

To prevent fetal and maternal complications

- Cotrimoxazole (PO) **plus** folic acid (PO) until 32 weeks' gestation

For pregnant women >32 weeks' gestation—seek expert advice

For chronic disease or endocarditis, seek expert advice

- Doxycycline (PO) **plus** rifampicin (**or** hydroxychloroquine) (PO) for 18 months (24 months if having prosthetic valves)

Cardiac surgery may be required
Serologically monitor for at least 5 years

Post-exposure prophylaxis

- Doxycycline (PO) for 7 days (for adult and child >8 years)
- Cotrimoxazole (PO) for 7 days (for child 2 months to 8 years)

Dosage of above antibiotics

- Doxycycline 100 mg (child: 2 mg/kg up to 100 mg) PO q12h
- Cotrimoxazole 160/800 mg (child: 4/20 mg/kg up to 160/800 mg) PO q12h
- Folic acid 5 mg PO daily
- Rifampicin 600 mg (child: 20 mg/kg up to 600 mg) PO daily
- Hydroxychloroquine (seek expert advice)

Vaccination

Recommended for:

- Abattoir workers, farmers, veterinarians, shearers, stockyard workers, animal transporters, wool sorters and shooters

Pre-vaccination testing

- Q fever serology and skin test must be done before vaccination
- Vaccination is given only if both serology and skin test are negative

Vaccination

- Q-VAX 0.5 mL SC as a single dose

RABIES AND AUSTRALIAN BAT LYSSAVIRUS

Other names: pteropid lyssavirus, PLV

Pathogens

- Rabies virus and Australian bat lyssavirus (ABLV) belong to a group of viruses called lyssaviruses

Distribution

Rabies

- Most countries of Europe (except the United Kingdom), Africa, the Middle East, most of Asia (including Indonesia) and the Americas
- It is absent from some islands, including Australia, New Zealand, Hong Kong, Japan, Singapore, Papua New Guinea and the Pacific Islands
- There have been human rabies cases in Australia following animal bites received overseas

Australian bat lyssavirus

- Distributed throughout Australia in a variety of bat species

Transmission

- Overseas mammals that carry rabies include dogs, bats, cats, raccoons, skunks, monkeys, foxes, jackals, mongooses and other mammals that can bite and scratch
- In Australia only bats (Australian fruit bats [flying foxes] and Australian insectivorous bats) have been found to carry ABLV
- Both viruses spread from infected mammals to humans or other mammals via bites or scratches
- ABLV is not spread by bat urine, faeces or blood
- There is no risk of ABLV infection from eating cooked flying foxes

Incubation

- From 1 week to several years

Clinical

- Early symptoms—flu-like: headache, fever and malaise
- Excitability, paraesthesia and/or fasciculations at or near the wound
- Aversion to fresh air and water, excessive salivation and difficulty in swallowing ('foaming at the mouth')
- Progress rapidly to paralysis, delirium, convulsions and coma
- Death from respiratory paralysis usually within 1 or 2 weeks after onset of symptoms

Diagnosis

Rabies and ABLV can be diagnosed by:

- Rabies virus or lyssavirus antigen detection and culture (from biopsy of brain or other neural tissue, skin snips from the nape of the neck, saliva or CSF)
- Rabies virus or lyssavirus RNA detection by PCR (saliva or CSF)
- Rabies virus or lyssavirus antibodies (serum or CSF)

Transport of specimens suspected to contain rabies virus or lyssavirus requires discussion with regional authorities

Management

1. Pre-exposure prophylaxis (PEP)

Prevent both rabies and ABLV infection

Indication for pre-exposure vaccination (high-risk people)
- People who handle or come into contact with bats in Australia (e.g. bat carers, wildlife officers and veterinarians)
- People travelling overseas who plan to handle any unvaccinated mammal that can bite and scratch or who will be spending prolonged periods in rural parts of rabies endemic areas (see www.who.int /zoonoses/diseases/en)
- Laboratory workers who work with live lyssaviruses and who perform ABLV or rabies diagnostic tests (should have rabies antibody titres measured every 6 months; if the titre is inadequate, a booster is recommended)
  - Rabies vaccine (Merieux, Rabipur, Verorab) 1 mL IM, 3 doses on days 0, 7 and 21–28, then single booster every 2 years if continue to be at risk

If previously (>2 years) vaccinated, give single booster

2. Post-exposure treatment

Indication
- After being bitten or scratched by a bat in Australia, or by a wild or unvaccinated animal overseas

Wound management
- Thoroughly wash the wound immediately with soap and water and then apply an antiseptic solution (e.g. povidone-iodine, iodine tincture or alcohol)
- Isolate the patient in an isolation room and disinfect all saliva-contaminated articles; healthcare workers should wear gowns, gloves and masks while attending the patient.

Blood and urine are not considered infectious

Bat ABLV test
- If possible send the offending bat for the ABLV test—contact state/ territory veterinary or health authorities to make sure the ABLV test result will be available within 48 hours of exposure

3. **Post-exposure vaccination**

- Before the onset of symptoms, both passive immunisation (human rabies immunoglobulin, HRIG) and active immunisation (rabies vaccine) are effective in the prevention of full-blown rabies or ABLV infection
- Following cleansing of the wound, give HRIG and rabies vaccine immediately. (administration of HRIG and rabies vaccine may be withheld for up to 48 hours of exposure if the bat's ABLV test result is likely to be available within the 48 hours)
  - HRIG* (e.g. IMOGRAM® Rabies) 20 IU/kg infiltration around wound (may give the rest of the dose by IM injection)
  - Rabies vaccine (e.g. Merieux, Rabipur, Verorab) 1 mL IM, 4 doses on days 0, 3, 7 and 14 (vaccine does not offer protection until after the 3rd dose is given)

If had full course of rabies vaccination in the past
  - Only need 2 further doses of vaccine

RETROPHARYNGEAL ABSCESS

Causes

- Secondary to lymphatic drainage or spread of upper respiratory or oral infections
- Pharyngeal trauma from endotracheal intubation, endoscopy, foreign body ingestion
- Patients who are immunocompromised or chronically ill (e.g. diabetes, cancer, alcoholism, or AIDS) are at increased risk of retropharyngeal abscess

Pathogens

- Aerobic organisms—*Streptococcus pyogenes* and *Staphylococcus aureus*
- Anaerobic organisms—*Bacteroide* spp and *Veillonella* spp
- Gram-negative organisms—*Haemophilus parainfluenzae* and *Bartonella henselae*

Clinical

- Sore throat, fever, dysphagia, poor oral intake or fails to eat or drink, drooling, trismus, neck stiffness/swelling, torticollis, cough, cervical adenopathy, retropharyngeal bulge, respiratory distress, dyspnoea and stridor
- Toxic symptoms usually out of proportion to the findings on physical examination

---

*Do not give HRIG later than 7 days after rabies vaccine started

Complications

- Airway obstruction, mediastinitis, aspiration pneumonia, epidural abscess, jugular venous thrombosis, necrotising fasciitis, sepsis and erosion into the carotid artery

Diagnosis

- Lateral x-ray of the neck shows soft-tissue swelling
- CT scan of the throat is diagnostic

Treatment

- Airway control (paramount)
- Surgical drainage
- IV antibiotics
  - Ceftriaxone (**or** cefotaxime) (IV) **plus** metronidazole (IV)

After clinical improvement, may change to oral
  - Amoxicillin/clavulanate (PO)

Dosage of above antibiotics

- Ceftriaxone 1 g (child: 25 mg/kg up to 1 g) IV daily
- Cefotaxime 1 g (child: 25 mg/kg up to 1 g) IV q8h
- Metronidazole 500 mg (child: 10 mg/kg up to 500 mg) IV q12h
- Amoxicillin/clavulanate 875 mg (child: 22.5 mg/kg up to 875 mg) PO q12h

RHEUMATIC FEVER

Pathogens

Acute rheumatic fever (ARF) is a sequela of group A streptococci (GAS) infection, usually of streptococcal pharyngitis.

Clinical

- Sudden onset of fever, polyarthritis 2–6 weeks after streptococcal pharyngitis
- Some ARF cases may be insidious or subclinical with mild carditis
- Children tend to develop carditis first; older patients tend to develop arthritis

Diagnosis

Clinical judgement + diagnostic test for GAS infection:

- Rapid strep test—positive
- Throat culture—growth of group A streptococci
- Streptococcal antibodies (e.g. antistreptolysin O, ASO)—elevated

Antibiotic treatment and prophylaxis

Against group A streptococci infection

Acute infection

To eradicate upper respiratory tract organisms

- Option 1: penicillin V (PO) for 10 days
- Option 2: benzathine penicillin (IM) single dose (if poor adherence)
- Option 3: cefalexin (PO) for 10 days (if non-immediate penicillin allergy)
- Option 4: azithromycin (PO) for 5 days (if immediate penicillin allergy)

After an attack of rheumatic fever to prevent recurrent ARF

- Option 1: benzathine benzylpenicillin (IM) q3–4 weeks
- Option 2: penicillin V (PO) q12h
- Option 3: erythromycin (PO) q12h (if penicillin allergy)

Duration of long-term prevention

- After recent episode of acute rheumatic fever—for at least 10 years
- Without carditis or valve disease—until 21 years of age
- With moderate valve disease—until 35 years of age
- With severe valve disease or valve surgery—until 40 years of age or for lifelong

Dosage of above antibiotics

Acute infection

- Penicillin V 500 mg (child: 15 mg/kg up to 500 mg) PO q12h
- Benzathine benzylpenicillin 900 mg (child 3–6 kg: 225 mg; 6–10 kg: 337.5 mg; 10–15 kg: 450 mg; 15–20 kg: 675 mg; >20 kg: 900 mg) IM st
- Cefalexin 1 g (child: 25 mg/kg up to 1 g) PO q12h
- Azithromycin 500 mg (child: 12 mg/kg up to 500 mg) PO daily

After an attack of rheumatic fever to prevent recurrent ARF

- Benzathine benzylpenicillin (adult and child >20 kg: 900 mg; child <20 kg: 450 mg) IM q3–4 weeks
- Penicillin V (all age) 250 mg PO q12h
- Erythromycin 250 mg (child >1 month: 10 mg/kg up to 250 mg) PO q12h

RICKETTSIA

Other names: typhus

Rickettsias are rod-shaped, spherical or pleomorphic Gram-negative organisms, which are smaller than true bacteria and only grow inside living cells (blood culture negative).

Transmission

- Rickettsias are natural parasites of arthropods (see Table 18.1)
- Infection is usually transmitted to humans through skin from arthropods or vector bites

TABLE 18.1

COMMON RICKETTSIAL INFECTIONS

Infection	Rickettsia	Reservoir (vector)	Distribution
Australian tick typhus*	R. australis	Rodents, dogs (ticks)	Qld
Endemic typhus	R. mooseri	Rat (flea)	Worldwide
Epidemic typhus	R. prowazekii	Man (louse)	Africa, South America
Flinders Island spotted fever*	R. honei	Possum, reptile (ticks)	Tas, Vic and NSW
Rickettsial pox	R. akari	Mouse (mites)	New York, Philadelphia
Rocky Mountain spotted fever	R. rickettsii	Rodents, dogs (ticks)	USA, South America
Scrub typhus*	O. tsutsugamushi	Rodents (mites)	Qld, Asia
Trench fever	R. quintana	Man (louse)	Europe

*Australian tick typhus (Australian spotted fever), scrub typhus and Flinders Island spotted fever, see Typhus (p. 415)

Diagnosis

- Species-specific antibodies (serology)
- Rickettsias may be isolated from the blood in the first week of illness by intra-peritoneal inoculation into mice or guinea pigs

Treatment

- All rickettsias respond to doxycycline or azithromycin:
  - Option 1: doxycycline (PO) for 7 days
  - Option 2: azithromycin (PO) for 4 days

Severe disease—see expert advice

Dosage of above antibiotics

- Doxycycline (child: 2 mg/kg up to 100 mg) PO q12h
- Azithromycin 500 mg (child: 10 mg/kg up to 500 mg) PO on day 1, then 250 mg (child: 5 mg/kg up to 250 mg) PO daily for a further 4 days

ROSEOLA INFANTUM

Other names: exanthem subitum

Roseola is one of the very common mild viral illnesses that can cause high fever and rash in babies and young children aged between 6 months and 3 years.

Pathogen

- Human herpes virus type 6 (HHV-6) and type 7 (HHV-7)

Transmission

- Via person-to-person oral secretions
- The virus has been found in the saliva of healthy adults

- Adult family members or older siblings appear to be the infective source

Incubation

- 5–15 days
- Most infectious while the child is unwell—from the start of the fever

Clinical

- High fever up to 40°C (possibly higher) usually lasts for a few hours to 3–5 days
- Febrile convulsions may occur
- After a few days the fever subsides and just as the child appears to be recovering, a maculopapular or erythematous rash appears, which usually begins on the trunk, spreading to the arms, legs and neck; the rash is non-pruritic and may last 1–2 days; it can sometimes be confused with measles or rubella
- The baby may also have diarrhoea or cough

Complications

- Roseola is usually a self-limiting illness with no sequelae
- Ear infections may occur
- Encephalitis, fulminant hepatitis, haemophagocytic syndrome and disseminated infection with HHV-6 are extremely rare

Treatment

- Children with roseola recover fully, usually within a week
- Supportive and symptomatic treatment
- It is best to keep the sick child home

ROSS RIVER VIRUS

Ross River virus (RRV) infection is one of the most common and widespread arboviruses that infect humans in Australia.

Pathogen

- Ross River virus

Distribution

- Throughout Australia
- Also in eastern Indonesia, Papua New Guinea and the nearby Pacific Islands

Transmission

- Mosquitoes transmit the virus between animals and humans
- Infection does not occur directly from person-to-person contact

Incubation

- 7–9 days

Clinical

- Most RRV infections have slight or no symptoms (70–90%)
- More severe patients have rash, fever, chills, headache and photophobia
- Tiredness is common and can persist or recur later
- Rheumatic symptoms (such as pain, tenderness, joint and muscle stiffness and difficulty in moving) can appear suddenly or develop gradually over the next 2 weeks

Diagnosis

- RRV serology
- Detection of RRV by nucleic acid testing
- Isolation of RRV

Treatment and progress

- Symptomatic treatment
- NSAIDs can give dramatic symptomatic relief
- The severity and extent of the symptoms gradually diminish
- Some people will recover fully in 3 months and most within 1 year

Prevention

- Mosquito reduction and avoidance (e.g. wearing loose-fitting light-coloured clothing, especially in the late afternoon and early evening, insect screening in the home, using insecticide and insect repellent)

Vaccination

- Vaccine against RRV has shown promise in clinical trial

ROTAVIRUS

Rotavirus infection is the most common cause of severe diarrhoea in infants and young children.

Pathogen

- Rotaviruses (wheel-shaped viruses)

Transmission

- Hand-to-mouth contact with faeces from an infected person
- Aerosol spread from vomitus has been suggested in outbreaks
- Children can spread rotavirus both before and after they develop symptoms
- High prevalence in winter months

Incubation

- 1–3 days

Clinical

- Vomiting and/or diarrhoea (usually watery), with or without fever
- Severe diarrhoea can rapidly cause dehydration
- Dissemination of infection to brain, liver, heart and lungs can cause death
- Rotavirus infection occurs principally in children
- In adults, symptoms tend to be mild or asymptomatic
- Infection in bottle-fed babies is more severe than in breastfed babies
- The infection generally lasts 3–9 days

Laboratory

- Faecal rotavirus antigen screen
- Faecal rotavirus PCR detection

Laboratory testing for rotavirus is recommended for all patients with significant infectious vomiting and/or diarrhoea requiring substantial rehydration

Treatment

- No antibiotics are indicated
- Most patients recover with oral fluid and supportive treatment
- Severe dehydration needs IV fluid and hospitalisation

Prevention

- Washing with soap or cleanser helps reduce the spread of infection
- Maintain strict hygienic practices at home and in day-care centres; wash hands after using the toilet, after helping a child to use the toilet, after changing a child's nappy and before preparing or serving food

Vaccination

- Can potentially result in significant reductions in the need for medical intervention
- Can potentially decrease the burden of rotavirus gastroenteritis on families and society
  - Rotavirus vaccine (e.g. Rotarix, RotaTeq®) 1.5 mL PO, at 2 and 4 months of age

1st dose should be given within 6–14 weeks of age
2nd dose should be within 10–24 weeks, at least 4 weeks intervals between doses

Note

- Rotavirus vaccine must not be given after 24 weeks of age due to the potential risk of intussusception

RUBELLA

Other names: German measles

Pathogen

- A rubivirus (an enveloped RNA virus)

Transmission

- Via droplets

Incubation

- 14–23 days
- Infectious from 1 week before to 4 days after onset of rash

Clinical

- Rash from face down to body (lasts <3 days) + post-auricular and suboccipital lymphadenopathy + conjunctivitis + arthralgia, malaise, fever

Rubella infection in pregnancy

Rubella virus affects fetus, causes congenital rubella syndrome (CRS):

- 8–10 weeks of pregnancy → 90% of CRS
- By 16 weeks of pregnancy → 10–20% of CRS
- After 20 weeks of pregnancy → CRS is rare

Complications

- Pneumonia
- Myocarditis
- Thrombocytopenia
- Encephalitis

Laboratory

- Rubella serology (IgM or IgG)—mother and infant (2 samples 2–4 weeks apart)
- Rubella virus detection and culture (blood, urine or saliva)—for CRS infant

Screen rubella serology for the following people:

1. All young women (not pregnant) with negative or very low antibody levels → revaccination
2. All healthcare and childcare staff, if seronegative → vaccination, recheck serology 2 months later, if still negative → revaccination
3. Women planning to conceive → check serology, if seronegative → vaccination, wait for at least 2 months to conceive
4. Pregnant women with negative or very low antibody levels in antenatal screen; do not give vaccine during pregnancy—vaccination after delivery

5. Pregnant women with suspected rubella or exposure to rubella →
serology test (irrespective of prior vaccination, rubella infection or a
positive rubella antibody) (blood sample should have the date of last
menstrual period and the date of presumed exposure)
   • If exposure is in early pregnancy and seronegative → discuss
   termination
   • If antibody level is below protective level and remains asymptomatic
   → 2nd serological test 28 days after exposure
   • If symptoms develop → 2nd blood test, if seropositive → discuss
   termination

Treatment

• Supportive

Vaccination

Live attenuated rubella vaccine, combined in MMR or MMRV

   • MMR (e.g. Priorix) **or** MMRV (e.g. Prioris Tetra®) (IM) 2 doses at 12,
   18 months of age or 1 dose booster IM outside pregnancy

S

SALMONELLA ENTERITIS

Other names: Salmonellosis, non-typhoidal *Salmonella* enteritis

Pathogen

- *Salmonella enteritica*, a rod-shaped gram-negative enterobacteria

Transmission

- Through faecal–oral route
- From handling or consuming contaminated foods
- May also result from handling infected poultry or reptiles
- Bacteria are shed in the faeces for months to a year

Incubation

- 8–48 hours

Clinical

- Acute illness lasting 1–2 weeks
- Fever with afternoon spikes, diarrhoea, abdominal pain, anorexia, weight loss and changed sensorium

Complications

- Septicaemia
- Intestinal perforation

Laboratory

- Faeces culture
- PCR testing—sensitivity 98–100%, result available in 24 hours

Treatment

- Symptomatic treatment, rehydration
- Mild cases and asymptomatic short-term carriers—antibiotics are not advisable
- Antibiotics are indicated for:
    - Neonates and children ≤3 months
    - Children aged 3–12 months with fever
    - Patients >65 years
    - Patients with severe illness, sepsis or bacteraemia, haemoglobinopathies, prosthetic grafts
    - Immunocompromised
    - Option 1: azithromycin (PO) for 7 days
    - Option 2: ciprofloxacin (PO) for 5–7 days

If intolerant of oral antibiotic or septicaemic

- Option 1: ceftriaxone (IV)
- Option 2: ciprofloxacin (IV)

IV therapy until significant improvement, then change to oral

Dosage of above antibiotics

- Azithromycin 1 g (child: 20 mg/kg up to 1 g) PO on day 1, followed by 500 mg (child: 10 mg/kg up to 500 mg) PO for a further 6 days
- Ciprofloxacin 500 mg (child: 12.5 mg/kg up to 500 mg) PO q12h
- Ceftriaxone 2 g (child ≥1 month: 50 mg/kg up to 2 g) IV daily
- Ciprofloxacin 400 mg (child: 10 mg/kg up to 400 mg) IV q12h

SARS (SEVERE ACUTE RESPIRATORY SYNDROME)

Pathogen

- SARS coronavirus

Transmission

- Mainly via respiratory droplets
- Possible fomite and faecal spread

Incubation

- 2–7 days

Clinical

- Symptoms usually appear 2–10 days following exposure
- Flu-like symptoms, high fever, cough, SOB and confusion

Alert case (in the absence of an alternative diagnosis)

Hospital acquired flu-like illness in ≥2 healthcare workers or ≥3 other hospital staff and/or patients and/or visitors in the same healthcare unit fulfilling the clinical case definition of SARS and with onset of illness in the same 10-day period

Diagnosis

- At least three of following are present:
1. **Symptoms and signs:** flu-like symptoms, cough and fever ≥38°C
2. **Contact history:** contact (sexual or casual) with someone with a diagnosis of SARS within the last 10 days or recent (within 14 days) travel to an area with current local transmission of SARS
3. **Chest x-ray:** atypical pneumonia (may be absent in early disease)
4. **Laboratory:** any of following tests for SARS becoming positive
   - SARS virus PCR—early detection of SARS virus from blood, nasopharyngeal aspirates, sputum, tissue samples and faeces (very specific but not very sensitive)
   - SARS serology (immunofluorescence)—detects antibodies to SARS, becomes positive 10 days after the onset of symptoms
   - SARS serology (ELISA)—detects antibodies to SARS, reliable but becomes positive 3 weeks after the onset of symptoms
   - Isolation of SARS-CoV

Management

- Send samples—viral swabs of both nostrils and throat in viral transport medium for SARS virus PCR, SARS virus serology; also send samples for *Mycoplasma* and *Chlamydia* (PCR and serology) and for *Legionella* antigen urine test
- Isolation—suspected cases of SARS must be isolated in negative-pressure rooms, with full barrier nursing precautions
- Supportive—symptomatic treatment, oxygen and ventilatory support as needed
- Antiviral drugs—ribavirin (but no published evidence supports this therapy)
  - Ribavirin (e.g. Virazide) solution, inhale for 12–18 hours/day for 3–7 days
    Reconstitute powder and dilute further with water for injection to final volume of 300 mL (final concentration is 20 mg/mL)
- Steroids—some benefit from using steroids and immune-modulating agents
- SARS vaccine has been developed and tested, still undergoing more studies

SCABIES

Pathogen

- Scabies mite—*Sarcoptes scabiei*

Risk groups

- School-aged children
- Indigenous communities
- Nursing home residents

Clinical and diagnosis

- Markedly itchy papules or nodules with scaly burrows on sides of fingers, in interdigital webs, wrist flexures, axillae, abdomen, buttocks or groin; itch is worse at night; itchy red penile or scrotal papules are virtually diagnostic
- Scraping of burrows or biopsy to identify the mites or eggs

Anti-scabetic treatment

Adult or child >6 months and in pregnancy and lactation

- Permethrin 5% cream/lotion (e.g. Quellada, Lyclear) top, repeat in 7 days

If allergic to permethrin or if permethrin fails

- Benzyl benzoate* 25% emulsion (e.g. Ascabiol, Benzemul) top, repeat in 7 days

---

*Benzyl benzoate is more irritating than permethrin, particularly to excoriated skin; it is cheaper and suitable for those with less severe infestation

Child <6 months

- Permethrin 5% cream (e.g. Quellada, Lyclear)—apply to entire skin surface, including scalp, avoiding eyes and mouth; cover hands with mittens; leave on for 8 hours

If the risk of using permethrin outweighs the benefit

- Option 1: sulfur 10% in white soft paraffin (child <2 months: sulfur 5% in white soft paraffin) top daily for 2–3 days
- Option 2: crotamiton* cream (e.g. Eurax) top daily for 2–3 days

Immunocompromised patient or if topical therapy fails

If topical therapy fails, consider wrong diagnosis, unidentified source of re-infestation or non-compliance with instructions

- Ivermectin (e.g. Stromectol) adult, child >5 years: 0.2 mg/kg PO with fatty food weekly until cleared

If secondary bacterial infection is present

- Treat as for impetigo (p. 183) simultaneously

Dosage of above preparations

- Permethrin 5% cream (e.g. Quellada, Lyclear)—apply to dry skin from neck down or including head and face if scabies affects the area; pay particular attention to hands, genitalia and nails (avoid eyes and mucous membranes); leave on skin overnight; the time may be increased to 24 hours if there has been a treatment failure (reapply to hands if they are washed)
- Benzyl benzoate 25% emulsion (e.g. Ascabiol, Benzemul)—dilute according to instructions, apply to dry skin from neck down (for children <2 years, older persons and persons in central and northern Australia, treatment should also include face, scalp and ears but avoid eyes, mouth and mucous membranes); pay particular attention to hands, genitalia and under nails; leave on skin for 24 hours (reapply to hands if they are washed)
- Crotamiton cream (e.g. Eurax)—rub over entire body surface except face and scalp after bathing, daily for 2–3 days depending on response

Note

- All family members and close contacts should be treated simultaneously
- In the nursing home, all patients and staff should be treated
- Clothes, bedding and towels should be washed with hot water and detergent the morning after each treatment, or heat-treated from an iron or hot clothes drier, or they can be stored for a week (as the mites survive for only 36 hours away from host)
- Spray insecticide thoroughly in rooms

---

*Crotamiton is less irritating but less effective than permethrin

- Contact tracing and notification are essential to prevent treatment failure
- School should be notified, but treatment of uninvolved children is not required
- Infected children may return to school after 2 treatments weekly
- Post-treatment itch can last for 1–2 weeks or longer; assess healing in 1 month

Crusted (Norwegian) scabies

- Occurs in physically incapacitated and immunocompromised (including HIV) patients and also in remote Indigenous communities
- Treatment is difficult and discussion with an expert is recommended

Oral ivermectin*

For less severe crusted scabies
- Ivermectin (Stromectol) 0.2 mg/kg (adult and child >5 years) PO on days 1, 2 and 8

For moderately severe crusted scabies
- Ivermectin (Stromectol) 0.2 mg/kg (adult and child >5 years) PO on days 1, 2, 8, 9 and 15

For severe crusted scabies
- Ivermectin (Stromectol) 0.2 mg/kg (adult and child >5 years) PO on days 1, 2, 8, 9, 15, 22 and 29

For HIV patients
- Ivermectin (Stromectol) 0.2 mg/kg PO weekly until scrapings are negative and no further evidence of infection is present

Frequent topical scabicide (together with oral ivermectin)

- Permethrin 5% cream/lotion (e.g. Quellada, Lyclear) top daily every 2nd day for the 1st week, then twice a week until cured

If allergic to permethrin or if permethrin fails
- Benzyl benzoate** 25% emulsion (e.g. Ascabiol, Benzemul) top daily every 2nd day for the 1st week, then twice a week until cured

If the risk of using permethrin outweighs the benefit
- Option 1: sulfur 10% in white soft paraffin (child <2 months: sulfur 5% in white soft paraffin) top daily every 2nd day for the 1st week, then twice a week until cured
- Option 2: crotamiton*** cream (e.g. Eurax) top daily every 2nd day for the 1st week, then twice a week until cured

---

*Ivermectin is not recommended in geriatric patients, particularly those on multiple medications, or in children under 5 years of age

**Benzyl benzoate is more irritating than permethrin, particularly to excoriated skin; it is cheaper and suitable for those with less severe infestation

***Crotamiton is less irritating but less effective than permethrin

Topical keratolytics (to reduce scaling)

- Salicylic acid 5–10% in sorbolene cream (e.g. Sorbolene Cream and Salicylic Acid 5%) top daily after washing, on days when scabicides are not applied
- Lactic acid 5% + urea 10% in sorbolene cream (e.g. Calmurid) top daily after washing, on days when scabicides are not applied

Note

- All family members and close contacts should be treated simultaneously
- In nursing homes, quarantine the affected ward and treat all patients, medical and nursing staff and their families; if staff from the affected ward have worked elsewhere, that area should also be treated
- Clothes, bedding and towels should be washed, or heat-treated from an iron or hot clothes drier, or they can be stored for a week (as the mites survive for only 36 hours away from the host)

SCARLET FEVER

Other names: Scarlatina

Pathogen

- Group A Streptococcus (produces erythrogenic toxin)

Incubation

- 1–3 days following a streptococcal infection (usually throat infection)

Clinical

- Mainly infects children
- Streptococcal pharyngitis
- Rash usually appears 2–4 days after the onset of illness, first on the neck and chest, then spreading over the body with sparing of the face, palms and soles; the rash is described as 'sandpapery' and lasts for up to 2–3 weeks; as the rash fades, desquamation may occur around the fingertips, toes and groin area
- A 'strawberry tongue' may also be present

Complications

- Acute rheumatic fever
- Otitis media
- Adenitis or abscess
- Peritonsillar or retropharyngeal abscess
- Pneumonia
- Sinusitis
- Meningitis
- Osteomyelitis or septic arthritis

- Hepatitis
- Glomerulonephritis

Diagnosis

- Isolation of group A beta-haemolytic streptococci in the presence of a clinically compatible illness
- High antistreptolysin O (ASO) and/or anti-DNase B titres in the presence of a clinically compatible illness; serial rising titres are more diagnostic

Treatment

- With proper antibiotic treatment, symptoms should resolve quickly
- Patient should not attend school or work to avoid infecting other individuals
  - Option 1: penicillin V (PO) for 10 days
  - Option 2: benzathine penicillin (IM) st

If allergic to penicillin

  - Roxithromycin (PO) for 10 days

Dosage of above antibiotics

  - Penicillin V 500 mg (child: 15 mg/kg up to 500 mg) PO q12h
  - Benzathine penicillin 900 mg (child 3–6 kg: 22 mg; 6–10 kg: 337.5 mg; 10–15 kg: 450 mg; 15–20 kg: 675 mg; >20 kg: 900 mg) IM st
  - Roxithromycin 300 mg PO daily (child: 4 mg/kg up to 150 mg PO q12h)

SEPSIS—EMPIRICAL THERAPY

Empirical therapy is usually for 24–48 hours only and should be changed to direct therapy as soon as pathogens and susceptibility are known

Initial management

- Resuscitation (oxygen, IV fluid, vasopressors)
- Obtain 2 sets of blood cultures and other cultures (e.g. urine, sputum, wounds)
- Serum procalcitonin test can be used as a marker of severe sepsis and generally grades well with the degree of sepsis; procalcitonin monitoring is also a fast and reliable diagnostic approach to assess septic complications and prognosis
- Administer appropriate antibiotics immediately after obtaining blood cultures (within 1 hour of ED presentation)
- Control the source of sepsis where possible (surgical drainage/debridement)

1. Empirical therapy for adults

Low-dose corticosteroid therapy (optional)

  - Hydrocortisone 50 mg IV q6h +/– fludrocortisone 0.1–0.2 mg PO daily

EMPIRICAL ANTIBIOTIC THERAPY

- Flucloxacillin (IV) **plus** gentamicin (IV)

If non-immediate penicillin allergy

- Cefazolin (IV) **plus** gentamicin (IV)

If immediate penicillin allergy or MRSA infection is suspected

- Vancomycin (IV) **plus** gentamicin (IV) (all septic shock patients need vancomycin)

If a multi-drug–resistant gram-negative organism is suspected

- Meropenem 1 g IV q8h

Dosage of above antibiotics

- Flucloxacillin 2 g IV q4h
- Gentamicin 4–7 mg/kg IV for the 1st dose (further dosing, see p. 459)
- Cefazolin 2 g IV q6h
- Vancomycin 25–30 mg/kg IV for the 1st dose (further dosing, see p. 462)

2. Empirical therapy for children

- Meningitis should be considered in all neonates precented with sepsis
- Antibiotic regimen should be modified as soon as pathogen and susceptibility result are available

CHILD <2 MONTHS

If meningitis is not excluded

- Ampi(amoxi)cillin (IV) **plus** cefotaxime*

If herpes simplex encephalitis is suspected **add**

- Aciclovir (IV)

If meningitis is excluded

- Ampi(amoxi)cillin (IV) **plus** gentamicin (IV)

CHILD ≥2 MONTHS

To cover *S. aureus* and gram-negative infection

IF NOT CRITICALLY ILL

- Option 1: cefotaxime (IV)
- Option 2: ceftriaxone (IV)

To cover MRSA **add**

- Vancomycin (IV)

If allergic to penicillin

- Ciprofloxacin (IV) **plus** vancomycin (IV)

---

*Cefotaxime is preferred to ceftriaxone for gram-negative septicaemia in neonates (ceftriaxone displaces bilirubin from albumin and may increase the risk of bilirubin encephalopathy in neonates)

If herpes simplex encephalitis is suspected **add**

- Aciclovir (IV)

If meningitis is suspected, see Meningitis—empirical therapy, p. 221

IF CRITICALLY ILL

- Cefotaxime (**or** ceftriaxone) (IV) **plus** gentamicin (IV) **plus** vancomycin (IV)

If immediate penicillin allergy

- Ciprofloxacin (IV) **plus** gentamicin (IV) **plus** vancomycin (IV)

If herpes simplex encephalitis is suspected **add**

- Aciclovir (IV)

If meningitis is suspected, see Meningitis—empirical therapy, p. 221

Dosage of above antibiotics

Child <2 months

- Ampi(amoxi)cillin 50 mg/kg IV q6h
- Cefotaxime 50 mg/kg IV q6h
- Aciclovir 20 mg/kg IV q8h
- Gentamicin 7.5 mg/kg IV for the 1st dose (further dosing, see p. 459)

Child ≥2 months

- Cefotaxime 50 mg/kg up to 2 g IV q6h
- Ceftriaxone 50 mg/kg up to 2 g IV q12h
- Vancomycin 30 mg/kg IV for the 1st dose (further dosing, see p. 462)
- Ciprofloxacin 10 mg/kg up to 400 mg IV q8h
- Aciclovir 20 mg/kg (child >5 years: 15 mg/kg) IV q8h
- Gentamicin 7.5 mg/kg IV for the 1st dose (further dosing, see p. 459)

SEPSIS—BILIARY OR GI TRACT SOURCE

Pathogens

- Enteric gram-negative rods
- Anaerobic cocci
- *Bacteroides fragilis*
- *Enterococcus faecalis*

Antibiotic treatment

1.   Biliary source is suspected

- Ampi(amoxi)cillin (IV) **plus** gentamicin (IV)

If gentamicin use >72 hours or is contraindicated

- Option 1: piperacillin/tazobactam (**or** ticarcillin/clavulanate) (IV)
- Option 2: ceftriaxone (**or** cefotaxime) (IV) (if penicillin allergy)
- Option 3: gentamicin (IV) (if immediate penicillin allergy)

If chronic biliary obstruction with anaerobic organisms **add**
- Metronidazole (IV) to above Option 2 and Option 3

After clinical improvement, switch to oral therapy
- Option 1: amoxicillin/clavulanate (PO)
- Option 2: cotrimoxazole (PO) **plus** metronidazole (PO) (if penicillin allergy)

Review therapy after results of susceptibility testing are available

Dosage of above antibiotics

- Ampi(amoxi)cillin 2 g (child: 50 mg/kg up to 2 g) IV q6h
- Gentamicin 4–7 mg/kg IV for the 1st dose (further dosing, see p. 459)
- Piperacillin/tazobactam 4 g (child: 100 mg/kg up to 4 g) IV q8h
- Ticarcillin/clavulanate 3 g (child: 50 mg/kg up to 3 g) IV q6h
- Ceftriaxone 1 g (child: 50 mg/kg up to 1 g) IV daily
- Cefotaxime 1 g (child: 50 mg/kg up to 1 g) IV q8h
- Metronidazole 500 mg (child: 12.5 mg/kg up to 500 mg) IV q12h
- Amoxicillin/clavulanate 875/125 mg (child: 22.5/3.2 mg/kg up to 875/125 mg) PO q12h
- Cotrimoxazole 160/800 mg PO q12h
- Metronidazole 400 mg (child: 10 mg/kg up to 400 mg) PO q12h

2. GI tract source is suspected

- Ampi(amoxi)cillin (IV) **plus** gentamicin (IV) **plus** metronidazole (IV)

If gentamicin use >72 hours or is contraindicated
- Option 1: piperacillin/tazobactam (**or** ticarcillin/clavulanate) (IV)
- Option 2: ceftriaxone (**or** cefotaxime) (IV) **plus** metronidazole (IV) (if penicillin allergy)
- Option 3: gentamicin (IV) **plus** clindamycin (IV) (if immediate penicillin allergy)

After clinical improvement, switch to oral therapy
- Option 1: amoxicillin/clavulanate (PO)
- Option 2: cotrimoxazole (PO) **plus** metronidazole (PO) (if penicillin allergy)

Review therapy after results of susceptibility testing are available

Dosage of above antibiotics

- Ampi(amoxi)cillin 2 g (child: 50 mg/kg up to 2 g) IV q6h
- Gentamicin 4–7 mg/kg IV for the 1st dose (further dosing, see p. 459)
- Metronidazole 500 mg (child: 12.5 mg/kg up to 500 mg) IV q12h

- Piperacillin/tazobactam 4 g (child: 100 mg/kg up to 4 g) IV q8h
- Ticarcillin/clavulanate 3 g (child: 50 mg/kg up to 3 g) IV q6h
- Ceftriaxone 1 g (child: 50 mg/kg up to 1 g) IV daily
- Cefotaxime 1 g (child: 50 mg/kg up to 1 g) IV q8h
- Clindamycin 600 mg (child: 15 mg/kg up to 600 mg) IV q8h
- Amoxicillin/clavulanate 875/125 mg (child: 22.5/3.2 mg/kg up to 875/125 mg) PO q12h
- Cotrimoxazole 160/800 mg PO q12h
- Metronidazole 400 mg (child: 10 mg/kg up to 400 mg) PO q12h

SEPSIS—FEMALE GENITAL TRACT SOURCE

Pathogens

- Anaerobes (particularly anaerobic cocci)
- Enteric gram-negative rods
- *Neisseria gonorrhoeae* (disseminated gonococcal sepsis)
- Streptococci, occasionally staphylococci
- Sepsis after caesarean section, commonly caused by *Staphylococcus aureus*
- *Mycoplasma hominis* or *Ureaplasma urealyticum*

Antibiotic treatment

- Ceftriaxone (**or** cefotaxime) (IV) **plus** azithromycin (IV) **plus** metronidazole (IV)

If immediate penicillin allergy

- Gentamicin (IV) **plus** azithromycin (IV) **plus** clindamycin (IV)

After improvement, change to oral to complete at least 2 weeks of treatment

- Doxycycline (**or** azithromycin) (PO) **plus** metronidazole (PO)

If recent caesarean section—*S. aureus* is common

- Option 1: flucloxacillin (IV)
- Option 2: cefalotin (**or** cefazolin) (IV) (if non-immediate penicillin allergy)
- Option 3: vancomycin (IV) (MRSA infection or immediate penicillin allergy)

Dosage of above antibiotics

- Ceftriaxone 2 g IV daily
- Cefotaxime 2 g IV q8h
- Azithromycin 500 mg IV daily
- Metronidazole 500 mg IV q12h
- Gentamicin 4–7 mg/kg IV for the 1st dose (further dosing, see p. 459)
- Clindamycin 600 mg IV q8h
- Doxycycline 100 mg PO q12h
- Azithromycin 1 g PO st
- Metronidazole 400 mg PO q12h

- Flucloxacillin 2 g IV q4–6h
- Cefalotin 2 g IV q4h
- Cefazolin 2 g IV q6–8h
- Vancomycin 25–30 mg/kg IV for the 1st dose (further dosing, see p. 462)

SEPSIS—INTRAVASCULAR DEVICE SOURCE

Pathogens

- Coagulase-negative staphylococci and *Staphylococcus aureus* (the most common)
- Gram-negative rods
- Fungi, especially *Candida* spp

Treatment

- Immediate removal of peripheral intravascular catheter—if sepsis is suspected, send the tip for culture together with blood cultures from another site
- Remove central venous catheter if there is tunnel infection, disseminated intravascular coagulation, shock or thromboembolism or infected by *Candida* spp (removal may be deferred if the central catheter is difficult to replace and the patient's condition is improving)

Antibiotic treatment

- Vancomycin (IV) **plus** gentamicin (IV)

Duration of treatment

- If sepsis quickly resolves after removal of the infected device and the infection is caused by low-virulence organism (e.g. coagulase-negative staphylococci), may cease treatment
- If infection is caused by more virulent organism (e.g. *S. aureus* or *Candida* spp), prolonged treatment is required

Dosage of above antibiotics

- Vancomycin 25–30 mg/kg IV for the 1st dose (further dosing, see p. 459)
- Gentamicin 4–7 mg/kg (child: 7.5 mg/kg up to 320 mg) IV for the 1st dose (further dosing, see p. 462)

SEPSIS—SKIN SOURCE

Pathogens

Skin infections

- *Staphylococcus aureus*
- *Streptococcus pyogenes*

Infected decubitus, ischaemic ulcers or diabetic foot infections

- *Staphylococcus aureus*
- *Streptococcus pyogenes* (the most common)

- Enteric gram-negative rods
- Beta-haemolytic streptococci
- Anaerobes

Water-related skin infection

- *Aeromonas* spp
- *Mycobacterium marinum*
- *Shewanella putrefaciens*
- *Vibrio* spp (e.g. *Vibrio vulnificus, Vibrio alginolyticus* and other non-cholera Vibrios)

Treatment

- Surgical debridement if indicated

Sepsis with skin infections

- Option 1: flucloxacillin (IV)
- Option 2: cefazolin (IV)

If immediate penicillin allergy

- Option 1: vancomycin (IV)
- Option 2: clindamycin (IV)

Sepsis with water-related skin wound infections

- Ciprofloxacin (IV) **plus** clindamycin (IV)

Sepsis with infected decubitus, ischaemic ulcers or diabetic foot infections

- Option 1: piperacillin/tazobactam (IV)
- Option 2: ticarcillin/clavulanate (IV)

If penicillin allergy

- Ciprofloxacin (IV) **plus** clindamycin (IVI)

Dosage of above antibiotics

- Flucloxacillin 2 g (child: 50 mg/kg up to 2 g) IV q6h
- Cefazolin 2 g (child: 50 mg/kg up to 2 g) IV q8h
- Vancomycin 25–30 mg/kg IV for the 1st dose (further dosing, see p. 462)
- Clindamycin 600 mg (child: 15 mg/kg up to 600 mg) IV q8h
- Ciprofloxacin 400 mg (child: 10 mg/kg up to 400 mg) IV q12h
- Piperacillin/tazobactam 4 g IV q8h
- Ticarcillin/clavulanate 3 g IV q6h
- Clindamycin[2] 900 mg IV q8h (slow infusion)

SEPSIS—URINARY TRACT SOURCE

Pathogens

- Enteric gram-negative rods
- *Enterococcus faecalis*
- Staphylococci (occasional)
- *Pseudomonas aeruginosa* (occasional)

Antibiotic treatment

- Ampi(amoxi)cillin (IV) **plus** gentamicin (IV)

If penicillin allergy

- Gentamicin (IV) alone (not cover enterococci)

If aminoglycoside is contraindicated

- Ceftriaxone (**or** cefotaxime) (IV) (does not cover enterococci and
  Pseudomonas)

To cover *Pseudomonas* sepsis

- Option 1: ceftazidime (IV) **plus** gentamicin (IV)
- Option 2: piperacillin/tazobactam (IV) **plus** gentamicin (IV)
- Option 3: ciprofloxacin (IV) **plus** gentamicin (IV)

Dosage of above antibiotics

- Ampi(amoxi)cillin 2 g (child: 50 mg/kg up to 2 g) IV q6h
- Gentamicin 4–7 mg/kg (child: 7.5 mg/kg up to 320 mg) IV for the 1st
  dose (further dosing, see p. 459)
- Ceftriaxone 1 g (child: 25 mg/kg up to 1 g) IV daily
- Cefotaxime 1 g (child: 25 mg/kg up to 1 g) IV q8h
- Ceftazidime 2 g (child: 50 mg/kg up to 2 g) IV q8h
- Piperacillin/tazobactam 4 g (child: 100 mg/kg up to 4 g) IV
  q6–8h
- Ciprofloxacin 400 mg (child: 10 mg/kg up to 400 mg)
  IV q8h

SEPSIS—DIRECT THERAPY

1. *STAPHYLOCOCCUS AUREUS* SEPSIS

Treatment

Penicillin-susceptible *S. aureus*

- Benzylpenicillin (IV)

Methicillin-susceptible *S. aureus*

- Flucloxacillin (IV)

If non-immediate penicillin allergy

- Cefalotin (**or** cefazolin) (IV)

MRSA infection or if immediate penicillin allergy

- Vancomycin (IV)

Duration of therapy

- For 2 weeks—if blood cultures become negative after 48–72 hours,
  rapid resolution of fever, source of infection has been removed, no
  valvular abnormality, no intravascular prosthetic material and no
  significant immunocompromise
- For ≥4 weeks—if all above criteria are not met

Dosage of above antibiotics

- Benzylpenicillin 1.8 g (child: 50 mg/kg up to 1.8 g) IV q4h
- Flucloxacillin 2 g (child: 50 mg/kg up to 2 g) IV q4–6h

- Cefalotin 2 g (child: 50 mg/kg up to 2 g) IV q4h
- Cefazolin 2 g (child: 50 mg/kg up to 2 g) IV q8h (child: q8h)
- Vancomycin 25–30 mg/kg IV for the 1st dose (further dosing, see p. 462)

2. *STREPTOCOCCUS PYOGENES* SEPSIS

Treatment

- If *S. pyogenes* sepsis is associated with necrotising fasciitis—surgical debridement +/– hyperbaric oxygen therapy
  - Benzylpenicillin (IV) **plus** clindamycin (IV)

If non-immediate penicillin allergy
  - Cefazolin (IV) **plus** clindamycin (IV)

If immediate penicillin allergy
  - Vancomycin (IV) **plus** clindamycin (IV)

Once clinically improved, change to oral
  - Amoxicillin (PO)

Duration of therapy

Usually for 7–10 days (IV + oral)

Dosage of above antibiotics

- Benzylpenicillin 1.8 g (child: 50 mg/kg up to 1.8 g) IV q4h
- Clindamycin 600 mg (child: 15 mg/kg up to 600 mg) IV q8h for first 72 hours
- Cefazolin 2 g (child: 50 mg/kg up to 2 g) IV q8h
- Vancomycin 25–30 mg/kg IV for the 1st dose (further dosing, see p. 462)
- Amoxicillin 1 g (child: 25 mg/kg up to 1 g) PO q8h

3. GRAM-NEGATIVE ENTERIC BACTERIAL SEPSIS

Pathogens

Enterobacteriaceae include

- *Citrobacter* (e.g. *C. freundii*)
- *Enterobacter* (e.g. *E. cloacae*)
- *Erwinia* (e.g. *E. amylovora*)
- *Escherichia* (e.g. *E. coli*)
- *Hafnia* (e.g. *H. alvei*)
- *Klebsiella* (e.g. *K. pneumoniae*)
- *Morganella* (e.g. *M. morganii*)
- *Proteus* (e.g. *P. vulgaris*)
- *Providencia* (e.g. *P. retteri*)
- *Serratia* (e.g. *S. marcescens*)

Antibiotic treatment

Usually the source of infection is the biliary or urinary tract

- Option 1: gentamicin 4–7 mg/kg IV for the 1st dose (further dosing, see p. 459)*
- Option 2: ceftriaxone 1 g (child: 25 mg/kg up to 1 g) IV q12h
- Option 3: cefotaxime 2 g (child: 50 mg/kg up to 2 g) IV q8h

Further treatment according to antibiotic susceptibility

If multi-drug–resistant gram-negative organisms is suspected or identified
- Meropenem 1 g (child: 40 mg/kg up to 1 g) IV q8h (seek expert advice)

4. PSEUDOMONAS AERUGINOSA SEPSIS

- Option 1: ceftazidime (IV) **plus** gentamicin (IV)**
- Option 2: piperacillin/tazobactam (IV) **plus** gentamicin (IV)**

If immediate penicillin allergy
- Ciprofloxacin (IV) **plus** gentamicin (IV)**

Further treatment according to antibiotic susceptibility

Duration of therapy

At least 7 days, total duration depends on the primary site of infection

Dosage of above antibiotics

- Ceftazidime 2 g (child: 50 mg/kg up to 2 g) IV q8h
- Gentamicin 4–7 mg/kg IV for the 1st dose (further dosing, see p. 459)
- Piperacillin/tazobactam 4 g (child: 100 mg/kg up to 4 g) IV q6h
- Ciprofloxacin 400 mg (child: 10 mg/kg up to 400 mg) IV q8h

5. PNEUMOCOCCAL SEPSIS

Pathogens

- *Streptococcus pneumoniae* (pneumococcus)
- Determine MICs of penicillin and ceftriaxone or cefotaxime for all *S. pneumoniae* isolates

Treatment

Susceptible to penicillin (MIC <0.125 mg/L)
- Benzylpenicillin (IV) for 10–14 days

Susceptible to ceftriaxone or cefotaxime (MIC <1.0 mg/L)
- Ceftriaxone (**or** cefotaxime) (IV) for 10–14 days

If penicillin MIC >0.125 mg/L and ceftriaxone/cefotaxime MIC 1.0–2.0 mg/L
- Ceftriaxone (**or** cefotaxime) (IV) **plus** vancomycin (IV) for 10–14 days

If immediate penicillin allergy
- Option 1: vancomycin (IV) **plus** ciprofloxacin (IV) for 10–14 days
- Option 2: moxifloxacin (IV) for 10–14 days

---

*Gentamicin should be ceased after 72 hours
**Gentamicin should be ceased after 72 hours

If resistant to ceftriaxone/cefotaxime (MIC >2.0 mg/L), seek expert advice

Dosage of above antibiotics

- Benzylpenicillin 2.4 g (child: 60 mg/kg up to 2.4 g) IV q4h
- Ceftriaxone 2 g (child: 50 mg/kg up to 2 g) IV q12h **or** 4 g (child: 100 mg/kg up to 4 g) IV daily
- Cefotaxime 2 g (child: 50 mg/kg up to 2 g) IV q6h
- Vancomycin 25–30 mg/kg IV for the 1st dose (further dosing, see p. 462)
- Ciprofloxacin 400 mg (child: 10 mg/kg up to 400 mg) IV q8h
- Moxifloxacin 400 mg (child: 10 mg/kg up to 400 mg) IV daily

6. MENINGOCOCCAL SEPSIS

Pathogen

- *Neisseria meningitidis*

Antibiotic treatment

For either acute or chronic meningococcaemia

- Option 1: benzylpenicillin (IV) for 5–7 days
- Option 2: ceftriaxone (**or** cefotaxime) (IV) for 5–7 days

If immediate penicillin allergy or cefalosporin allergy

- Option 1: ciprofloxacin (IV) for 5–7 days
- Option 2: chloramphenicol (IV) for 5–7 days (if ciprofloxacin is not available)

Prophylaxis for close contacts

- Option 1: ciprofloxacin (PO) st (preferred for women taking OCP)
- Option 2: ceftriaxone (IM)* st (preferred for pregnant women)
- Option 3: rifampicin** 600 mg (PO) for 2 days (preferred for children)

Dosage of above antibiotics

For either acute or chronic meningococcaemia

- Benzylpenicillin 1.8 g (child: 50 mg/kg up to 1.8 g) IV q4h
- Ceftriaxone 2 g (child: 50 mg/kg up to 2 g) IV q12h
- Cefotaxime 2 g (child: 50 mg/kg up to 2 g) IV q6h
- Ciprofloxacin 400 mg (child: 10 mg/kg up to 400 mg) IV q8h
- Chloramphenicol 1 g (child: 25 mg/kg up to 1 g) IV q6h

Prophylaxis for close contacts

- Ciprofloxacin 500 mg (child <5 years: 30 mg/kg up to 125 mg; 5–12 years: 250 mg) PO st
- Ceftriaxone 250 mg (child >1 month: 125 mg) IM st

---

*IM injection of ceftriaxone needs to be reconstituted with 1% lidocaine (lignocaine)

**Rifampicin is associated with multiple drug interactions and is contraindicated in pregnancy, alcoholism and severe liver disease

- Rifampicin 600 mg (neonate: 5 mg/kg; child: 10 mg/kg up to 600 mg) PO q12h for 2 days

7. *NEISSERIA GONORRHOEAE* (GONOCOCCAL SEPSIS)

Treatment

- Option 1: ceftriaxone 2 g IV daily
- Option 2: cefotaxime 2 g IV q8h

If immediate penicillin allergy, seek expert advice

Duration of therapy

- Continue for 48 hours after becoming afebrile then switch to oral regimen based on culture and susceptibility results
- Total duration of therapy should be ≥7 days

SEPTIC ARTHRITIS/BURSITIS AND OPEN FRACTURE

Other names: pyogenic arthritis

1. STAPHYLOCOCCAL SEPTIC ARTHRITIS AND BURSITIS

Pathogens

- MSSA (methicillin-susceptible S. *aureus*)
- MRSA (methicillin-resistant *S. aureus*)
- MS-CNS (methicillin-sensitive, coagulase-negative staphylococci, e.g. *S. epidermidis*)
- MR-CNS (methicillin-resistant, coagulase-negative staphylococci, e.g. *S. epidermidis*)

Clinical

- Haematogenous invasion
- Infection follows penetrating trauma or joint aspiration/injection
- Predominantly monoarticular (80–90%)
- Blood cultures, joint aspiration for Gram stain and culture—prior to antibiotic use
- Acute crystal arthropathies and acute rheumatic fever should be firmly excluded

Treatment

- Urgent treatment to prevent further joint damage
- Drainage of pus with joint irrigation, debridement and washout plays a critical part in limiting further damage.
- Infected bursa may need repeated aspiration/drainage or surgical excision

Antibiotic therapy for septic arthritis

Empirical therapy (should be guided by Gram stain of joint aspiration)
- Flucloxacillin (IV)

- Cefazolin (IV) (if non-immediate penicillin allergy)
- Vancomycin (IV) (if immediate penicillin allergy)

If gram-negative infection is suspected, or child <5 years has not received Hib

- Flucloxacillin (IV) **plus** ceftriaxone (**or** cefotaxime) (IV)

Continue treatment until the bacteria are isolated; adjust therapy according to susceptibility

Duration of therapy for septic arthritis

- Neonate—IV therapy for total 3 weeks
- Child—IV therapy for 3 days, followed by oral therapy, total 3 weeks
- Adult—IV therapy for 2 weeks, followed by oral therapy, total 4 weeks

Dosage of above antibiotics

- Flucloxacillin 2 g (child: 50 mg/kg up to 2 g) IV q6h
- Cefazolin 2 g (child: 50 mg/kg up to 2 g) IV q8h
- Vancomycin 25-30 mg/kg IV for the 1st dose (further dosing, see p. 462)
- Ceftriaxone 2 g (child: 50 mg/kg up to 2 g) IV daily
- Cefotaxime 2 g (child: 50 mg/kg up to 2 g) IV q8h

Antibiotic therapy for septic bursitis

- Usually caused by *S. aureus*
- Often follows local trauma
- Usual sites are pre-patellar bursae and olecranon bursae

Penicillin-susceptible *S. aureus*

- Benzylpenicillin (IV)

Methicillin-susceptible *S. aureus*

- Option 1: flucloxacillin (IV)
- Option 2: cefazolin (IV) (if non-immediate penicillin allergy)

MRSA infection or if immediate penicillin allergy

- Vancomycin (IV)

Duration of therapy

- 2–3 weeks

Dosage of above antibiotics

- Benzylpenicillin 1.8 g (child: 50 mg/kg up to 1.8 g) IV q4h
- Flucloxacillin 2 g (child: 50 mg/kg up to 2 g) IV q6h
- Cefazolin 2 g (child: 50 mg/kg up to 2 g) IV q8h
- Vancomycin 25–30 mg/kg IV for the 1st dose (further dosing, see p. 462)

2. GONOCOCCAL ARTHRITIS

Pathogens

- *Neisseria gonorrhoeae*

Clinical

- More common in young women
- Typically migratory polyarthritis
- Joint aspiration/blood culture and sensitivity test for *Neisseria gonorrhoea*—prior to antibiotic treatment

Treatment

- Joint washout is usually unnecessary
  - Option 1: ceftriaxone 1 g IV daily for at least 7 days
  - Option 2: cefotaxime 1 g IV q8h for at least 7 days
If immediate penicillin allergy, seek expert advice

3. OPEN FRACTURE (COMPOUND FRACTURE)

- Urgent orthopaedic consultation
- Thorough debridement, irrigation and fracture stabilisation
- Tetanus immunisation assessment (see p. 393)

Antibiotic prophylaxis—if no severe tissue damage or evidence of infection

  - Option 1: cefazolin 2 g (child: 50 mg/kg up to 2 g) IV q8h
  - Option 2: clindamycin (IV **or** PO) (if immediate penicillin allergy)

Duration

- If debridement within 8 hours of injury—for 24–72 hours
- If debridement ≥8 hours of injury—for 7 days

Dosage of above antibiotics

  - Cefazolin 2 g (child: 50 mg/kg up to 2 g) IV q8h
  - Clindamycin 600 mg (child: 15 mg/kg up to 600 mg) IV q8h
  - Clindamycin 450 mg (child: 10 mg/kg up to 450 mg) PO q8h

Empirical therapy—if there is severe tissue damage or evidence of infection

  - Option 1: piperacillin/tazobactam (IV)
  - Option 2: ticarcillin/clavulanate (IV)
If non-immediate penicillin allergy
  - Cefazolin (IV) **plus** metronidazole (IV)
If immediate penicillin allergy or if water exposure of the wound
  - Ciprofloxacin (IV) **plus** clindamycin (IV)

For established bone infection, continue with oral therapy

  - Amoxicillin/clavulanate (PO)
If non-immediate penicillin allergy
  - Cefalexin (PO) **plus** metronidazole (PO)
If immediate penicillin allergy or if water exposure of the wound
  - Ciprofloxacin (PO) **plus** clindamycin (PO)

Dosage of above antibiotics

- Piperacillin/tazobactam 4 g (child: 100 mg/kg up to 4 g) IV q6h
- Ticarcillin/clavulanate 3 g (child: 50 mg/kg up to 3 g) IV q6h
- Cefazolin 2 g (child: 50 mg/kg up to 2 g) IV q8h
- Metronidazole 500 mg (child: 12.5 mg/kg up to 500 mg) IV q12h
- Ciprofloxacin 400 mg (child: 10 mg/kg up to 400 mg) IV q8h
- Clindamycin 600 mg (child: 15 mg/kg up to 600 mg) IV q8h

Oral therapy

- Amoxicillin/clavulanate 875/125 mg (child: 22.5/3.2 mg/kg up to 875/125 mg) PO q12h
- Cefalexin 1 g (child: 25 mg/kg up to 1 g) PO q6h
- Metronidazole 400 mg (child: 10 mg/kg up to 400 mg) PO q12h
- Ciprofloxacin 750 mg (child: 20 mg/kg up to 750 mg) PO q12h
- Clindamycin 450 mg (child: 10 mg/kg up to 450 mg) PO q8h

SHIGELLOSIS

Other names: bacillary dysentery

Pathogens

Shigella spp including:
- *Shigella sonnei* ('group D' *Shigella*)—accounts for over 60% of shigellosis
- *Shigella flexneri* ('group B' *Shigella*)—accounts for almost all the rest

Transmission

- Faecal–oral route
- Person-to-person

Incubation

- 12–50 hours

Clinical

- Abdominal cramps; diarrhoea; fever; vomiting; blood, pus or mucus in faeces; tenesmus; and dehydration

Complications

- Reiter's disease, haemolytic uraemic syndrome and post-infectious arthritis (about 2% of *S. flexneri* infection)

Laboratory

- Stool culture—isolation or detection of *Shigella* spp
- Faecal multiplex PCR testing—sensitivity 98–100%, result available in 24 hours

Treatment

Treatment reduces disease transmission and is recommended for:

1. Children <6 years
2. People who are institutionalised
3. Men who have sex with men
4. People who are immunosuppressed
5. Food handlers

- Oral or IV rehydration
- Mild cases usually resolve within 4–8 days
- Severe infections may last 3–6 weeks

Antibiotic therapy is recommended in all above cases due to the risk to public health

Empirical treatment

- Option 1: ciprofloxacin (PO) for 5 days
- Option 2: norfloxacin (PO) for 5 days
- Option 3: cotrimoxazole (PO) for 5 days

If quinolone resistance
- Azithromycin (PO) for 5 days

Adjust treatment according to stool culture and susceptibility tests

For severe cases (hospitalised, septicaemic or immunocompromised)
- Ciprofloxacin (IV)

Switch to oral after improvement

Dosage of above antibiotics

- Ciprofloxacin 500 mg (child: 12.5 mg/kg up to 500 mg) PO q12h
- Norfloxacin 400 mg (child: 10 mg/kg up to 400 mg) PO q12h
- Cotrimoxazole 160/800 mg (child: 4/20 mg/kg up to 160/800 mg) PO q12h
- Azithromycin 500 mg (child: 10 mg/kg up to 500 mg) PO on day 1, then 250 mg (child: 5 mg/kg up to 250 mg) PO daily for a further 4 days
- Ciprofloxacin 500 mg (child: 10 mg/kg up to 500 mg) IV q12h

Prevention

- Wash hands with soap and water carefully and frequently, especially after going to the bathroom, after changing nappies and before preparing foods or beverages
- Dispose of soiled nappies properly and disinfect nappy-changing areas after use
- Keep children with diarrhoea out of childcare
- Supervise handwashing of toddlers and small children after they use the toilet
- Do not prepare food for others while ill with diarrhoea
- Avoid drinking water from dams, lakes or untreated pools

SINUSITIS

Other names: rhinosinusitis
Most sinus infections are caused by viruses, antibiotics are not indicated.

1. ACUTE BACTERIAL SINUSITIS

Pathogens

- *S. pneumoniae*
- *H. influenzae*
- *Moraxella catarrhalis*

Causes

- As a complication of acute viral rhinosinusitis
- Being immunocompromised
- Secondary to odontogenic infection
- Deficient mucociliary clearance
- Mechanical nasal obstruction (e.g. nasal foreign body in children)

Clinical

- Nasal blockage
- Purulent nasal discharge
- Facial pain or pressure, maxillary toothache, sinus tenderness
- May have fever

Treatment

- Steam inhalation, saline nasal drops or spray and nasal decongestant

Indication for antibiotic therapy

At least three of the following features present:
- Persistent mucopurulent nasal discharge (>5–7 days)
- Unilateral facial pain (or maxillary toothache)
- Poor response to decongestants
- Tenderness over the sinuses, especially unilateral maxillary sinus
- Tenderness on percussion of maxillary molar and premolar teeth

Urgent ENT specialist referral

- Diplopia or impaired vision
- Periorbital oedema
- Fungal sinus infections
- Mental status deterioration

Antibiotic treatment

- Amoxicillin (PO) for 5 days

If no improvement within 2–3 days*
- Amoxicillin/clavulanate (PO) for 7–14 days

---

*High dose of amoxicillin/clavulanate (q8h) for penicillin-resistant *S. pneumoniae* or beta-lactamase–producing *H. influenza*

If allergic to penicillin
  • Cefuroxime (PO) for 5 days
If immediate penicillin allergy
  • Option 1: doxycycline (PO) for 5 days
  • Option 2: cotrimoxazole (PO) for 5 days

Dosage of above antibiotics

  • Amoxicillin 500 mg (child: 15 mg/kg up to 500 mg) PO q8h
  • Amoxicillin/clavulanate 875 mg (child: 22.5 mg/kg up to 875 mg) PO q8h
  • Cefuroxime 500 mg (child 3 months–2 years: 10 mg/kg up to 125 mg; >2 years: 15 mg/kg up to 500 mg) PO q12h
  • Doxycycline 100 mg (child >8 years: 2 mg/kg up to 100 mg) PO q12h
  • Cotrimoxazole 160/800 mg (child: 4/20 mg/kg up to 160/800 mg) PO q12h

2. CHRONIC SINUSITIS

Causes

• Chronic infection
• Allergy
• Structural abnormalities (e.g. nasal polyps or anatomical variation)
• Mucociliary impairment
• Cystic fibrosis
• Immune deficiency
• Prolonged use of nasal decongestant sprays

Treatment

• Acute exacerbation of chronic sinusitis—treat as acute bacterial sinusitis (see above) with a longer course of antibiotic therapy
• Chronic rhinosinusitis >3 months with yellow/green nasal discharge (without acute exacerbation)—nasal swabs for culture and antibiotic treatment based on culture results; antibiotic course may take up to 4 weeks
• Saline nasal douches
• Intranasal corticosteroids if allergy is the cause
• Short course of oral corticosteroids for symptoms uncontrolled by saline douches, topical corticosteroids and short-term antibiotics
  • Prednisone 0.5 mg/kg PO daily for 5–10 days
• Chronic rhinosinusitis with nasal polyps—a short, reducing course of oral corticosteroids (if does not respond to saline nasal douches and topical corticosteroids)

'Medical polypectomy'

  • Prednisone 25 mg PO daily for 1 week, then 12.5 mg PO daily for 1 week, then 12.5 mg every second day for 1 week

- Fungal rhinosinusitis with nasal polyps may require longer medical and surgical treatment; oral antifungals may be tried
- Referral to an ENT specialist for polypectomy, endoscopic sinus surgery

SMALLPOX

Other names: variola
Smallpox may be used as a potential biological warfare agent.

Pathogen

- Variola virus

Two forms of smallpox

- **Variola major**—severe and most common form, with more extensive rash and higher fever; fatality rate about 30%
- **Variola minor**—less common and much less severe disease (1%)

Transmission

- Via droplets and direct contact with infected bodily fluids or contaminated objects
- Infections are highest during the winter and spring
- Smallpox patients become infectious from the first appearance of fever until all scabs have separated

Incubation

- 7–17 days

Clinical

- Sudden onset of fever, malaise, headache, nausea, vomiting and back pain, followed by rash characterised by firm, deep-seated vesicles or pustules
- Crusts (or scabs) form after pustules have deflated and depressed de-pigmented scars are left following the crusts flaking off

Diagnosis

- Distinctive rash
- Electron microscopic examination of pustular fluid or scabs
- Variola virus culture
- Variola serology testing
- Variola PCR

Complications

- Pneumonia, encephalitis, eye complications (conjunctivitis, keratitis, corneal ulcer, iritis, iridocyclitis, optic atrophy and blindness), osteomyelitis, arthritis, limb deformities, ankylosis, malformed bones, flail joints and stubby fingers

Treatment and post-exposure prophylaxis

- Notification by phone to state/territory public health authority
- Isolation (home or hospital) and supportive treatment
- Antiviral drug
  - Cidofovir (adult and child) 5 mg/kg IV weekly for 2 weeks
- Smallpox vaccination up to 4 days (possibly up to 7 days) after exposure and before rash appears—will prevent or significantly lessen the severity of the disease; vaccination usually prevents smallpox infection for at least 10 years
- Vaccinia immune globulin—co-administration with smallpox vaccine to pregnant women and patients with eczema
- Close contacts should be vaccinated or placed on daily fever watch for up to 18 days from the last day of contact

STAPHYLOCOCCAL FOOD POISONING

Cause

- The staphylococci bacteria grow in food and produce toxins (heat-stable staphylococcal enterotoxins A, B, C, D and E in varying combinations)
- Typical contaminated foods include custard, cream-filled pastries, milk, processed meats and fish
- Ingestion of the contaminated food with enterotoxins causes the symptoms
- The risk of an outbreak is high when food handlers with skin infections contaminate foods that are undercooked or left at room temperature

Clinical

- Sudden onset of severe nausea, vomiting, abdominal pain and diarrhoea
- Starts 2–8 hours after ingestion of contaminated food
- Severe fluid loss can cause dehydration, electrolytes disturbance and shock
- Symptoms usually resolve in 12 hours
- Occasionally, staphylococcal food poisoning is fatal, especially in the very young, the very old and people with chronic illness

Diagnosis

- May be suspected when other people who ate the same food develop similar symptoms
- To confirm the diagnosis, a laboratory analysis must identify staphylococci in the suspected food (not usually performed)

Treatment

- Symptomatic treatment
- Oral or IV fluids for dehydration

Prevention

- Careful food preparation
- Anyone who has a skin infection should not prepare food
- Food should be consumed immediately or refrigerated

STAPHYLOCOCCAL SCALDED SKIN SYNDROME

Other names: Ritter disease, Lyell disease, Staphylococcal epidermal necrolysis

Pathogen

- *S. aureus* (some toxigenic strains)

Transmission

- Outbreaks often occur in childcare facilities; adult carriers (15–40% of healthy humans) introduce the bacteria into the nursery

Clinical

- Children <6 years, particularly neonates, are most susceptible
- Patients who are immunocompromised or have renal failure are at risk
- Fever, irritability and widespread redness and wrinkling of the skin; blisters develop within 24–48 hours, then rupture, with peeling of the skin, leaving a moist, red and tender area like a burn

Laboratory

- Nasal swab, wound swab for culture
- Skin biopsy may be indicated

Treatment

Most patients require admission and IV antibiotic
- Flucloxacillin (IV **then** PO) for 7–10 days

If non-immediate penicillin allergy
- Cefazolin (IV **then** cefalexin (PO) for 7–10 days

If immediate penicillin allergy
- Clindamycin (IV **then** PO) for 7–10 days

For methicillin-resistant *S. aureus* (MRSA) infection
- Vancomycin (IV)

Dosage of above antibiotics

- Flucloxacillin 2 g (child: 50 mg/kg up to 2 g) IV or PO q6h
- Cefazolin 2 g (child: 37.5 mg/kg up to 2 g) IV q8h
- Cefalexin 500 mg (child: 25 mg/kg up to 500 mg) PO q6h
- Clindamycin 450–600 mg (child: 10 mg/kg up to 600 mg) IV q6h
- Clindamycin 300–450 mg (child: 7.5-10 mg/kg up to 450 mg) PO q8h
- Vancomycin 25–30 mg/kg IV for the 1st dose (further dosing, see p. 462)

Prevention

- If there is an outbreak in childcare facility, childcare workers, parents or visitors should have swabs from nose and skin cultured; the

identified carriers should be treated with oral antibiotic (see above) and total body eradication after all acute lesions have healed
- To prevent further infection, strict handwashing with antibacterial soap/gel should be employed

STAPHYLOCOCCAL SKIN INFECTION—RECURRENT

Treatment

Total body eradication of carriage of *S. aureus*

- Indication: recurrent boils, carbuncles, furunculosis or impetigo (school sores)
- Diabetes, HIV and background skin conditions should be excluded
- Start total body eradication only after all acute lesions have healed

Confirm chronic carriage of pathogenic S. aureus
- Take swabs from nose, axilla and groin/perinea for culture

To eradicate nasal carriage

Use either of the following:

- Mupirocin 2% nasal ointment (e.g. Bactroban) intranasal bid for 5 days
- Chlorhexidine 0.3% nasal cream (e.g. Nasalate) intranasal q8h for 7 days

To eradicate skin colonisation (antiseptic total body wash)

Wash whole body daily for 5 days with either of the following:

- Chlorhexidine 2% solution (e.g. Microshield 2)
- Triclosan 1% solution (e.g. pHisoHex) or soap (e.g. Cetaphil Antibacterial Bar)

Pay particular attention to hair-bearing areas
Wash clothes, towels and sheets in hot water (>60°C) on two separate occasions

If lesions continue to recur
- Take swabs from nose, axilla and groin/perinea for culture
- Eradication treatment for whole family and close contacts
- Repeat above total body eradication, together with oral antibiotics according to the susceptibility of the organism
  - Option 1: rifampicin (PO) **plus** flucloxacillin (PO) for 7 days
  - Option 2: rifampicin (PO) **plus** fusidate sodium (PO) for 7 days
  - Option 3: rifampicin (PO) **plus** cotrimoxazole (PO) for 7 days

Dosage of above antibiotics
- Rifampicin 300 mg (child: 7.5 mg/kg up to 300 mg) PO q12h
- Flucloxacillin 500 mg (child: 12.5 mg/kg up to 500 mg) PO q6h
- Cotrimoxazole 160/800 mg (child: 4/20 mg/kg up to 160/800 mg) PO q12h
- Fusidate sodium 500 mg (child: 12 mg/kg up to 500 mg) PO q8–12h

Note

- Ensure the MRSA strains are susceptible to both medications in above regimens
- If the strains are resistant to mupirocin or any of the antibiotics prescribed, successful eradication is unlikely—seek expert advice

STAPHYLOCOCCAL TOXIC SHOCK SYNDROME

Diagnosis

Diagnosis of staphylococcal toxic shock syndrome (STSS) is based on the following criteria:

- Fever >38.9°C
- Systolic BP <90 mmHg
- Diffuse rash, erythroderma, subsequent desquamation, especially on palms/soles
- Multi-organ (≥3 organ systems) involvement:
  - GI (vomiting, diarrhoea)
  - Mucous membrane hyperaemia (vaginal, oral, conjunctival)
  - Renal failure (serum creatinine >2 times of normal)
  - Hepatic inflammation (AST, ALT >2 times of normal)
  - Thrombocytopenia (platelet count <100,000/mm^3)
  - CNS involvement (confusion without any focal neurological findings)

Treatment

- Aggressive resuscitation
- Culture of all potential infected sites prior to antibiotic therapy
- Hydrocortisone and normal immunoglobulin may be required
- Antibiotic therapy to eradicate the toxin-producing staphylococci

Penicillin-susceptible *S. aureus*
  - Benzylpenicillin (IV) **plus** clindamycin (IV)

Methicillin-susceptible *S. aureus*
  - Flucloxacillin (IV) **plus** clindamycin (IV)

If non-immediate penicillin allergy
  - Cefalotin (**or** cefazolin) (IV) **plus** clindamycin (IV)

MRSA infection or if immediate penicillin allergy
  - Vancomycin (IV) **plus** clindamycin (IV)

After improvement, change to oral for additional 10–14 days
  - Option 1: flucloxacillin (**or** cefalexin) (PO) **plus** clindamycin (PO)
  - Option 2: cotrimoxazole (PO)
- Normal immunoglobulin may be added:
  - Normal immunoglobulin (adult and child) 1–2 g/kg IV for 1 or 2 doses during first 72 hours

Dosage of above antibiotics

  - Benzylpenicillin 1.8 g (child: 50 mg/kg up to 1.8 g) IV q4h

- Clindamycin 600 mg (child: 15 mg/kg up to 600 mg) IV q8h for first 72 hours
- Flucloxacillin 2 g (child: 50 mg/kg up to 2 g) IV q4–6h
- Cefalotin 2 g (child: 50 mg/kg up to 2 g) IV q4h
- Cefazolin 2 g (child: 50 mg/kg up to 2 g) IV q8h
- Vancomycin 25–30 mg/kg IV for the 1st dose (further dosing, see p. 462)
- Flucloxacillin 500 mg (child: 25 mg/kg up to 500 mg) PO q6h
- Cefalexin 500 mg (child: 25 mg/kg up to 500 mg) PO q6h
- Clindamycin 300 mg (child: 7.5 mg/kg up to 300 mg) PO q8h
- Cotrimoxazole 160/800 mg (child: 4/20 mg/kg up to 160/800 mg) PO q12h

STREPTOCOCCAL TOXIC SHOCK SYNDROME

Other names: toxic shock-like syndrome (TSLS)

Pathogen

- *Streptococcus pyogenes* (Group A streptococcus)

Clinical

- Soft-tissue infection rapidly progresses to gas invasive infections (necrotising fasciitis or myositis)
- Hypotension does not respond to fluid resuscitation
- Multi-organ involvement
- Coagulopathy
- Hyperbilirubinaemia
- Adult respiratory distress syndrome
- Higher mortality rate than STSS

Diagnosis

- As STSS (p. 384)

Treatment

- Treat shock
- Prompt and aggressive exploration and debridement, fasciotomy or amputation
- Antibiotic therapy
  - Benzylpenicillin (IV) **plus** clindamycin (IV)

If non-immediate penicillin allergy
  - Cefazolin (IV) **plus** clindamycin (IV)

If immediate penicillin allergy
  - Vancomycin (IV) **plus** clindamycin (IV)

After improvement, change to oral for additional 10–14 days
  - Option 1: flucloxacillin (**or** cefalexin) (PO) **plus** clindamycin (PO)
  - Option 2: cotrimoxazole (PO)

- Normal immunoglobulin may be added:
  - Normal immunoglobulin (adult and child) 1–2 g/kg IV for 1 or 2 doses during first 72 hours

Dosage of above antibiotics

- Benzylpenicillin 1.8 g (child: 50 mg/kg up to 1.8 g) IV q4h
- Clindamycin 600 mg (child: 15 mg/kg up to 600 mg) IV q8h for the first 72 hours
- Cefazolin 2 g (child: 50 mg/kg up to 2 g) IV q8h
- Vancomycin 25–30 mg/kg IV for the 1st dose (further dosing, see p. 462)
- Flucloxacillin 500 mg (child: 25 mg/kg up to 500 mg) PO q6h
- Cefalexin 500 mg (child: 25 mg/kg up to 500 mg) PO q6h
- Clindamycin 300 mg (child: 7.5 mg/kg up to 300 mg) PO q8h
- Cotrimoxazole 160/800 mg (child: 4/20 mg/kg up to 160/800 mg) PO q12h

STREPTOCOCCUS AGALACTIAE

Other names: Group B streptococcus (GBS)

Pathogen

- *Streptococcus agalactiae*

Clinical

- GBS is a commensal organism and should be ignored
- Up to 30% of pregnant women carry GBS in their vagina or rectum
- Rarely, GBS can cause vaginitis (symptoms + heavy growth of predominantly GBS)
- GBS can infect the neonate during delivery and cause serious illness in the newborn
- The mother may also be infected during and after delivery
- GBS can occasionally cause symptomatic vulvovaginitis

GBS screen

- Low vaginal and anal swabs for culture at 35–37 weeks' gestation
- Screening pregnant women for GBS and subsequent antibiotic treatment can reduce the incidence of early-onset neonatal infections with GBS and maternal postpartum infections

Indication for antibiotic treatment

- Pregnant women with GBS carriage (positive GBS screen)
- Previous neonate invasive GBS infection
- GBS UTI or bacteriuria
- Breaking or leaking of the amniotic membrane before 37 weeks
- Pre-term onset of labour (<37 weeks' gestation)
- Prolonged (>18 hours) rupture of membrane
- Maternal fever (>38°C) during labour
- Symptomatic vulvovaginitis

Intrapartum antibiotic therapy

- Option 1: benzylpenicillin 3 g IV for the 1st dose, then 1.8 g IV q4h until delivery
- Option 2: cefazolin 2 g IV q8h until delivery

If immediate penicillin allergy

- Clindamycin 600 mg IV q8h until delivery

For prolonged rupture of membrane or maternal fever (chorioamnionitis)

- Amp(amox)icillin (IV) **plus** gentamicin (IV) **plus** metronidazole (IV)

For symptomatic vulvovaginitis

- Option 1: clindamycin 2% vaginal cream intravaginally at bedtime for 14 days
- Option 2: phenoxymethylpenicillin 500 mg PO q12h for 10 days

Dosage of above antibiotics

- Amp(amox)icillin 2 g IV q6h
- Gentamicin 4–7 mg/kg IV for the 1st dose (further dosing, see p. 459)
- Metronidazole 500 mg IV q12h

SWINE INFLUENZA

Other names: swine flu, influenza A (H1N1)
Swine influenza is a highly contagious acute respiratory disease of pigs. H1N1 has established person-to-person transmission and caused a pandemic.

Pathogens

- Swine influenza A viruses, most commonly H1N1 subtype
- Other subtypes are also circulating in pigs (e.g. H1N2, H3N1, H3N2)

Transmission

- The virus is transmitted among pigs by aerosols or direct and indirect contact
- People get swine influenza initially from close contact with the infected pigs
- Person-to-person transmission occurs by droplets or direct and indirect contact

Incubation

- 3–7 days
- Infectious period from 1 day prior to until 7 days after the onset of symptoms or until acute respiratory symptoms have resolved

Implications for human health

- Pigs and humans can be infected with more than one virus type at a time (e.g. swine influenza viruses, human seasonal influenza viruses or avian influenza viruses)

- The co-infection enables the genes from these viruses to mix
- People will probably have little or no immunity to the novo virus that can cause a pandemic

Clinical

- Symptoms are similar to human seasonal influenza: fever, rhinorrhoea, nasal congestion, sore throat, cough, headache, fatigue, diarrhoea and vomiting
- H1N1 influenza A virus seems to be more commonly associated with a severe form of myocarditis than seasonal influenza
- Clinical presentation ranges broadly from asymptomatic infection to severe pneumonia resulting in death

Diagnosis

If the patient is outside the swine flu–affected area:

- An acute febrile respiratory illness or pneumonia **plus** a history of travel to swine flu–affected area or close contact with a confirmed case of swine flu infection within last 7 days **plus** laboratory confirmation of swine influenza

If the patient is in the swine flu–affected area:

- An acute febrile respiratory illness or pneumonia **plus** laboratory confirmation of swine influenza

Laboratory confirmation of swine influenza infection

- Nasal/throat viral swabs (or tracheal aspirate/bronchoalveolar lavage from intubated patient) should be sent to the state/territory reference laboratory for one or more of following tests:
    - H1N1 viral sequencing
    - H1N1 viral RT-PCR
    - H1N1 viral culture
- H1N1 virus serology—if presentation is >7 days after the onset

Management

- Stay in a separate room or section in the house; remain >1 m away from other people at all times; improve airflow in the house
- Patients and family members should wear face masks at home
- Quarantine at home until well (confirmed cases) or until swine flu infection has been excluded (suspected cases) or for 7 days (asymptomatic contacts)
- If a contact develops symptoms at home, Public Health Unit should be notified immediately and assessment in an emergency department may be arranged
- In hospital, patient should be isolated in a single room and face masks should be worn

- All healthcare staff contacting symptomatic patients should wear face masks, eye protection (goggles or face shield), long-sleeved gown and gloves

Antiviral

Start ASAP within 2 days of onset of symptoms

- For mild to moderate uncomplicated infection—only treat **at-risk groups** (infants, children <5 years; adults >65 years; Indigenous Australians; pregnant women; patients with chronic comorbid diseases and the immunosuppressed)
- For severe or progressive infection, treat all patients
- When multiple influenza A subtypes are co-circulating, treat all patients
  - Oseltamivir (e.g. Tamiflu) 75 mg (child: ≤15 kg: 30 mg; 15–23 kg: 45 mg; 23–40 kg: 60 mg; >40 kg: 75 mg) PO bid for 5 days*
  - Zanamivir (e.g. Relenza) adult, child >5 years: 10 mg inh via disc inhaler q12h for 5 days**

Antiviral prophylaxis

- For contacts, particularly in at-risk groups who have contacted suspected cases (positive influenza A) or confirmed cases (positive swine influenza A infection)
  - Oseltamivir (e.g. Tamiflu) 75 mg (child: ≤15 kg: 30 mg; 15–23 kg: 45 mg; 23–40 kg: 60 mg; >40 kg: 75 mg) PO daily for 10 days

Vaccination

Swine influenza vaccine (Panvax H1N1):

- Panvax: adult, child ≥10 years: 0.5 mL IM st
- Panvax Junior: child 6 months–3 years: 0.25 mL IM, 2 doses at least 4 weeks apart
- Panvax Junior: child 3–10 years: 0.5 mL IM, 2 doses at least 4 weeks apart

Provides protection after 2 weeks and lasting for at least 2 years

SYPHILIS

Pathogen

- *Treponema pallidum* (a spirochaete)

Transmission

- Direct contact with a syphilis sore during vaginal, anal or oral sex
- From infected pregnant woman to her unborn baby

---

*Depending on the clinical response, higher doses of up to 150 mg twice daily and longer duration of treatment may be indicated

**Zanamivir is indicated when oseltamivir is not available or not possible to use, or when the virus is resistant to oseltamivir but susceptible to zanamivir

Incubation

- From 10 days to 3 months

Tests for screening of syphilis

- Venereal disease research laboratory (VDRL) test (blood or CSF)
- Non-treponemal rapid plasma reagin (RPR) test (blood or CSF)

High titres usually indicate active infection, provided the syphilis serology is also positive
Both are not very useful for detecting early or advanced syphilis

Tests for diagnosis of syphilis

- Syphilis serology (TPPA, TPHA, FTA-Abs)—positive after first 3–4 weeks of exposure; it can confirm a syphilis infection if VDRL or RPR is also positive (high titres)
- Syphilis serology may stay positive for life after infection
- Syphilis PCR (swab from lesion, biopsy or CSF)—the most sensitive test
- Dark ground microscopy—to examine exudate or tissue from an open sore (chancre) for syphilis spirochaetes; it is only for early syphilis diagnosis

Tests for treatment or re-infection monitoring

- VDRL or RPR

1. EARLY SYPHILIS (INFECTIOUS)

Definition

- Early syphilis of less than 2 years duration, including:
1. **Primary syphilis (chancre)**—painless anogenital or oral ulcers
2. **Secondary syphilis**—acute systemic illness with rash, anogenital condylomata lata (soft and moist lumps in skin folds), lymphadenopathy, hepatitis, meningitis etc
3. **Early latent syphilis**—infection less than 2 years' duration with no symptoms

Treatment

- Option 1: benzathine penicillin 1.8 g IM st
- Option 2: procaine penicillin 1.5 g IM daily for 10 days

If penicillin allergy
- Doxycycline 100 mg PO q12h for 14 days
  (ceftriaxone may be effective for early syphilis)

Pregnant patients who are allergic to penicillin
- Penicillin desensitisation and then treat with penicillin

HIV-infected patients with early syphilis
- Benzathine penicillin 1.8 g IM weekly for 3 doses

Concomitant steroid may reduce Jarisch-Herxheimer reaction
- Prednisone 20 mg PO q12h for 3 doses

- RPR or VDRL testing at 3, 6, 12 and 24 months after therapy
- Avoid sexual activity until lesions are healed
- Contact tracing—inform sexual partners to have test and treatment

Treatment of contacts (same regimen as above)

- For patients with primary syphilis—all sexual contacts within the last 3 months should be treated, even if their serology is negative
- For patients with secondary syphilis—all sexual contacts within the last 6 months should be treated, even if their serology is negative
- For patients with early latent syphilis—all sexual contacts within the last 12 months should be treated, even if their serology is negative

Prevention

- Low-dose doxycycline for high-risk men could prevent new infections
  - Doxycycline 100 mg PO daily for long term

2. LATE LATENT SYPHILIS (NON-INFECTIOUS)
Definition

- Asymptomatic syphilis (positive syphilis serology) of longer than 2 years or unknown duration

Treatment

- Lumbar puncture and CSF should be checked before treatment to exclude neurosyphilis
- If CSF is consistent with neurosyphilis, treat for neurosyphilis
- Antibiotic treatment
  - Option 1: benzathine penicillin 1.8 g IM weekly for 3 weeks
  - Option 2: procaine penicillin 1.5 g IM daily for 15 days

3. TERTIARY SYPHILIS (NON-INFECTIOUS)
Definition

- Syphilis of longer than 2 years or unknown duration with organ involvement, including:
1. **Late benign syphilis (gummatous syphilis)**—granulomatous inflammatory response to spirochaetes, forming gumma in any organ system
2. **Cardiovascular syphilis**—endarteritis obliterans, aortic regurgitation and coronary artery stenosis
3. **Neurosyphilis**—syphilis with any neurological signs or symptoms + positive CSF testing

Treatment

Seek expert advice

  - Benzylpenicillin 1.8 g IV q4h for 15 days

Concomitant steroid may reduce Jarisch-Herxheimer reaction
- Prednisone 20 mg PO q12h for 3 doses

4. PREGNANCY AND CONGENITAL SYPHILIS

- All pregnant women should be screened (syphilis serology) early in pregnancy
- In high-prevalence communities, pregnant women should have a repeated syphilis serology test at 28 weeks' gestation
- The pregnant patient and her partner should be treated with penicillin (≥4 weeks before delivery)
- A pregnant patient who is allergic to penicillin should be desensitised and then treated with penicillin
- The placenta should be examined by syphilis PCR testing, direct immunofluorescence and silver stains
- All newborn infants of mothers with syphilis should be checked for congenital syphilis

Diagnosis of congenital syphilis

Diagnosis is suggested by any one of the following tests of the newborn infant:

- Syphilis serology—IgM positive
- Syphilis serology—IgG titres are four-fold higher than the mother's
- Syphilis PCR (swabs, biopsy, tissue or CSF or placenta)—positive

Treatment of congenital syphilis

- Benzathine penicillin 50 mg/kg IV q12h for 10 days

Seek expert advice

5. ENDEMIC SYPHILIS (BEJEL)

The infection may be seen in central and north Australia.

Pathogen

- *Treponema endemicum*

Transmission

- Direct contact, usually within family and not sexually

Clinical

- The early and late lesions resemble those of secondary and tertiary syphilis (see above), but cardiovascular and neurological manifestations are rare

Treatment

- Benzathine penicillin 900 mg IM st

If allergic to penicillin

- Doxycycline 100 mg PO q12h for 14 days

TETANUS

Pathogen

- *Clostridium tetani*, a gram-positive rod that forms endospores
- Spores can enter the wound, grow anaerobically and produce a toxin, which has two components: neurotoxin and haemolysin

Incubation

- 3–21 days

The shorter the incubation period, the more severe the disease

Clinical

- Trismus (lockjaw), dysphagia, stiffness or pain in the neck, shoulder and back muscles
- Progress to paroxysmal, violent, painful, generalised muscle spasms and laryngospasm or apnoea
- Mental state is unimpaired

Complications

- Pneumonia, muscle rupture, fracture, DVT, pulmonary emboli, decubitus ulcers and rhabdomyolysis
- Death results from respiratory failure, circulation failure or cardiac arrest

Neonatal tetanus

- Poor feeding, rigidity and spasms during the first 2 weeks of life
- It is frequently due to non-sterile treatment of the umbilical cord stump
- It develops in babies born to inadequately immunised mothers

Diagnosis

Diagnosis is bases on clinical features

- Microscopy and culture for *Clostridium tetani* (tissue from wound excision or debridement)—the organism is rarely isolated

Treatment

- Surgical treatment of tetanus-prone wounds
- Supportive treatment
- Tetanus immunoglobulin—for the treatment of clinical tetanus:
  - Tetanus immunoglobulin-VF 4000 IU slow IV infusion

Prophylaxis (see Table 20.1)

Adults who have not received primary course of tetanus vaccination
  - dTpa (e.g. Adacel, Boostrix) **or** dT (e.g. ADT) 0.5 mL IM, followed by 2 doses of dT (ADT) 0.5 mL IM, at least 4 weeks apart

TABLE 20.1

TETANUS PROPHYLAXIS

Tetanus prophylaxis	Last tetanus vaccine (≥3 doses) >5 years but ≤10 years	>10 years	Had <3 doses of tetanus vaccine*
Tetanus booster[1]	Dirty wounds	All wounds	All wounds
Tetanus Ig[2]	No need	No need	Dirty wounds

*Include those with uncertain tetanus vaccination history
[1]Dose of tetanus booster:
dTpa is preferred to dT as it also boosts pertussis
  • dTpa (e.g. Adacel, Boostrix) **or** dT (e.g. ADT) 0.5 mL IM st
[2]Dose of tetanus immunoglobulin (TIG)
  • Tetanus immunoglobulin-VF (TIG) 250 IU (500 IU if injury >24 hours) IM as soon as practicable after injury
Tetanus booster and TIG should be given in opposite limbs

Antibiotic prophylaxis

Indicated for following high-risk wounds:

• Wounds presented ≥8 hours after injury
• Wounds on face, hands or feet
• Clenched fist injuries and occlusive human bites
• Puncture wounds
• Wounds involving bones, joints or tendons
• Wounds in immunocompromised patients
  • Amoxicillin/clavulanate (PO) for 5 days
May give a dose of procaine penicillin injection for early cover
  • Procaine penicillin (IM) st
If penicillin allergy
  • Option 1: doxycycline (PO) **plus** metronidazole (PO) for 5 days
  • Option 2: cotrimoxazole (PO) **plus** metronidazole (PO) for 5 days
  • Option 3: ciprofloxacin (PO) **plus** metronidazole (PO) for 5 days
If wound infection has developed
  • Antibiotic treatment, see Wound infection (pp. 448, 451)

Dosage of above antibiotics

  • Amoxicillin/clavulanate 875 mg (child: 22.5 mg/kg up to 875 mg) PO q12h
  • Procaine penicillin 1.5 g (child: 50 mg/kg up to 1.5 g) IM st
  • Doxycycline 200 mg (child >8 years: 4 mg/kg up to 200 mg) PO on day 1, then 100 mg (child >8 years: 2 mg/kg up to 100 mg) PO daily
  • Metronidazole 400 mg (child: 10 mg/kg up to 400 mg) PO q12h
  • Cotrimoxazole 160/800 mg (child: 4/20 mg/kg up to 160/800 mg PO q12h
  • Ciprofloxacin 500 mg (child: 10–15 mg/kg up to 500 mg) PO q12h

Tetanus vaccination

  • Primary course: DTPa 0.5 mL IM, 3 doses at 2, 4 and 6 months of age
  • 1st booster: DTPa 0.5 mL IM, at 4 years of age, st

- 2nd booster: dTpa (e.g. Adacel, Boostrix) **or** dT (e.g. ADT) 0.5 mL IM, at 12–17 years of age
- Further booster: every 5–10 years (5 years if tetanus-prone wounds)
- Booster at age of 50 (if no booster received in last 10 years): dTpa **or** dT IM, st

THROMBOPHLEBITIS—SUPERFICIAL

Risk factors

- IV cannulation
- Pregnancy
- Malignancy
- Varicose veins
- Other causes of venous stasis and venous trauma

Pathogens

- Spontaneous superficial thrombophlebitis—no pathogen
- IV-catheter associated infection—*Staphylococcus aureus*

Complication

- Deep vein thrombosis (DVT)
- Pulmonary embolism (PE)

Treatment

Spontaneous superficial thrombophlebitis

- Non-steroidal anti-inflammatory drug (NSAID)
- Low dose of low-molecular-weight heparin (LMWH):
  - Option 1: dalteparin 5000 units SC daily for 4 weeks
  - Option 2: enoxaparin 40 mg SC daily for 4 weeks
  - Option 3: unfractionated heparin (10000 units SC bid for 4 weeks

IV-catheter related superficial thrombophlebitis

- Remove the infected catheter and send the tip for culture
- Blood culture from another site
- Try NSAID:
  - Option 1: diclofenac 75 mg PO bid
  - Option 2: diclofenac 1% gel top tds
- Surgical drainage of purulent material and/or removal of the infected clot may sometimes be required
- Antibiotic therapy if bacterial infection is suspected:
  - Flucloxacillin (IV) **plus** gentamicin (IV)

If non-immediate penicillin allergy
  - Cefazolin (IV) **plus** gentamicin (IV)

If immediate penicillin allergy or possible MRSA infection
  - Vancomycin (IV) **plus** gentamicin (IV)

Change to oral after significant improvement

Dosage of above antibiotics

- Flucloxacillin 2 g (child: 50 mg/kg up to 2 g) IV q6h
- Cefazolin 2 g (child: 30 mg/kg up to 2 g) IV q8h
- Gentamicin 4–7 mg/kg (child: 7.5 mg/kg up to 320 mg) IV for the 1st dose (further dosing, see p. 459)
- Vancomycin 25–30 mg/kg IV for the 1st dose (further dosing, see p. 462)

TINEA

A superficial fungal infection of skin, hair or nails.

Pathogens

- *Epidermophyton*, *Trichophyton* and *Microsporum* (dermatophytes)— cause skin/scalp infections
- *Trichophyton rubrum*—causes onychomycosis
- *Trichophyton mentagrophytes*—causes superficial onychomycosis

1. TINEA CORPORIS AND TINEA CRURIS

- Tinea corporis (ringworm)—tinea on body
- Tinea cruris—tinea in groin

Laboratory

- Skin scrapings, subungual debris—for KOH and fungal culture (prior to treatment)

Treatment

Topical antifungal therapy (for localised tinea)

- Effect of topical antifungal agents: Terbinafine (fungicidal) > Azoles (e.g. bifonazole, clotrimazole, econazole, ketoconazole, miconazole) (fungistatic) > Tolnaftate
  - Option 1: terbinafine 1% (e.g. Lamisil, SolvEasy) top daily for 1 week
  - Option 2: bifonazole1% (e.g. Mycospor) top daily for 2–3 weeks
  - Option 3: clotrimazole 1% (e.g. Canesten) top bid or tds for 2–4 weeks, continued for 2 weeks after symptoms resolve
  - Option 4: econazole 1% (e.g. Pevaryl Topicals) top bid, continued for 1 week after symptoms resolve
  - Option 5: ketoconazole 2% (e.g. Nizoral, DaktaGOLD) top daily, continued for 1 week after symptoms resolve
  - Option 6: miconazole 2% (e.g. Daktarin) top bid for 4 weeks

Combination with hydrocortisone

Use when there is severe inflammation; stop using once inflammation subsides

- Clotrimazole + hydrocortisone (e.g. Hydrozole) top bid or tds
- Miconazole + hydrocortisone (e.g. Resolve Plus) top bid

Oral antifungal therapy

Indicated for:

- Widespread or chronic tinea that fails to respond to repeated topical therapy
- Tinea in hair-bearing areas and on palms and soles
- Tinea previously treated with corticosteroids
  - Option 1: griseofulvin fine particle 500 mg (child >2 years: 10–20 mg/kg up to 500 mg) PO daily for 4–6 weeks (take with fatty food)
  - Option 2: terbinafine 250 mg (child <20 kg: 62.5 mg; 20–40 kg: 125 mg) PO daily for 2–6 weeks until resolution
  - Option 3: fluconazole 150 mg PO weekly for 2–6 weeks until resolution
  - Option 4: itraconazole 200 mg PO daily for 1 week (fungal culture 3–4 weeks post therapy)

2. TINEA CAPITIS, KERION AND TINEA BARBAE

- Tinea capitis (ringworm of scalp, tinea tonsurans)—tinea on scalp, eyebrows and eyelashes
- Kerion—a large, boggy scalp mass due to severe reaction to tinea capitis
- Tinea barbae (barber's itch)—tinea around bearded area of men

Laboratory

- Skin scrapings and plucked hairs—for KOH and fungal culture (prior to treatment)

Antifungal treatment

- Topical therapy is ineffective for tinea of scalp
  - Option 1: griseofulvin fine particle (PO) for 4–8 weeks (take with fatty food)
  - Option 2: terbinafine (PO) for 4 weeks

Repeat fungal culture at the end of treatment

Dosage of above agents

- Griseofulvin fine particle 500 mg (child >2 years: 20 mg/kg up to 500 mg) PO daily
- Terbinafine 250 mg (child <20 kg: 62.5 mg; 20–40 kg: 125 mg) PO daily

3. TINEA PEDIS AND TINEA MANUUM

- Tinea pedis (athlete's foot)—tinea on foot
- Tinea manuum—tinea on palm of the hand

Laboratory

- Skin scrapings—for KOH and fungal culture (prior to treatment)
  - Option 1: terbinafine 250 mg (child <20 kg: 62.5 mg; 20–40 kg: 125 mg) PO daily for 2–6 weeks
  - Option 2: itraconazole 100 mg PO daily for 4 weeks

- Option 3: fluconazole 150 mg PO once weekly for 2–6 weeks
- Option 4: griseofulvin 1 g (child: 10–20 mg/kg up to 1 g) PO daily (with fatty food) for 4–8 weeks

Prevention

- Dry between toes after showering
- Dust the feet regularly with an antifungal powder
- Spray shoes regularly with an antifungal spray

4. TINEA OF NAILS

- Tinea on fingernails or toenails (tinea unguium, onychomycosis)

Pathogens

- *Trichophyton rubrum*—causes distal subungual onychomycosis (DSO) and total dystrophic onychomycosis (TDO), also involves the soles of the foot (thick skin)
- *Trichophyton mentagrophytes* var. *interdigitale*—causes toe web and soft sole infection, also causes white superficial onychomycosis (WSO)

Laboratory

- Nail clippings, subungual debris —for KOH and fungal culture (prior to treatment)
- Nail clippings (sent in formalin)—for PAS stain (more sensitive than culture)
- Nail plate histology—if nail-clipping culture is negative, a clipping of the distal nail plate can be sent

Treatment

Topical nail lacquers
Effective for WSO, limited efficacy on DSO
- Amorolfine 5% nail lacquer (e.g. Loceryl) top once weekly until resolved (for up to 12 months)
Oral antifungal therapy
- Terbinafine (PO) 6 weeks for fingernails, 12 weeks for toenails
If terbinafine is not tolerated
- Itraconazole (PO) as pulse treatment for 2–4 months (see below)
- Fluconazole (PO) 3–6 months for fingernails and 6–12 months for toenails

Dosage of above agents

- Amorolfine 5% nail lacquer (e.g. Loceryl) top 1–2 times per week until resolved (may require up to 12 months)
- Terbinafine 250 mg (child <20 kg: 62.5 mg; 20–40 kg: 125 mg) PO daily

- Itraconazole (pulse treatment): 200 mg bid for 1 week, then 3-week drug-free interval (2 courses for fingernail infection and 3–4 courses for toenail infection)
- Fluconazole 150–300 mg PO weekly

TONSILLITIS AND PERITONSILLAR ABSCESS

Other names: peritonsillar cellulitis, quinsy, Lemierre's syndrome

Pathogens

- Bacterial infections—*Streptococcus pyogenes* (most common), *Fusobacterium necrophorum* (gram-negative anaerobe, may cause life-threatening complications)
- EB virus ('glandular fever')—can present with severe sore throat with exudation
- Diphtheria—may occur in patients recently returned from overseas travel
- *Neisseria gonorrhoeae*—can cause exudative pharyngitis
- Herpes simplex virus types I and II—can cause ulcerative eruptions in throat
- Some strains of enterovirus—can cause vascular or ulcerative eruptions in throat
- Secondary syphilis—can present with mucosal lesions in throat

Indications for antibiotic therapy

- Tonsillitis with the following features (suggestive of *S. pyogenes* infection):
  - Fever >38°C
  - Tonsillar exudate
  - Tender cervical lymphadenopathy
  - Absence of nasal symptoms
  - Absence of cough

Children aged 3–14 years old are more likely to have bacterial tonsillitis

- Peritonsillar cellulitis or abscess (quinsy), Lemierre's syndrome—caused by *Fusobacterium necrophorum* with bacteraemia, suppurative thrombophlebitis of the internal jugular vein and metastatic lung abscesses
- Rheumatic fever—2–25 years in communities with high incidence of rheumatic fever (e.g. in Indigenous communities in central and northern Australia)
- Existing rheumatic heart disease
- Scarlet fever—fever/shivers + generalised punctate red rash with facial sparing

Treatment

For acute tonsillitis

- Penicillin V 500 mg (PO) for 10 days

If poorly compliant
  - Benzathine penicillin (IM) single dose
If non-immediate penicillin allergy
  - Cefalexin (PO) for 10 days
If immediate penicillin allergy
  - Azithromycin (PO) for 10 days (does not cover *F. necrophorum*)

For quinsy (aspiration or drainage + antibiotics)

  - Option 1: benzylpenicillin (IV) **plus** metronidazole (IV or PO)
  - Option 2: clindamycin (IV or PO) (if penicillin allergy)
If restricted swallowing and drooling **add** corticosteroid
  - Option 1: dexamethasone 10 mg IV or PO st, may repeat next day
  - Option 2: prednisone 60 mg PO st, may repeat next day

Dosage of above antibiotics

  - Penicillin V 500 mg (child: 15 mg/kg up to 500 mg) PO q12h
  - Benzathine penicillin 900 mg (child 3–6 kg: 225 mg; 6–10 kg: 337.5 mg; 10–15 kg: 450 mg; 15–20 kg: 675 mg; >20 kg: 900 mg) IM st
  - Cefalexin 1 g (child: 25 mg/kg up to 1 g) PO q12h
  - Azithromycin 500 mg (child: 12 mg/kg up to 500 mg) PO daily
  - Benzylpenicillin 1.2 g (child: 30 mg/kg up to 1.2 g) IV q6h
  - Metronidazole 500 mg (child: 12.5 mg/kg up to 500 mg) IV q12h **or** metronidazole 400 mg (child: 10 mg/kg up to 400 mg) PO q12h
  - Clindamycin 450 mg (child: 10 mg/kg up to 450 mg) IV or PO q8h

TOXOPLASMA GONDII

Other names: toxoplasmosis, toxoplasma encephalitis

Pathogen

- *Toxoplasma gondii*—an intracellular protozoan parasite

Transmission

- Adult parasites live in a cat's gut and produce cysts in faeces; humans, cattle, sheep and pig get infection from the contaminated faeces
- Humans can also get infection from eating undercooked infected beef, lamb or pork
- Seronegative woman infected during pregnancy may transmit toxoplasma to fetus
- The infection may also be transmitted from blood transfusion or organ transplantation

Clinical

- **Congenital toxoplasmosis**—usually fatal; if the patient survives, they are frequently disabled and blind

- **Acquired infection in immunocompetent people**—may be asymptomatic; acute form may have fever, rash and pneumonia; chronic form may only have enlarged lymph nodes with increased atypical mononuclear cells similar to glandular fever
- **Immunocompromised patients (especially AIDS)**—infection usually from reactivation of latent toxoplasmosis; it causes encephalitis and brain abscess

Laboratory

- Toxoplasma serology (may be negative in ocular toxoplasmosis)
- PCR for *Toxoplasma gondii* DNA (in CSF of immunocompromised patients)
- MRI brain—multiple ring-enhancing brain lesions

Prophylaxis

Toxoplasmosis prophylaxis is required for:

- Allogeneic GSCT recipients with positive *Toxoplasma gondii* IgG pre-transplant
- Heart transplant recipients receiving an organ from an IgG-positive donor
  - Cotrimoxazole 80/400 mg PO daily **or** 160/800 mg PO 3 times weekly

If unable to take cotrimoxazole
  - Dapsone 200 mg **plus** pyrimethamine 75 mg **plus** calcium folinate 15 mg PO weekly

Treatment

- Most patients—spontaneously resolve, no specific treatment required
- Infants, immunocompromised people and those with eye involvement—need treatment
- Toxoplasma encephalitis/brain abscess—common in AIDS patients, use:
  - Sulfadiazine (PO)* **plus** pyrimethamine (PO)

If allergic to sulfonamides
  - Option 1: clindamycin (IV)** **plus** pyrimethamine (PO)
  - Option 2: atovaquone (PO) **plus** pyrimethamine (PO)

If sulfonamides not available and clindamycin not tolerated
  - Cotrimoxazole (PO) or (IV) **plus** pyrimethamine (PO)

To reduce bone marrow suppression
  - **Add** calcium folinate 15–30 mg PO daily

---

*Sulfadiazine is available via Special Access Scheme <www.tga.gov.au/hp/access-sas.htm>

**Clindamycin 600 mg orally q6h is rarely tolerated by patients; IV is preferred

Duration of therapy
- For at least 6 weeks

Maintenance with reduced dosages

Take the following three medications together:

- Sulfadiazine 1 g (child: 25 mg/kg up to 1 g) PO q12h
- Pyrimethamine 25 mg (child: 1 mg/kg up to 25 mg) PO daily
- Calcium folinate 5 mg PO every 3 days

Duration of maintenance for AIDS patients

When CD4 cell count >200 for >6 months

Dosage of above agents
- Sulfadiazine 1–1.5 g (child: 25 mg/kg up to 1 g) PO q6h
- Pyrimethamine 50–200 mg (child: 2 mg/kg up to 50 mg) PO for the 1st day, then 25–75 mg (child: 1 mg/kg up to 25 mg) PO daily
- Clindamycin 600 mg (child: 15 mg/kg up to 600 mg) IV q6h
- Atovaquone 1500 mg PO q12h (with food)(adults only)
- Cotrimoxazole adult and child >1 month: 5/25 mg/kg PO **or** IV q12h

TRAVELLER'S DIARRHOEA

Pathogens

- Enterotoxigenic *Escherichia coli* (ETEC) (the most common cause)
- *Campylobacter jejuni* (an important cause in Asia)
- *Cyclospora cayetanensis*
- *Dientamoeba fragilis*
- *Salmonella enterica*
- *Shigella* spp
- *Giardia intestinalis*
- *Yersinia* spp
- *Norovirus* (the predominant cause on cruise ships)

Treatment

Mild diarrhoea

Oral fluid +/– anti-motility drug (avoid in children)
- Loperamide 4 mg PO initially, then 2 mg PO after each loose bowel movement up to 16 mg/day

Moderate to severe diarrhoea

Oral antibiotic +/– anti-motility drug

- Option 1: azithromycin (PO) as a single dose
- Option 2: norfloxacin (PO) as a single dose
- Option 3: rifaximin (PO) for 3 days (do not use if fever or bloody diarrhoea)

With fever or bloody stools

Do not use anti-motility drug
- Option 1: azithromycin (PO) for 2–3 days
- Option 2: norfloxacin* (PO) for 2–3 days
- Option 3: ciprofloxacin* (PO) for 2–3 days

Dosage of above antibiotics

Moderate to severe diarrhoea
- Azithromycin 1 g (child: 20 mg/kg up to 1 g) PO st
- Norfloxacin 800 mg (child: 20 mg/kg up to 800 mg) PO st
- Rifaximin adult and child >12 years: 200 mg PO tds

With fever or bloody stools
- Azithromycin 500 mg (child: 10 mg/kg up to 500 mg) PO daily
- Norfloxacin 400 mg (child: 10 mg/kg up to 400 mg) PO q12h
- Ciprofloxacin 500 mg (child: 12.5 mg/kg up to 500 mg) PO q12h

Persistent diarrhoea in returned travellers
- Stool microscopy and cultures (may need multiple samples)
- Serology for amoebiasis, schistosomiasis, strongyloidiasis

If no clear diagnosis identified, try empirical therapy for giardiasis
- Option 1: tinidazole 2 g (children: 50 mg/kg up to 2 g) PO, as a single dose
- Option 2: metronidazole 400 mg (child: 10 mg/kg) PO q8h for 5–7 days

If symptoms persist, consider lactose intolerance, coeliac disease or irritable bowel syndrome; specialist referral may be required

Prevention

- Food hygiene: eat fresh, cooked or tinned foods; eat fruits that can be peeled; drink bottled or boiled water
- Travelan (antibodies against ETEC for prevention):
  - Travelan 1 cap PO tds before meals
- Chemoprophylaxis is considered only for patients with:
  - Immunodeficiency
  - Active inflammatory bowel disease
  - Type I diabetes
  - Heart or kidney failure
  - High dose of antacid medicine (e.g. PPI)
- Option 1: norfloxacin 400 mg (child: 10 mg/kg up to 400 mg) PO daily
- Option 2: ciprofloxacin 500 mg (child: 12.5 mg/kg up to 500 mg) PO daily

Duration

- For up to 3 weeks until 1–2 days after leaving the risk area

---

*Quinolone resistance is high in South Asia

TRICHOMONIASIS

Trichomoniasis is a common sexually transmitted infection that affects both women and men, although symptoms are more common in women.

Pathogen

- *Trichomonas vaginalis*, single-celled protozoan parasite

Transmission

- Sexually transmitted infection

Incubation

- 4–28 days

Clinical

- Most men do not have signs or symptoms
- Some men have irritation or pruritus inside penis, urethral discharge, dysuria, slight burning after urination or ejaculation
- Many women experience no symptoms
- Some women have vaginal discharge (fishy smell, frothy yellow-green, pH >4.5), vulvovaginal itching and soreness, dyspareunia and dysuria
- In pregnant women, may cause premature rupture of membranes, preterm delivery and low birth weight baby

Complications

- In women—vaginitis, cervicitis and pelvic inflammatory disease (PID)
- In men—urethritis, urethral stricture, epididymitis, prostatitis and infertility

Diagnosis

- Vaginal or urethral swab (urethral discharge in men)—for microscopy and culture (visually observing the trichomonads)
- Vaginal or urethral swab—for trichomonas PCR testing (more sensitive)
- Screen for other sexual transmitted infections such as *Chlamydia* and gonorrhoea (first-void urine PCR) and HIV (serology)
- Sexual partners also need to be checked

Treatment

- Treat both patient and sexual partners at the same time
  - Option 1: metronidazole 2 g PO st (category B2)
  - Option 2: tinidazole 2 g PO st (category B3)

If relapse
  - Metronidazole 400 mg PO q12h for 5 days (category B2)

Following successful treatment, the person can still be susceptible to reinfection

TUBERCULOSIS

Australian doctors must consider tuberculosis (TB) when treating migrants from developing countries and when caring for Indigenous Australians.

Pathogen

- *Mycobacterium tuberculosis* (an acid-fast bacillus)

Transmission

- By airborne droplets from persons with infectious tuberculosis
- By direct invasion through mucous membranes or skin breaks
- By indirect contact with contaminated articles
- By eating meat infected with TB

Incubation

- 2–10 weeks

Management

- Promptly notify the state public authorities
- Refer to a specialist with the appropriate training and experience
- Contact tracing by public health nurses liaising closely with the treating doctors
- Make sure patient has good adherence to anti-TB therapy

Pre-therapy screening

- Check baseline weight, visual acuity and colour vision
- Check FBC, liver function, kidney function, hep B, C and HIV serology
- Check hepatotoxic medication and alcohol consumption
- Contraceptive advice for fertile females (reduced effect of OCP while on TB therapy)

Direct observed therapy (DOT)

Recommended for all TB patients if possible, particularly for:

- Patients known or suspected to be non-adherent
- Child patients
- Patients with multiple-resistant TB

Patients usually become non-infectious

- After 2 weeks of daily standard short-course therapy with clinical improvement (if the TB is fully drug susceptible)
- Longer than 2 weeks of therapy is required if patients are HIV positive, have large cavitation, laryngeal TB or positive smear with high risk of drug resistance

BCG (bacillus Calmette-Guerin) vaccination

Recommended for (Mantoux test must be negative):

- Aboriginal and Torres Strait Island neonates living in regions of high TB risk (e.g. NT, far north Qld, some regions of WA and SA)
- Neonates born to parents with leprosy or with a family history of leprosy
- Children <5 years of age who are going to stay in developing countries >3 months
- Healthcare workers involved in conducting autopsies, and embalmers

Monitoring anti-TB therapy

- Check adherence (if not under DOT)—pill counting, urine colour check, monthly sputum culture
- Check visual acuity and colour vision monthly
- Monitor liver function (minor impairment does not require cessation of therapy)

1.   Pulmonary tuberculosis

Laboratory

- FBC, ESR, LFT, U/E, hep B and C serology, and HIV serology
- Sputum microscopy for acid-fast bacilli (three samples)—the least sensitive
- Tuberculin testing (Mantoux test) or interferon-gamma release assay (IGRA)
- Mycobacterial culture and susceptibility (sputum, bronchial brush/wash, or bronchoalveolar lavage)—results available in 1–3 weeks
- Rapid testing for rifampicin resistance—if there is a risk of multidrug resistant TB
- TB-PCR—less sensitive than culture
- CXR

Treatment

Standard short-course (6 months) therapy (initial cure rate: 98%)

Indication for standard short-course therapy:

- Organisms are susceptible to isoniazid, rifampicin and pyrazinamide
- Patient tolerates all drugs in the regimen and is adherent to treatment
- No extensive cavitation on initial chest x-ray
- No evidence of miliary or central nervous system TB
- Good response to initial treatment

If standard short-course (6 months) therapy is unsuitable, 9–12 months of therapy is required

Daily regimen

- Isoniazid **plus** rifampicin **plus** pyrazinamide* **plus** ethambutol** (PO) daily for 2 months, continue isoniazid **plus** rifampicin for further 4 months
- Pyridoxine (vitamin B$_6$) 25 mg PO daily with each dose of isoniazid

3-times-weekly regimen (after at least 2 weeks of daily regimen)#

- Isoniazid **plus** rifampicin **plus** pyrazinamide* **plus** ethambutol** (PO) 3 times weekly for 2 months, continue isoniazid **plus** rifampicin for further 4 months
- Pyridoxine (vitamin B$_6$) 25 mg PO daily with each dose of isoniazid

Note: As the patient's weight may change during therapy, dose adjustment may be necessary

Dosage of above agents

Daily regimen

- Isoniazid 300 mg (child <14 years: 10 mg/kg up to 300 mg) PO daily for 6 months
- Rifampicin 600 mg (adult <50 kg: 450 mg; child <50 kg: 15 mg/kg up to 450 mg; child ≥50 kg: 600 mg) PO daily for 6 months
- Ethambutol 15 mg/kg up to 1.2 g (child <14 years: 20 mg/kg up to 1.2 g) PO daily for 2 months
- Pyrazinamide 25–40 mg/kg up to 2 g (child <14 years: 35 mg/kg up to 2 g) PO daily for 2 months

3-times-weekly regimen

- Isoniazid (adult and child) 15 mg/kg up to 900 mg PO 3 times weekly for 6 months
- Rifampicin (adult and child) 15 mg/kg up to 600 mg PO 3 times weekly for 6 months
- Ethambutol (adult and child ≥6 years) 30 mg/kg up to 2.4 g PO 3 times weekly for 2 months
- Pyrazinamide (adult and child) 50 mg/kg up to 3 g PO 3 times weekly for 2 months

---

*Pyrazinamide can only be discontinued at or after 2 months of treatment when the organism is known to be susceptible to isoniazid and rifampicin; pyrazinamide is available through the Special Access Scheme <www.tga.gov.au/hp/access-sas.htm>

**Discontinue ethambutol once the organism is known to be sensitive to isoniazid and rifampicin, even if this is prior to 2 months; continue ethambutol if susceptibility results are not available at 2 months; ethambutol should not be used in young children due to difficulties in assessing optic neuritis

#Only under DOT and if the patient is HIV negative

2. EXTRAPULMONARY TUBERCULOSIS (EPTB)

Extrapulmonary sites of infection

- Lymph nodes, particularly cervical lymph nodes
- Pleura—causing pleural effusion
- Bones and joints (spine is affected in 50% of cases)
- Genitourinary tract—uterus, epididymis, prostate, kidney, ureter or bladder
- Abdomen—bowel and peritoneum
- CNS, including meninges
- Pericardium—causing constrictive pericarditis
- Skin
- Miliary (disseminated) tuberculosis

Laboratory

- Tuberculin testing (Mantoux test) or IGRA
- Smear for acid-fast bacillus, biopsy for histological examination and *M. tuberculosis* culture (negative results do not exclude the infection)
- Urine for mycobacteria (3 early morning fully passed urine collections)
- Adenosine deaminase levels and PCR

Management

- Treatment duration may need to be extended for CNS and skeletal tuberculosis, depending on drug resistance, and in patients who have a delayed or an incomplete response
- Adjunctive surgical management may be required (e.g. for relief of spinal cord compression or ureteric obstruction)

For most forms of extrapulmonary TB

- Treat with standard short-course (6 months) therapy (see Pulmonary TB)

For miliary TB, CNS TB or skeletal TB

- Treat as standard short-course regimen but for 12 months (see Pulmonary TB)

Corticosteroids should be used in tuberculous meningitis, pericarditis, pleural effusion (if febrile) and miliary tuberculosis

- Prednisone 40–60 mg (child 1 mg/kg up to 40 mg) PO daily for 2–3 weeks then taper the dose gradually

3. LATENT TUBERCULOSIS

Definition

Mycobacterium tuberculosis infection without active disease.

- Positive tuberculin (Mantoux) skin test (≥5 mm induration at 48–72 hours) **plus** no evidence of active TB (false positive tuberculin skin test may be seen in people with past BCG vaccination or with immunodeficiency)

- Positive TB-specific IGRA **plus** no evidence of active TB (TB-specific IGRA is not affected by previous BCG vaccination, but may be false negative in people with immunodeficiency)

Indication for chemoprophylaxis of latent TB

- Patients with HIV infection
- Close contacts of a patient with smear-positive pulmonary TB
- Recent tuberculin converters
- Patients less than 35 years of age with no known TB contact
- Patients who are immunocompromised or are receiving immunosuppressive drugs

Treatment of latent TB

- Isoniazid 300 mg (child: 10 mg/kg up to 300 mg) PO daily for 6–9 months
- Pyridoxine (vitamin B_6) 25 mg PO daily with each dose of isoniazid

If isoniazid cannot be used or the organism is likely to be isoniazid-resistant, seek expert advice

4. TUBERCULOSIS IN CHILDREN

- Usually acquired from contact with an adult
- Usually not infectious
- Children who have not received BCG vaccination are susceptible to miliary and meningeal TB

Treatment

For primary pulmonary TB
  Child ≤6 years of age
- Standard short-course regimen with omission of ethambutol for ≥9 months
  Child >6 years of age
- Standard short-course regimen for 6 months (if acquired in a country with low incidence of drug resistance)
For 'adult-type' pulmonary TB (upper lobe infiltration and cavity)
- Standard short-course regimen for 6 months
For miliary and meningeal TB (more in infant and children ≤5 years)
- Standard short-course regimen for 12 months

BCG vaccination is recommended for:

(Mantoux test must be negative)

- Aboriginal and Torres Strait Island neonates living in regions of high TB risk (e.g. NT, far northern Qld, some regions of WA and SA)
- Neonates born to parents with leprosy or with a family history of leprosy

- Children <5 years of age who are going to stay in developing countries >3 months
  - BCG vaccine 0.1 mL (infant <12 months: 0.05 mL) intradermal inj st

BCG should be given at an authorised travel or BCG vaccination clinic

Isolation and school exclusion

- Children with primary pulmonary TB are not infectious and do not need to be isolated or excluded from school
- Children with adult-type pulmonary TB or disseminated TB should be isolated and excluded from school until the infection is under control

5.   TUBERCULOSIS IN PREGNANT AND BREASTFEEDING WOMEN

Treatment

Pregnant women
  - Treat with standard short-course therapy for 6 months
Breastfeeding women
  - Treat with standard short-course therapy for 6 months (continue breastfeeding during treatment)
  - Breastfed baby should be given pyridoxine 5 mg* on the day when mother receives isoniazid
Baby of mother with smear-positive pulmonary TB
  - Isoniazid 10 mg/kg PO daily for 6–9 months **plus** pyridoxine 5 mg* PO daily

6.   DRUG-RESISTANT TUBERCULOSIS

- Isoniazid-resistant TB (7–10% of TB cases in Australia)
- Multidrug-resistant TB (MDRTB)—resistant to both isoniazid and rifampicin (1–3% of TB cases in Australia)
- Extensively drug-resistant TB (XDRTB)—MDRTB + resistant to quinolones and second-line injectable drugs
- MDRTB is increasing in Australia and should be suspected in:
  - Migrants from high-risk areas (e.g. China, Indian subcontinent, Eastern Europe, Papua New Guinea, Southeast Asia, sub-Sahara Africa, Russia and South Africa)
  - Patients who have previously failed treatment or who fail to respond within 2–3 months of treatment
  - Contacts of patients with MDRTB
- Rapid identification of cases is important to prevent transmission

Treatment

Should be under the supervision of an expert

Isoniazid-resistant TB
  - Extend the duration of standard short-course therapy to 18–24 months

---

*For 5 mg dose, crush a 25 mg tablet, make up to 5 mL with water, give 1 mL

Multidrug-resistant TB
  * Use second-line anti-TB drugs (e.g. moxifloxacin, ethambutol, streptomycin* or amikacin)

Directly observed therapy should be provided

TULARAEMIA

Other names: rabbit fever, deer fly fever, Ohara's fever
Tularaemia is a bacterial infection that is transferred from an animal to a human. It may be used as a possible biological warfare agent. Any traveller to areas where tularaemia is endemic is at risk.

Pathogens

* *Francisella tularensis* (a gram-negative, non-motile coccobacillus)
* *Francisella tularensis palaearctica*

Transmission

* Through tick or mosquito bites
* Direct contact with the tissues or secretions of infected animals
* Inhalation or ingestion of the bacteria
* Dissemination methods as a biological warfare agent: aerosol, vectors

Incubation

* 1–21 days (average 4 days)

Clinical

Six forms of tularaemia:

* **Ulceroglandular tularaemia** (80%)—an infected scratch or abrasion becomes ulcerated with painful regional lymphadenopathy
* **Typhoidal (septicaemic) tularaemia** (10–15%)—fever, chills, septic shock
* **Glandular tularaemia**—painful regional lymphadenopathy with no skin lesion
* **Oculoglandular tularaemia** (1–2%)—unilateral purulent conjunctivitis with submandibular, preauricular and cervical lymphadenopathy
* **Oropharyngeal tularaemia** (rare)—from eating poorly cooked meat of an infected rabbit; sore throat (pharyngotonsillitis), abdominal pain (mesenteric lymphadenopathy), vomiting, diarrhoea and occasionally frank PR bleeding
* **Pneumonic tularaemia**—may develop after septicaemic tularaemia; adult respiratory distress syndrome may develop

---

*Streptomycin is available via Special Access Scheme <www.tga.gov.au/hp/access-sas.htm>

Diagnosis

- Tularaemia serology—may cross-react with *Salmonella*, *Brucella*, *Yersinia* and *Legionella* spp
- Tularaemia PCR test—allows early diagnosis
- Blood culture—requires special media containing cysteine (cultivation poses a hazard for laboratory staff)
- Skin testing—may detect a cellular immune response and is sensitive and specific (but skin test antigens are not commercially available)

Complications

Pneumonia, lung abscess, respiratory failure, rhabdomyolysis, renal failure, haemoptysis, meningitis and endocarditis

Treatment

- Symptomatic and supportive care
- Antibiotic treatment
  - Option 1: gentamicin (IV) for 10 days
  - Option 2: doxycycline (IV* then PO) for a total of 14 days
  - Option 3: ciprofloxacin (IV then PO) for a total of 14 days

Dosage of above antibiotics

- Gentamicin 4–7 mg/kg (child: 7.5 mg/kg up to 320 mg) IV for the 1st dose (further dosing, see p. 459)
- Doxycycline 200 mg (child >8 years: 5 mg/kg up to 200 mg) IV for 1 dose, then 100 mg (child >8 years: 2.5 mg/kg up to 100 mg) IV q12h
  When improved, switch to oral: 100 mg (child >8 years: 2.5 mg/kg up to 100 mg) PO q12h
- Ciprofloxacin 400 mg (child: 15 mg/kg up to 400 mg) IV q12h
  When improved, switch to oral: 500 mg (child: 15 mg/kg up to 500 mg) PO q12h

Post-exposure prophylaxis

- Option 1: doxycycline (PO) for 14 days
- Option 2: ciprofloxacin (PO) for 14 days

Dosage of above antibiotics

- Doxycycline 100 mg (child >8 years: 15 mg/kg up to 100 mg) PO q12h
- Ciprofloxacin 500 mg (child: 15 mg/kg up to 500 mg) PO q12h

Prognosis

- If treated, the overall mortality rate of tularaemia is 1–3%
- In untreated cases, the mortality rate ranges from 4% to 30–60% in more serious disease

---

*IV doxycycline is available via Special Access Scheme <www.tga.gov.au/hp/access-sas.htm>

Prevention

- Vaccine is not available in Australia
- Travellers should take care to avoid tick bites, ensuring their surroundings are kept clean, so as not to encourage rats and other potential carriers
- Water should be boiled and food should be protected from animals and cooked thoroughly

TYPHOID AND PARATYPHOID FEVERS

Other name: enteric fevers
Almost all typhoid and paratyphoid fevers are acquired outside Australia. The infection should be considered in febrile returned travellers.

Pathogens

- *Salmonella typhi*
- *Salmonella paratyphi* A, B and C

Transmission

- Contact with contaminated food or water, an infected individual or an asymptomatic carrier

Incubation

- 10–14 days (range 3–21 days)

Clinical

- Chills, high fever, relative bradycardia (pulse-temperature dissociation), diaphoresis, malaise, myalgia, arthralgia, cough, headache, rose spots (faint salmon-coloured maculopapular rash on the trunk and abdomen), loss of appetite, abdominal pain/distension, jaundice, constipation followed by diarrhoea (may be bloody), attention deficit, confusion, delirium, fluctuating mood and hallucinations
- Low platelets with high or low WBC count
- Children often present with vomiting and diarrhoea

Complications

- Intestinal bleeding or perforation

Diagnosis

- Relative bradycardia (pulse-temperature dissociation), rose spots and attention deficit may suggest the disease
- Microscopy, culture with quinolone susceptibility test (blood, faeces, urine, bone marrow or rose spots)
- *Salmonella typhi* antigen detection (blood, faeces, urine)
- Salmonella serology (Widal test or ELISA)—positive results may represent previous infection

- CSF analysis in all neonates and children <3 months to exclude neurological disease

Treatment

- Hospital admission
- Close monitoring for complications
- Antibiotic treatment
  - Option 1: azithromycin (PO) **or** (IV then PO) for 5 days

Neonates and infants <3 months IV treat for 10 days; infants 3–12 months treat for 7 days

If susceptibility is confirmed (MIC <0.125 mcg/mL)*
  - Option 2: ciprofloxacin (PO) **or** (IV then PO) for total of 7 days

If clinical response is delayed (fever >7 days)
  - Option 3: ceftriaxone (IV) daily

After improvement, switch to oral according to susceptibilities

  - Azithromycin (**or** ciprofloxacin) (PO) for a further 7 days

For severe disease (delirium, septic shock, stupor or coma)
  - **Add** dexamethasone 3 mg/kg IV, then 1 mg/kg IV q6h for 48 hours

Dosage of above antibiotics

  - Azithromycin 500 mg (child: 10 mg/kg up to 500 mg) IV daily
  - Azithromycin 1 g (child: 20 mg/kg up to 1 g) PO daily
  - Ciprofloxacin 400 mg (child: 10 mg/kg up to 400 mg) IV q12h
  - Ciprofloxacin 500 mg (child: 12.5 mg/kg up to 500 mg) PO q12h
  - Ceftriaxone 2 g (child >1 month: 50 mg/kg up to 2 g) IV daily

Typhoid vaccination

Provides 70% protection

Indications for typhoid vaccination
- Travellers ≥2 years of age going to endemic regions
- Laboratory personnel routinely working with *Salmonella typhi*
Choice of typhoid vaccines
- Vaccination should be completed at least 2 weeks before travel
Oral live attenuated vaccine**
  - Vivotif Oral—adult, child ≥6 years: 1 cap PO (1 hour before food) 3-dose course on days 1, 3 and 5 (or 4-dose course on days 1, 3, 5

---

*Quinolone-resistant organisms are common in the Indian subcontinent and Southeast Asia
**Oral live attenuated vaccine should not be taken with antibiotics but may be taken concurrently with mefloquine or Malarone (atovaquone/proguanil). It should not be used during pregnancy and should not be given to individuals with impaired immunity. It should be separated from oral cholera vaccine by at least 8 hours.

and 7), repeat 3-dose course after 3 years (or repeat 4-dose course after 5 years) if needed

Parenteral vaccines

- Typherix **or** Typhim Vi—adult, child ≥2 years: 0.5 mL IM st, booster after 3 years if needed

Combined vaccine

- Vivaxim (Typhoid + hep A)—adult, child ≥2 years: 1 mL IM st, booster after 3 years if needed

TYPHUS

Pathogens

- Australian tick typhus: *Rickettsia australis*
- Scrub typhus: *Orientia tsutsugamushi*
- Flinders Island spotted fever: *Rickettsia honei*

Distribution

- Australian tick typhus—Qld
- Scrub typhus—Qld, South Pacific Islands, Indonesia, India, Pakistan, Bangladesh, Burma and Far East
- Flinders Island spotted fever—Tas, SA, Vic and NSW

Reservoir and vector

- Australian tick typhus—*Ixodid* ticks
- Scrub typhus—*Trombiculid* mites
- Flinders Island spotted fever—*Australian paralysis tick*

Transmission

- Infected ticks may be picked up by walking in grassy/bushy areas
- Dogs may bring ticks into the house

Incubation

- 7–10 days

Clinical

- Eschar (single skin lesion at the site of inoculation, which goes on to ulcerate and form a black scar) with enlarged regional lymph nodes, fever and rash
- History of recent tick bites
- Delirium and meningeal signs possible in severe cases

Diagnosis

- Serology (early and convalescent serum samples)
- PCR for rickettsial DNA (from skin petechial lesions or inoculation eschar biopsy or WBCs)
- Rickettsial culture (takes 3–7 days)

Treatment

- Most patients recover spontaneously in 1–3 weeks without treatment
- Antibiotic treatment may shorten the course
  - Option 1: doxycycline (PO) for 7–10 days
  - Option 2: azithromycin (PO) for 5 days

Severe disease, seek expert advice

Dosage of above antibiotics

- Doxycycline (child >8 years: 2 mg/kg up to 100 mg) PO q12h
- Azithromycin 500 mg (child: 10 mg/kg up to 500 mg) PO on day 1, then 250 mg (child: 5 mg/kg up to 250 mg) PO q12h for further 4 days

TYPHUS—MURINE TYPHUS

Other names: endemic typhus

Pathogens

- *Rickettsia typhi*
- *Rickettsia felis* (less often)

Transmission

- Transmitted (bitten) by rat fleas that infest rats
- Less often, transmitted by cat fleas or mouse fleas carried by cats or possums

Incubation

- 7–10 days

Clinical

- Murine typhus is an under-recognised entity, as it is often confused with viral illnesses; most people who are infected do not realise that they have been bitten by fleas
- Headache, fever, muscle and joint pain, nausea and vomiting
- A discrete rash (eschar) appears 6 days after the onset of symptoms (40–50%)
- Neurological signs e.g. confusion, stupor, seizures or imbalance (45%)

Laboratory

- Serology for murine typhus (early and convalescent serum samples)
- PCR for rickettsial DNA (from skin petechial lesions or inoculation eschar biopsy or WBCs)
- Rickettsial culture (takes 3–7 days)

Treatment

- Most people recover fully in 1–3 weeks, but death may occur in the elderly, people with severe disabilities or patients with immunosuppression

- Antibiotic treatment:
  - Option 1: doxycycline (PO) for 7–10 days
  - Option 2: azithromycin (PO) for 5 days

Severe disease, seek expert advice

Dosage of above antibiotics

- Doxycycline (child >8 years: 2 mg/kg up to 100 mg) PO q12h
- Azithromycin 500 mg (child: 10 mg/kg up to 500 mg) PO on day 1, then 250 mg (child: 5 mg/kg up to 250 mg) PO q12h for further 4 days

U

UREAPLASMA

Pathogens

Ureaplasma is a member of the family *Mycoplasmataceae*.
There are two species of *Ureaplasma* that can infect the lower genital tract:

- *Ureaplasma urealyticum*
- *Ureaplasma parvum*

Transmission

- Sexual contact—through genital-to-genital, oral-to-genital or oral-to-oral contact
- Vertically—from mother to baby (either in uterus or at birth)
- Hospital-acquired—through transplanted tissues

Incubation

- 10–20 days after sexual transmission

Clinical

- It is estimated that 40–80% of sexually active women may harbour *Ureaplasma urealyticum* in their genital tract with no symptoms
- In women it may cause vaginosis (abnormal vaginal discharge, odour), salpingitis, endometritis, chorioamnionitis, postpartum fever and pelvic inflammatory disease
- In men it may cause non-gonococcal, non-chlamydia urethritis, epididymitis, orchitis and prostatitis; may be linked with abnormal sperm morphology and decreased sperm motility
- In neonate and fetus it may cause spontaneous abortion, stillbirth, premature delivery, low-birth-weight baby, neonatal pneumonia, neonatal sepsis and neonatal meningitis
- It may cause reactive arthritis and chronic fatigue

Diagnosis

- *Ureaplasma* species are frequently found in the genital tract of asymptomatic men and women
- Routine testing is recommended for men with urethral symptoms but gonococcal and *Chlamydia* testing are negative (non-gonococcal, non-*Chlamydia* urethritis)
  - *Ureaplasma* PCR (urine, urethra swab)
  - *Ureaplasma* culture

Treatment

- Some *Ureaplasma urealyticum* cases have developed resistance to some antibiotics
- Sexual partners should be taking antibiotics simultaneously

- Safe sex should be implemented by both partners until treatment is finished
- A repeat test should be taken 1 month after treatment to ensure the infection has been eradicated
  - Option 1: azithromycin 1 g PO as a single dose, may repeat in 14 days
  - Option 2: doxycycline 100 mg PO q12h for 10 days

For resistant *Ureaplasma* infection
  - Moxifloxacin 400 mg PO daily for 5 days

URETHRITIS

Pathogens

- *Chlamydia trachomatis* (D-K serovars)—the commonest cause
- *Neisseria gonorrhoeae*—other important cause
- *Mycoplasma genitalium*—a significant minority of cases
- *Ureaplasma urealyticum*—a potential opportunistic pathogen
- Herpes simplex—potential cause
- *Trichomonas vaginalis*—potential cause
- Adenoviruses—potential cause

Transmission

- Via sexual transmission

Clinical

- Often asymptomatic, may have urinary frequency, dysuria and urethral discharge
- May lead to epididymo-orchitis (male) or pelvic inflammatory disease (female)

Laboratory

- Urine—for *C. trachomatis* and *N. gonorrhoeae* PCR testing
- Urethral or vaginal swab—for Gram stain, microscopy and culture for *N. gonorrhoeae* (susceptibility testing is required on any isolated gonococci)
- Urethral or vaginal swab—for *C. trachomatis* and *N. gonorrhoeae* PCR testing
- Urethral or vaginal swab—microscopy for trichomonas
- Urethral or vaginal swab or urine—for *Mycoplasma genitalium* PCR testing
- APTIMA assay for both *Chlamydia* and gonorrhoea—more sensitive and specific than PCR (requires green-topped urine container and APTIMA swab collection kit)

Treatment

Empirical treatment—covers both *Chlamydia* and gonococci
  - Ceftriaxone (IM **or** IV) **plus** azithromycin (**or** doxycycline) (PO) (doses see below)

If *Chlamydia* infection only
- Option 1: azithromycin 1 g PO st
- Option 2: doxycycline 100 mg PO q12h for 7 days

If gonococci infection only
- Ceftriaxone 500 mg in 2 mL 1% lidocaine (lignocaine) IM st **or** 500 mg IV st

If gonococci resistant to ceftriaxone* seek expert advice

In remote Australia where penicillin-resistant *N. gonorrhoeae* is low
- Amoxicillin 3 g **plus** probenecid 1 g **plus** azithromycin 1 g PO st

If no response to above treatment or *Mycoplasma genitalium* infection
- Option 1: doxycycline 100 mg PO q12h for 10 days
- Option 2: moxifloxacin 400 mg PO daily for 10 days

For disseminated gonococcal sepsis
- Ceftriaxone 1 g IV daily (**or** cefotaxime 1 g IV q8h)

Continue for 48 hours after defervescence, then switch to oral based on culture and susceptibility results

Total duration
- 7 days or 14 days (if symptoms persist)

Note
- If symptoms persist or recur—requires a second course of antibiotics and further investigation of aetiology (e.g. urine/urethral or vaginal swabs for *Mycoplasma genitalium* PCR)
- Sexual partners should be examined, investigated and treated empirically to prevent reinfection
- Post-treatment follow-up is recommended: a test of cure at 1 month; a test of reinfection at 3–6 months

UTI—CYSTITIS

Pathogens

In uncomplicated urinary tract infections (UTIs)
- *Escherichia coli* (70–95% infections)
- *Staphylococcus saprophyticus* (5–10% infections)

In complicated UTIs
- *Escherichia coli* (20–50% infections)
- Other gram-negative bacteria (e.g. *Proteus*, *Klebsiella*)
- Enterococci
- Group B streptococci (*Streptococcus agalactiae*)

---

*As cefalosporin-resistant gonorrhoea emerges, any suggestion of possible treatment failure in gonorrhoea should be reported to public health authorities and advice from a sexual health practitioner needs to be sought

Diagnosis

Urine cultures—for following patients:

- Pregnant women
- Men
- Recurrent UTIs
- Nursing home residents
- International travel within last 6 months (particularly in South and East Asia)

Treatment

Antibiotic treatment

- UTIs cannot be treated effectively without antibiotics
- Antibiotic treatment should be started ASAP
- Delay in taking or not taking antibiotics may result in relapse or development of pyelonephritis

Urine alkalisation (e.g. Ural)

- Can relieve the symptoms of UTIs
- Should not be used with quinolones (increased risk of crystalluria)

High fluid intake and complete bladder emptying

Help resolution of UTIs

1. Cystitis in non-pregnant women

- Option 1: trimethoprim 300 mg PO daily for 3 days
- Option 2: cefalexin 500 mg PO q12h for 5 days
- Option 3: amoxicillin/clavulanate 500 mg PO q12h for 5 days
- Option 4: nitrofurantoin 100 mg PO q12h for 5 days
- Option 5: fosfomycin* 3 g PO as a single dose

Do not use amoxicillin unless susceptibility is confirmed

For *Pseudomonas aeruginosa* or for other multi-resistant bacteria
- Norfloxacin 400 mg PO q12h for 3 days

Longer course (7–14 days) for following
- UTI associated with incontinence
- UTI associated with diabetes
- UTI in patients with immunosuppression
- UTI acquired in hospital or aged care facilities

Note: trimethoprim is as effective as cotrimoxazole, which is not recommended for empirical treatment of UTIs due to its rare but serious adverse effects

---

*Fosfomycin is available via Special Access Scheme <www.tga.gov.au/hp/access-sas. htm> or from compounding chemist

If relapse occurs
- Pyelonephritis should be considered and treatment given for 10–14 days

If treatment failure, usually due to:
- A resistant organism infection—treat according to susceptibility
- Re-infection with a similar organism—treat for 10–14 days
- Underlying abnormality of urinary tract—further investigation

2.   Cystitis in pregnant women

- Urine cultures and susceptibility test should be sent for pregnant women with UTIs

Empirical therapy
  - Option 1: cefalexin 500 mg PO q12h for 5 days (category A)
  - Option 2: nitrofurantoin 100 mg PO q12h for 5 days (category A)
  - Option 3: amoxicillin/clavulanate 500 mg PO q12h for 5 days (category B1)

Do not use amoxicillin unless susceptibility is confirmed
Modify therapy according to cultures and susceptibility testing
Repeat urine culture 1–2 weeks after the course of antibiotic

Pregnant women with recurrent UTIs, consider prophylaxis
  - Option 1: cefalexin 250 mg PO nocte for rest of pregnancy
  - Option 2: trimethoprim 150 mg PO nocte for rest of pregnancy (avoid 1st trimester)

3.   Cystitis in men

- All males with UTI should be investigated to exclude an underlying abnormality (e.g. STI, non-gonococcal urethritis, prostatitis or epididymitis)

Empirical therapy

While awaiting results of urine culture or STI screen or both

  - Option 1: trimethoprim 300 mg PO daily for 7 days
  - Option 2: cefalexin 500 mg PO q12h for 7 days
  - Option 3: amoxicillin/clavulanate 500 mg PO q12h for 7 days
  - Option 4: nitrofurantoin 100 mg PO q12h for 7 days (does not cover prostatitis)

If pathogen is resistant to above antibiotics and is susceptible to quinolones
  - Norfloxacin 400 mg PO q12h for 7 days

To treat *Chlamydia* trachomatis infection
  - Option 1: azithromycin 1 g PO st
  - Option 2: doxycycline 100 mg PO q12h for 7 days

To treat gonococcal infection
  - Ceftriaxone 500 mg in 2 mL 1% lidocaine (lignocaine) IM st **or** 500 mg IV st

f chronic prostatitis is suspected or diagnosed (in patients with recurrent **b** wer UTIs with the same organism)
- Treat as Chronic prostatitis (p. 339)

4. Cystitis in children

- Urine for microscopy and culture (urine sample should be obtained from 'clean catch', suprapubic aspiration or catheterisation)

Child >1 month with no sepsis
- Option 1: trimethoprim 4 mg/kg up to 150 mg PO q12h
- Option 2: cotrimoxazole 4/20 mg/kg up to 160/800 mg PO q12h
- Option 3: cefalexin 12.5 mg/kg up to 500 mg PO q6h
- Option 4: amoxicillin/clavulanate 22.5 mg/kg up to 875 mg PO q12h

f resistant to all above drugs or if *Pseudomonas aeruginosa* infection
- Norfloxacin 10 mg/kg up to 400 mg PO q12h

Duration of treatment
- Child <1 year—treat for 5 days
- Child ≥1 year—treat for 3 days

Child ≤1 month

V therapy only—dosing is complex—seek expert advice

Child >1 month with sepsis or acute pyelonephritis—see *Pyelonephritis* (p. 425)

Follow-up of children with UTI
- Ultrasound KUB—should be considered in all infants and in children with severe, atypical or recurrent UTI; if the ultrasound is normal, further imaging is not indicated
- If ultrasound finding suggests vesicoureteral reflux, particularly in male infants, refer to a specialist for further investigations (e.g. micturating cystourethrogram, MCUG)

Prophylaxis for recurrent UTIs in children
- Antibiotic prophylaxis is not recommended for children after 1st episode of UTI

Prophylaxis may be considered for children with severe or recurrent UTIs
- Occasionally, surgical intervention is necessary to reduce the recurrence
  - Option 1: trimethoprim 4 mg/kg up to 150 mg PO nocte
  - Option 2: cotrimoxazole (child >1 month) 2/10 mg/kg up to 80/400 mg PO nocte
  - Option 3: cefalexin 12.5 mg/kg up to 250 mg PO nocte
  - Option 4: nitrofurantoin* (child >1 month) 1 mg/kg up to 50 mg PO nocte

---

*Long-term use of nitrofurantoin may cause pulmonary toxicity (persistent cough or dyspnoea)

Duration of prophylaxis
- Trial prophylaxis for 6 months, then review the need for ongoing prophylaxis

Above antibiotics may be used in rotation to reduce the risk of antibiotic resistance

5.   Cystitis in elderly people
- Typical urinary symptoms are often absent. Patient may present with atypical symptoms—e.g. confusion, delirium or behavioural disturbance
- Asymptomatic bacteriuria (common in the elderly)—does not require treatment
- Cloudy or malodorous urine without other symptoms of UTI—do not investigate or treat
- Urethra syndrome (in women)—does not require antibiotic treatment
- It is important to obtain a urine sample before starting antibiotic treatment
- If mid-stream urine sample is difficult to obtain, collect urine sample by an in–out catheter (for women), or a new condom catheter (for men), or collect the urine sample through a new catheter or from the port in the drainage system (for patient with a catheter in situ)
- Symptomatic UTI (new or worsening urinary urgency or incontinence, urinary frequency, suprapubic pain/tenderness, gross haematuria) requires antibiotic treatment.
- Antibiotic choice and dosage are the same as Cystitis in women (p. 421) and Cystitis in men (p. 422)

UTI—ACUTE PYELONEPHRITIS

Pathogens
- Bowel organisms—e.g. *E. coli* (70–80%) and *Enterococcus faecalis*
- Hospital-acquired infections—e.g. coliforms, enterococci, *Klebsiella* spp *Pseudomonas aeruginosa*

Risk factors
- Structural abnormalities of the kidneys and urinary tract
- Vesicoureteral reflux (VUR) especially in young children
- Renal calculi
- Urinary tract catheterisation, urinary tract stents
- Pregnancy
- Neurogenic bladder (e.g. due to spinal cord damage, spina bifida or multiple sclerosis)
- Prostate disease (e.g. benign prostatic hyperplasia)
- Diabetes mellitus and immunosuppression
- Positive family history of frequent UTIs

Laboratory

- Urine and blood (inpatient) for culture and susceptibility test—sent before starting treatment
- Ultrasound or CT KUB—if a renal calculus is suspected
- Voiding cystourethrography and kidney ultrasound scan—for recurrent ascending UTIs, to exclude vesicoureteral reflux or polycystic kidney disease

Treatment

1. Mild infection (low-grade fever, no nausea or vomiting)

- Option 1: amoxicillin/clavulanate (PO) for 10–14 days
- Option 2: cefalexin (PO) for 10–14 days
- Option 3: trimethoprim (PO) for 10–14 days

If resistant to all above drugs or *Pseudomonas aeruginosa* infection

- Option 1: ciprofloxacin (PO) for 7 days
- Option 2: norfloxacin (PO) for 7 days

A follow-up urine culture at least 48 hours after the course

Dosage of above antibiotics

- Amoxicillin/clavulanate 875 mg (child: 22.5 mg/kg up to 875 mg) PO q12h
- Cefalexin 500 mg (child: 12.5 mg/kg up to 500 mg) PO q6h
- Trimethoprim 300 mg PO daily (child: 4 mg/kg up to 150 mg PO q12h)
- Ciprofloxacin 500 mg (child: 12.5 mg/kg up to 500 mg) PO q12h
- Norfloxacin 400 mg (child: 10 mg/kg up to 400 mg) PO q12h

2. Severe infection (with fever, rigors or vomiting)

- All acute cases with spiking fevers and leucocytosis should be admitted to the hospital for IV fluids hydration and IV antibiotic treatment
- Consider investigations to exclude abnormality of urinary tract
- Exclude upper urinary tract obstruction

Empirical treatment

- Ampicillin (IV) **plus** gentamicin (IV)

If penicillin allergy

- Gentamicin (IV) alone

If aminoglycoside is contraindicated

- Ceftriaxone (**or** cefotaxime)* (IV)

If multidrug-resistant gram-negative organisms is suspected

- Meropenem 12.5–25 mg/kg up to 500–1000 mg IV q8h

---

*If enterococci or *Pseudomonas aeruginosa* infection is suspected or confirmed, these antibiotics cannot be used

- Reassess after 48 hours of treatment
- Modify therapy based on result of cultures and susceptibility testing

Switch to oral therapy when significantly improved

- Option 1: cotrimoxazole 4/20 mg/kg up to 160/800 mg PO q12h
- Option 2: cefalexin 12.5 mg/kg up to 500 mg PO q6h
- Option 3: amoxicillin/clavulanate 22.5 mg/kg up to 875 mg PO q12h

If resistant to all above drugs or if *Pseudomonas aeruginosa* infection

- Option 1: ciprofloxacin 12.5 mg/kg up to 500 mg PO q12h
- Option 2: norfloxacin 10 mg/kg up to 400 mg PO q12h

Duration of treatment and follow-up

- Continue IV antibiotics until afebrile for 24–48 hours, switch to oral antibiotic (see above Mild infection) for a total of 10–14 days (3 weeks if delayed response)
- A follow-up urine culture 1–2 weeks after completion of therapy

Dosage of above antibiotics

- Ampicillin 2 g (child: 50 mg/kg up to 2 g) IV q6h
- Gentamicin 4–7 mg/kg IV for the 1st dose (further dosing see p. 459)
- Ceftriaxone 1 g (child>1 month: 50 mg/kg up to 1 g) IV daily
- Cefotaxime 1 g (child: 50 mg/kg up to 1 g) IV q8h

UTI—RECURRENT

Recurrent UTIs occur either as relapse of previous infection or reinfection.

Clinical

- Urine culture (M/C/S) is required in all patients
- Investigations should be done to identify underlying abnormalities or causes e.g. bladder dysfunction, bladder stones, diabetes, vesicoureteral reflux, prostatitis (men), prostate hypertrophy (men), STI or urethral stricture

Treatment

- Relapses of UTIs—treated as for acute pyelonephritis (p. 424)
- Reinfections—treated as for Cystitis (p. 420) or Acute pyelonephritis (p. 424)

Prophylaxis

Indication for prophylaxis

- Frequent symptomatic UTIs (≥2 UTIs over 6 months or ≥3 UTIs over 12 months)

Methods of prophylaxis

- Pass urine straight away after intercourse (female)
- Cranberry products, blueberry juice and probiotic bacteria may reduce the incidence of UTIs

- Intravaginal oestrogen in postmenopausal women may reduce recurrent UTIs
- Intermittent self-treatment—at the onset of symptoms, self-treat with one of the antibiotics used in treating Acute cystitis (p. 420) for 3 days, if symptoms do not resolve within 2–3 days after the treatment, seek medical attention
- Intermittent prophylaxis—e.g. take antibiotic within 2 hours post sexual intercourse
- Continuous prophylaxis—especially for frequent, severe and complicated recurrent UTIs

Treat a recurrent UTI (see Cystitis, p. 420 or Acute pyelonephritis, p. 424), for 10 days

Start prophylaxis following the successful treatment:
- Option 1: trimethoprim 150 mg PO nocte
- Option 2: cefalexin 250 mg PO nocte

Duration of prophylaxis

- Continue for 3–6 months or longer
- If recurrences continue to occur—seek expert advice

Recurrent UTIs in children

- Antibiotic prophylaxis is not recommended for children after 1st episode of UTI
- Prophylaxis may be considered for children with severe or recurrent UTIs
- Occasionally, surgical intervention is necessary to reduce the recurrence

Prophylaxis for recurrent UTIs in children
- Option 1: trimethoprim 4 mg/kg up to 150 mg PO nocte
- Option 2: cotrimoxazole (child >1 month) 2/10 mg/kg up to 80/400 mg PO nocte
- Option 3: cefalexin 12.5 mg/kg up to 250 mg PO nocte
- Option 4: nitrofurantoin* (child >1 month) 1 mg/kg up to 50 mg PO nocte

Duration of prophylaxis

- Trial prophylaxis for 6 months, then review the need for ongoing prophylaxis
- Above antibiotics may be used in rotation to reduce the risk of antibiotic resistance

UTI—ASYMPTOMATIC BACTERIURIA

Asymptomatic bacteriuria—significant number of bacteria in the urine without UTI symptoms

---

*Long-term use of nitrofurantoin may cause pulmonary toxicity (persistent cough or dyspnoea)

Treatment

- Asymptomatic bacteriuria does not usually require antibiotic treatment
- Antibiotic treatment is only indicated for the following conditions

1. Pregnant women with asymptomatic bacteriuria

- Routine screening for asymptomatic bacteriuria at the first antenatal visit
- Asymptomatic bacteriuria increases the risk of developing pyelonephritis and adverse pregnancy outcomes
  - Option 1: cefalexin 500 mg PO q12h for 5 days (category A)
  - Option 2: nitrofurantoin 100 mg PO q12h for 5 days (category A)
  - Option 3: amoxicillin/clavulanate 500 mg PO q12h for 5 days (category B1)

Do not use amoxicillin unless susceptibility is confirmed
Modify therapy according to cultures and susceptibility testing
Repeat urine culture 1–2 weeks after the course of antibiotic

2. Patients with asymptomatic bacteriuria before urological procedures (e.g. TURP)

ADULT
  - Option 1: trimethoprim 300 mg PO daily for 3 days
  - Option 2: cefalexin 500 mg PO q12h for 5 days
  - Option 3: amoxicillin/clavulanate 500 mg PO q12h for 5 days
  - Option 4: nitrofurantoin 100 mg PO q12h for 5 days
For *Pseudomonas aeruginosa* or multi-resistant bacteriuria
  - Norfloxacin 400 mg PO q12h for 3 days

CHILD
  - Option 1: trimethoprim 4 mg/kg up to 150 mg PO q12h for 3 days
  - Option 2: cotrimoxazole 4/20 mg/kg up to 160/800 mg PO q12h for 3 days
  - Option 3: cefalexin 12.5 mg/kg up to 500 mg PO q6h for 3 days
  - Option 4: amoxicillin/clavulanate 22.5 mg/kg up to 875 mg PO q12h for 3 days
If resistant to all above drugs or if *Pseudomonas aeruginosa* infection
  - Norfloxacin 10 mg/kg up to 400 mg PO q12h for 3 days

UTI—CATHETER-ASSOCIATED

1. Asymptomatic patients with urinary catheters

No need to check urine if no symptoms

2. Asymptomatic patients with urinary catheters who are high risk (pregnant women, organ transplant recipients, those with neutropenia and prior to urological or pelvic surgery)

Need urine culture (through a newly inserted catheter or from the port in the drainage system) and antibiotic treatment

3. Symptomatic patients with urinary catheters (fever, rigors, unwell, agitation or confusion in the elderly)

Need urine culture (through a newly inserted catheter or from the port in the drainage system) and antibiotic treatment

Antibiotic treatment

Empirical treatment (before culture results are available)

- Option 1: cefalexin (PO) for 7–14 days
- Option 2: amoxicillin/clavulanate (PO) for 7–14 days
- Option 3: trimethoprim (**or** cotrimoxazole) (PO) for 7–14 days

Adjust antibiotics according to culture results

Dosage of above antibiotics

- Cefalexin 500 mg (child: 12.5 mg/kg up to 500 mg) PO q6h
- Amoxicillin/clavulanate 875 mg (child: 22.5 mg/kg up to 875 mg) PO q12h
- Trimethoprim 300 mg PO daily (child: 4 mg/kg up to 150 mg PO q12h)
- Cotrimoxazole 160/800 mg (child: 4/20 mg/kg up to 160/800 mg) PO q12h (if trimethoprim liquid formulation is not available)

Note

- Permanent removal of the catheter whenever possible is the best way to cure the infection
- Antibiotics should not be routinely used at the time of catheter change
- Bladder irrigation containing antibiotics should not be used

Prevention

For short-term catheters

- Limit the duration of use as short as possible (the most effective prevention)
- Insert catheter using aseptic technique
- Ensure unobstructed flow of urine, maintain a closed drainage system
- Adhere to appropriate catheter care techniques

For long-term catheters

- Avoid catheter blockage, twisting or urethral trauma
- Treat bacteriuria prior to any invasive urological or pelvic surgery
- Consider suprapubic catheters for long-term use
- There may be a benefit in using prophylactic antibiotics at removal of the catheter after urological procedures in some high-risk patients

UTI—REFLUX NEPHROPATHY

Other names: chronic pyelonephritis, recurrent pyelonephritis

Causes

- Congenital vesicoureteral reflux (VUR) and recurrent UTIs (pyelonephritis) result in progressive kidney damage and scarring

Pathogens

- *Escherichia coli* (common)
- Other gram-negative bacteria

Clinical

- Girls are at greater risk of developing reflux nephropathy because of a higher rate of UTIs
- Children with reflux nephropathy may be asymptomatic, may only have nonspecific symptoms (e.g. failure to thrive, fever, poor food intake), may be acutely ill with acute pyelonephritis or may present with renal failure

Diagnosis

- Renal ultrasonography (RUS)
- Voiding cystourethrography (VCUG)
- Radionuclide renal scan
- Intravenous pyelogram (IVP)

Treatment for recurrent UTIs

- Treat each recurrent infection as acute cystitis (p. 420) or acute pyelonephritis (p. 424)

Prophylaxis

- Start prophylaxis after successful control of acute infection
- Prophylaxis may continue until puberty occurs or surgical correction is performed
  - Option 1: cefalexin 250 mg (child: 12.5 mg/kg up to 250 mg) PO nocte
  - Option 2: trimethoprim 150 mg (child: 4 mg/kg up to 150 mg) PO nocte
  - Option 3: nitrofurantoin 50 mg (child: 1 mg/kg up to 50 mg) PO nocte

Duration of prophylaxis

- 3–6 months or longer
- Antibiotics may be used in rotation to reduce the risk of antibiotic resistance

General management

- Early detection of VUR is essential
- Empty bladder completely, but never strain when passing urine
- Never let bladder fill to full with urine
- Double voiding: pass urine and then pass again soon after, to ensure complete emptying of the bladder, particularly before going to sleep
- Treat hypertension to protect the kidneys from further damage
- First-degree relatives should be investigated for VUR

V

VAGINITIS

Other names: vaginosis, vulvovaginitis

Pathogens

Pre-pubertal girls

- *Streptococcus* spp (common)
- *Staphylococcus*
- *Haemophilus*
- *Shigella* spp (rare)
- Sexually transmitted pathogens may be involved in cases of sexual assault

Women of reproductive age

- *Gardnerella vaginalis*
- *Atopobium vaginae*
- Anaerobic bacteria (e.g. *Mobiluncus* spp)
- *Mycoplasma hominis*

Postmenopausal women

- Atrophic vaginitis or dermatoses is more common than bacterial infections

Preschool girls

- Pinworms may be a cause
- A foreign body in the vagina should always be excluded

1. BACTERIAL VAGINOSIS (BV)

Pathogens

Normal vaginal *Lactobacillus* species are replaced by:

- *Gardnerella vaginalis*
- *Atopobium vaginae*
- Anaerobic bacteria (e.g. *Mobiluncus* spp)
- *Mycoplasma hominis*

Clinical

- Around 50% of women with BV are asymptomatic
- Offensive vaginal discharge with fishy odour

Laboratory

- Vaginal fluid pH > 4.5
- Gram stain smear or wet preparation of a vaginal swab—'clue cells'
- Fishy odour when adding 10% potassium hydroxide to discharge
- Vaginal swab for culture is not necessary and may show heavy growth of *Gardnerella vaginalis*

Screening

- Prior to termination of pregnancy or vaginal hysterectomy to reduce postoperative infectious complications

Treatment

Symptomatic patients and women with a positive screening result

- Option 1: metronidazole 400 mg PO q12h for 5 days*
- Option 2: metronidazole 0.75% vaginal gel (Zidoval) intravaginally for 5 nights
- Option 3: clindamycin 2% vaginal cream (Dalacin V) intravaginally for 7 nights
- Option 4: clindamycin 300 mg PO q12h for 7 days
- Option 5: metronidazole 2 g PO as a single dose
- Option 6: tinidazole 2 g PO as a single dose

Pregnant women

- Option 1: clindamycin 300 mg PO q12h for 7 days (category A)
- Option 2: clindamycin 2% vaginal cream (Dalacin V) intravaginally for 7 nights (before 20 weeks)
- Option 3: metronidazole 400 mg PO q12h for 5 days* (category B2)
- Option 4: metronidazole 0.75% vaginal gel (Zidoval) intravaginally for 5 nights

Failure of treatment

Treat possible *Mycoplasma hominis*

- Option 1: azithromycin 1 g PO weekly for 2 weeks
- Option 2: doxycycline 100 mg PO q12h for 14 days

2.   CANDIDA VAGINITIS

See candida vaginitis (p. 37)

3.   TRICHOMONIASIS

See Trichomoniasis (p. 404)

VARICOSE OR DECUBITUS ULCERS

Other names: venous leg ulcer

Pathogens

- Mixed aerobes and anaerobes

Complications

- Cellulitis, deep-tissue necrosis, bacteraemia and sepsis, osteomyelitis and septic thrombophlebitis

---

*Probiotics (e.g. oral lactobacillus) plus metronidazole may improve the outcome

Treatment

- Graduated compression therapy—improves ulcer healing and reduces recurrence
- Debridement and wound care (most important)
- Surgery (ligation and stripping) and sclerotherapy—may enhance healing of a resistant ulcer
- Antibiotic therapy is indicated when:
  - There is surrounding cellulitis or other complications (see above)
  - There are systemic symptoms (fever, rigor and high WBC count)

Mild to moderate infection (no evidence of osteomyelitis or sepsis)

- Option 1: amoxicillin/clavulanate (PO) for at least 5 days
- Option 2: cefalexin (PO) **plus** metronidazole (PO) for at least 5 days
- Option 3: ciprofloxacin (PO) **plus** clindamycin (PO) for at least 5 days

Severe infection (deep tissue necrosis or sepsis)

- Option 1: piperacillin/tazobactam (IV)
- Option 2: ticarcillin/clavulanate (IV)
- Option 3: meropenem (IV)
- Option 4: ciprofloxacin (IV or PO) **plus** clindamycin (**or** lincomycin) (IV)

If penicillin allergy

- Choose above Option 4

Patients with evidence of osteomyelitis

- See Osteomyelitis (p. 255)

Adjust antibiotic therapy according to the organism isolated from deep tissue specimens or blood culture
Change to oral therapy after substantial improvement

Dosage of above antibiotics

- Amoxicillin/clavulanate 875 mg PO q12h
- Cefalexin 500 mg PO q6h
- Metronidazole 400 mg PO q12h
- Ciprofloxacin 500 mg PO q12h
- Clindamycin 600 mg PO q8h
- Piperacillin/tazobactam 4 g IV q8h
- Ticarcillin/clavulanate 3 g IV q6h
- Meropenem 500 mg IV q8h
- Ciprofloxacin 400 mg IV q12h or ciprofloxacin 750 mg PO q12h
- Clindamycin 600-900 mg IV q8h (slow infusion required)
- Lincomycin 600 mg IV q8h (slow infusion required)

VIBRIO PARAHAEMOLYTICUS

Pathogens

- *Vibrio parahaemolyticus*—a curved, rod-shaped gram-negative bacterium found in brackish saltwater.
- Other non-cholera *Vibrio*

Transmission

- Faecal–oral—ingestion of bacteria from raw or undercooked seafood
- Direct contact—infections of eyes, ears, open cuts and wounds after contacting warm seawater in affected areas (less common than seafood-borne disease)

Incubation

- 24 hours

Clinical

1. Gastroenterocolitis

- Explosive watery diarrhoea, nausea, vomiting, abdominal cramps and fever
- Occasionally, a dysentery-like illness with bloody or mucoid faeces, high fever and high WBC count
- Systemic infection and death are rare
- Symptoms typically resolve within 72 hours, but can persist for up to 10 days in immunocompromised patients

2. Water-related wound infection

See Wound infection—water related (p. 451)

Diagnosis

- For diarrhoea after seafood ingestion—faeces and seafood for *Vibrio* culture
- For salt-water related wound infection—wound swab for *Vibrio* culture
- If febrile and septic—blood culture for *Vibrio*

(Write '*Vibrio* culture' on the request forms for use of special culture medium)

Treatment

- Most cases of food infection are self-limiting—antibiotic are not necessary
- Fluid and electrolyte replacement
- Antibiotic treatment is indicated for severe or prolonged illnesses— antibiotic choice should be based on the susceptibilities of the bacteria
  - Option 1: doxycycline (PO) daily for 10 days
  - Option 2: ceftriaxone (IV) daily for 5–7 days
  - Option 3: ciprofloxacin (PO or IV) q12h for 10 days

Dosage of above antibiotics

  - Doxycycline 100 mg (child >8 years: 2 mg/kg up to 100 mg) PO q12h
  - Ceftriaxone 1 g (child: 25 mg/kg up to 1 g) IV daily
  - Ciprofloxacin 500 mg (child: 10 mg/kg up to 500 mg) PO q12h **or** ciprofloxacin 400 mg (child: 10 mg/kg up to 400 mg) IV q12h

VIRAL ARTHRITIS

Pathogens

- Hepatitis A, B and C viruses
- Parvovirus B19
- Rubella/rubella vaccine
- Ross River virus (RRV)
- Barmah Forest virus (BFV)
- Chikungunya virus
- Sindbis virus
- HIV
- EBV
- Varicella zoster virus (VZV)
- Mumps virus
- Adenovirus or coxsackieviruses
- Echovirus
- Herpes simplex virus (HSV)
- Cytomegalovirus (CMV)

Clinical

- Acute oligoarthritis or polyarticular disease
- Mild and self-limiting, usually last no longer than a few weeks
- Joint pain usually resolving within 3–6 months
- Acute polyarticular synovitis may cause severe pain and disability

Diagnosis

- FBC (WBC usually not elevated), LFT, U/E
- Tests for suspected viral infection based on clinical clues
- Exclude reactive arthritis and acute rheumatic fever (in Indigenous peoples)
- Aspiration of the joint—rule out crystal arthropathy or bacterial infection

Treatment

- No effective antiviral drugs
- Symptomatic treatment with anti-inflammatory drugs and analgesics

WART

Pathogen

- Human papillomaviruses (HPVs)

Clinical

- **Common wart** (*Verruca vulgaris*)—a raised wart with a roughened surface, most common on hands and knees
- **Plantar wart** (*Verruca pedis*)—a hard lump, sometimes painful, often with multiple black specks in the centre; usually on pressure points on the soles
- **Plane wart or flat wart** (*Verruca plana*)—a small, smooth flattened wart, tan or flesh coloured, which can occur in large numbers, most common on the face, neck, hands, wrists and knees
- **Filiform or digitate wart**—a thread- or finger-like wart, most common on the face, especially near eyelids and lips
- **Subungual wart**—a wart under the finger or toe nails
- **Genital wart or venereal wart** (*Condyloma acuminatum*, *Verruca acuminata*)—a wart that occurs on the genitalia (see Wart—genital, p. 438)

Treatment

- Cryotherapy with liquid nitrogen to each wart q2–4 weeks until resolved
- Podophyllin paint: 2–3 drops to dry warts bid; oint: top 2–3 times a week
- Salicylic acid (e.g. Duofilm) top bid (remove dead skin with a pumice stone or emery board)
- Podophyllotoxin 0.5% (e.g. Condyline Paint, Wartec Cream, Wartec solution) top bid, 3 days per week for 4 weeks (for anogenital warts)
- Imiquimod (Aldara) (a topical immunomodifier) top daily 3 times a week (max 16 weeks) (for anogenital warts)
- Tretinoin 0.05% cream (e.g. ReTrieve) top daily until resolved (for plane warts on face—very difficult to treat, best left untreated)
- Fluorouracil cream (e.g. Efudix) top with tape cover (for plantar warts)
- Bleomycin 1 or 2 local injections
- Surgical curettage
- Infrared coagulator
- Silver nitrate cautery
- Laser treatment (requires 1–4 treatments)
- Duct tape occlusion therapy (DTOT): place a piece of duct tape over the wart(s) for 6 days, followed by soaking the area in water and scraping it with a pumice stone or emery board

WART—GENITAL

Other names: *Condylomata acuminata*, *Verruca acuminata*, venereal wart

Pathogen

- Human papillomavirus (HPV) types 6 and 11 (90%); also types 16, 18, 31, 33 (oncogenic)

Transmission

- Non-sexual and sexual transmission
- Most HPV infections are transient, but can reactivate many years later

Clinical

- Vulval warts are more common than vaginal or cervical warts
- May involve perineal and anal area
- Usually asymptomatic, may have vulval itching, burning, dyspareunia and cauliflower growths of varying sizes

Acetowhitening examination

- Small lesions can be seen after covering with gauze soaked with 5% acetic acid for 5 mins (tiny white papules)

Treatment

- Genital warts may disappear without treatment
- Child with suspected anogenital warts—seek expert advice
- Topical treatment of genital warts—use one of the following:
  - Cryotherapy (periodically)
  - Imiquimod 5% cream (e.g. Aldara)* top
  - Podophyllotoxin 0.15% cream (e.g. Wartec)* **or** 0.5% paint (e.g. Condyline)* top
  - Electrodesiccation **or** electrocautery
  - Laser cauterisation
  - Surgical removal of large warts (if failed with other treatments)

Use of above preparations

  - Imiquimod 5% cream (e.g. Aldara)—apply to each wart at bedtime, wash off after 6–10 hours, 3 times a week (usually 8–16 weeks) (avoid using in pregnant or breastfeeding women and in children; avoid contact with mucous membranes and inflamed skin; use precaution on uncircumcised penis)
  - Podophyllotoxin 0.15% cream (e.g. Wartec) or 0.5% paint (e.g. Condyline)—apply to each wart, twice daily for 3 days, repeat weekly for 4–6 weeks until warts disappear (avoid using in pregnant or breastfeeding women; avoid contact with mucous membranes and healthy skin; total area of application should not be >4 cm^2)

---

*Do not use on vaginal or cervical warts

Prognosis

- Although treatments can remove the warts, they cannot eliminate HPV virus from the body, so genital warts may recur after treatment
- May develop into cervical or genital SCC (HPV types 16, 18, 31 and 33 are oncogenic)

Prevention

- Male circumcision reduces the incidence of HPV infection
- HPV vaccination:
  - Female 9–45 years old—4vHPV or 9vHPV vaccine (for prevention of genital warts and cervical cancer)
  - Male 9–26 years old—4vHPV or 9vHPV vaccine (for prevention of genital warts and penile cancer)
  - 4vHPV vaccine (e.g. Gardasil) 0.5 mL IM, 3 doses at 0, 2 and 6 months
  - 9vHPV vaccine (e.g. Gardasil9) 0.5 mL IM, 2 doses at 0 and 6–12 months

WEST NILE VIRUS

Other names: West Nile fever, West Nile encephalitis

Pathogens

- West Nile virus (WNV)—a virus of the family *Flaviviridae*, closely related genetically to the Kunjin virus, the most common flavivirus in Australia
- It is an arbovirus, mainly infects birds, but also infects humans, horses, dogs, cats, bats, chipmunks, skunks, squirrels and domestic rabbits

Distribution

- In both tropical and temperate regions—eastern Mediterranean, southern European countries and North America

Transmission

- Birds are the reservoir of the virus
- Via the bites of infected mosquitoes—most common
- Via organ transplantation or blood transfusion—rarely
- Intrauterine transmission to fetus
- Via breastfeeding
- Occupational (including conjunctival) exposure to infected blood

Incubation

- 3–14 days

Clinical

- Most WNV infections have no symptoms or only mild flu-like symptoms
- **West Nile fever** (20% of infected)—sudden-onset fever, malaise, headache, anorexia, myalgia, nausea, vomiting, maculopapular or morbilliform rash, lymphadenopathy and retro-orbital pain, lasts 3–6 days

- **West Nile encephalitis** (1 in 150 cases)—severe muscle weakness and flaccid paralysis that may result in death; older people are at greater risk

Diagnosis

WNV should be seriously considered in adults >50 years old who have onset of unexplained encephalitis in late summer or early autumn

- Blood—WNV serology (specific IgM and neutralising antibodies)
- Blood—viral culture (within the first 2 weeks of disease)
- CSF—WNV-specific IgM and neutralising antibodies
- CSF—PCR for West Nile virus DNA
- Biopsy or autopsy tissue—histopathology and virus culture

Treatment

- Supportive treatment
- Ribavirin, immunoglobulin or alpha interferon may be tried
- Blocking angiotensin II—may treat 'cytokine storm' of West Nile encephalitis
- People with prior exposure to Kunjin virus may be protected

Prevention

- Mosquito control—eliminate mosquito-breeding areas
- Personal protection—use mosquito repellents, wear long-sleeved, covered clothing
- Infected women should avoid breastfeeding

WORM (HELMINTH)

1. PINWORM/THREADWORM (*ENTEROBIUS VERMICULARIS*)

Pinworm—the most common worm infection in Australia.

Life cycle

Adult worms reside in colon → females migrate to anus area to deposit ova → ova are eaten through contaminated food → reach colon → hatch and mature into adult worms → (new cycle)

Clinical

- Intense itching inside and around anus, especially at night, with irritability
- Reduced appetite, sometimes complicated with vaginitis

Diagnosis

- Observe worms around anus
- Apply a piece of clear adhesive tape to perianal region and examine for ova microscopically

Treatment

- Option 1: mebendazole 100 mg (child ≤10 kg: 50 mg) PO st, repeat after 2 weeks
- Option 2: pyrantel (adult and child) 10 mg/kg up to 1 g PO st, repeat after 2 weeks
- Option 3: albendazole 400 mg (child ≤10 kg: 200 mg) PO st, repeat after 2 weeks
- Patient should shower each morning, cut finger nails short; wash nightwear and bed linen daily for several days and wash hands thoroughly before preparing or eating food
- The infection may not be easily eradicated due to autoinfection (hosts reinfect themselves); if infection recurs, treat all family members

2. ROUNDWORM (*ASCARIS LUMBRICOIDES*)

Life cycle

Pet ingests ova from an infected source (e.g. rodent, soil) → ova hatch into larvae in pet's stomach → travel to small intestine and mature into adult worms → lay ova in pet's faeces → human eats ova-contaminated food → ova hatch inside duodenum → larvae migrate through the lungs and moult → ascend the bronchial tree and are swallowed → travel to small intestine and mature into adult worms → lay ova in faeces → (new cycle)

Clinical

- Larvae in lungs can cause pulmonary eosinophilia
- Adult worms may cause abdominal pain, vomiting, bowel obstruction, obstructive jaundice, pancreatitis, appendicitis and malnutrition

Diagnosis

- Faeces OCP—find ova or adult worm

Treatment

- Option 1: albendazole 400 mg (child ≤10 kg: 200 mg) PO st
- Option 2: mebendazole 100 mg (child ≤10 kg: 50 mg) PO q12h for 3 days
- Option 3: pyrantel (adult & child) 10 mg/kg up to 1 g PO st (repeat after 7 days if heavy infection)

3. HOOKWORM (*ANCYLOSTOMA DUODENALE*, *NECATOR AMERICAMUS*)

Life cycle

Adult hookworms in small intestine → pass ova into soil from faeces → hatch into infective larvae → penetrate human skin and migrate into lungs and moult → reach small intestines and mature into adult worms → (new cycle)

Incubation

- 4–7 weeks after the 'entry' of the larvae into the body

Clinical

- Cutaneous larva migrans—the site of skin penetration may be swollen and red; may last 1 month if untreated
- Visceral larva migrans—larvae in lungs can cause pulmonary eosinophilia
- GI symptoms—vomiting, abdominal pain, diarrhoea and loss of appetite
- Anaemia and malnutrition—caused by heavy adult worm infestation

Diagnosis

- Faeces OCP—find the ova

Treatment

- Option 1: albendazole 400 mg (child ≤10 kg: 200 mg) PO st
- Option 2: mebendazole 100 mg (child ≤10 kg: 50 mg) PO q12h for 3 days
- Option 3: pyrantel (adult and child) 10 mg/kg up to 1 g PO daily for 3 days

For cutaneous larva migrans

- Option 1: ivermectin (adult and child ≥15 kg) 200 mcg/kg PO with fatty food, st
- Option 2: albendazole 400 mg (child ≤10 kg: 200 mg) PO with fatty food, daily for 3 days

4.   DOG HOOKWORM (*ANCYLOSTOMA CANINUM*)

- Dog hookworm primarily infect animals (e.g. cats, dogs)
- Humans are accidental hosts; in human it causes eosinophilic enterocolitis

Life cycle

Larvae of *A. caninum* enter a human host by skin penetration or by oral ingestion → larvae reach the gut, mature into adult worms → secrete various potential allergens into the intestinal mucosa

Clinical

- In most of people, the larvae remain dormant in skeletal muscles and create no symptoms
- Increasingly severe recurrent abdominal pain; extreme cases may mimic appendicitis or intestinal perforation
- Peripheral eosinophilia (100%) and leucocytosis (75% of patients)

Laboratory

- Eosinophilia and raised serum IgE levels
- No eggs are found in stool (adult worms do not produce eggs in human hosts)

Treatment

- Option 1: albendazole 400 mg (child ≤10 kg: 200 mg) PO st
- Option 2: mebendazole 100 mg (child ≤10 kg: 50 mg) PO q12h for 3 days
- Endoscopic removal of the worm may be used

5. Pork tapeworm (*Taenia solium*) and 6. Beef tapeworm (*Taenia saginata*)

Life cycle

Human eats undercooked beef containing larvae of beef tapeworm or undercooked pork containing larvae of pork tapeworm → larvae reach small intestine and mature into adult worms → tapeworm segments (proglottids) are passed in faeces → eaten by animals such as cows or pigs → in the animal's body the juvenile forms migrate into muscles and become larvae (cysts) → human eats undercooked meat → (new cycle)

Humans may also have self-infection by ingesting tapeworm eggs in stools

Clinical

- **Intestinal tapeworm** (ingestion of encysted larvae in undercooked meat)—few or no symptoms, but seeing tapeworm segments in faeces may distress patient
- **Cysticercosis** (ingestion of eggs of pork tapeworm in contaminated food or water)—causes **neurocysticercosis** (epilepsy, headaches, strokes, hydrocephalus, and aseptic meningitis), ocular cysticercosis or systemic cysticercosis (parasites in subcutaneous tissue, muscle, liver, spleen or heart)

Diagnosis

- Tapeworm segments seen in faeces or on underclothing by patients
- Stool examination—cysts and ova may be found
- Cysticercosis serology—may be positive
- CT or MRI of brain
- Brain biopsy

Treatment

- Surgical treatment—remove parasites from tissue
- Anticysticercal treatment—if the parasite is viable and the patient has vasculitis, arachnoiditis or encephalitis
- A course of steroid or immunosuppressant is recommended before anticysticercal drugs

For pork tapeworm or unknown tapeworm

- Niclosamide* 2 g (child: 50 mg/kg up to 2 g) PO st

---

*Available via Special Access Scheme <www.tga.gov.au/hp/access-sas.htm> or from compounding chemist

For beef tapeworm

- Option 1: praziquantel (adult and child) 10 mg/kg PO st
- Option 2: niclosamide* 2 g (child: 50 mg/kg up to 2 g) PO st

7. DWARF TAPEWORM (*HYMNOLOGIES NANA*)

Life cycle

Human eats ova in contaminated food or infected grain beetles → ova hatch into larva (ionospheres) in duodenum → penetrate into villa and develop into cysticercoids → adult worms shed gravid terminal segments → disintegrate in the intestine, releasing ova in the faeces → human eats ova → (new cycle)

Clinical

- Often asymptomatic
- Heavy infections can cause enteritis (diarrhoea)

Diagnosis

- Inspecting faeces for ova

Treatment

- For symptomatic patients with persisting diarrhoea use:
  - Praziquantel (adult and child) 25 mg/kg PO st (repeat after 1 week if heavy infection)

8. LIVER FLUKE (TREMATODE)

- *Fasciola hepatica* (sheep liver fluke)
- *Clonorchis sinensis* (Chinese liver fluke or Oriental liver fluke)
- *Opisthorchis viverrini* (Southeast Asian liver fluke)

Life cycle

- ***Fasciola hepatica***: adult worms live in human bile ducts and produce eggs → eggs in bile are passed out from faeces → fall into water and develop into miracidia → invade snails, develop into cercariae (larvae) and are then encysted into cysts (metacercariae) on water vegetation → ingested by human → excysted in human's duodenum → penetrate into peritoneal cavity and find their way to liver → mature in bile ducts and produce eggs → (new cycle)
- ***Clonorchis sinensis*** and ***Opisthorchis viverrini***: adult worms live in human bile ducts and produce eggs → eggs in bile are passed out from faeces → fall into water and develop into miracidia → invade snails and develop into cercariae (larvae) → penetrate freshwater fish and form cysts → undercooked fish containing the cysts are ingested by human → excysted in human's duodenum → penetrate into peritoneal cavity and find their way to liver → mature in bile ducts and produce eggs → (new cycle)

Clinical

- During the migration of larvae (acute phase, lasts many weeks)—diarrhoea, eosinophilia, urticaria, fever, nausea/vomiting and abdominal pain
- In the chronic phase—worms cause liver inflammation and biliary tract obstruction—epigastric pain, jaundice, anaemia and weight loss
- Late complications—cirrhosis, carcinoma of intrahepatic bile ducts

Diagnosis

- Faeces OCP—eggs in stool; false positive can be due to patient eating infected liver and eggs passing through the faeces; liver-free diet and then re-examining the faeces will unmask the false diagnosis
- Serology test—detect anti-hepatica antibodies in serum, milk or faecal samples

Treatment

For *Fasciola hepatica*

  - Option 1: triclabendazole* (adult and child) 10 mg/kg PO st (with food)(repeat after 12–24 hours if heavy infection)
  - Option 2: bithionol* (adult and child) 30–50 mg/kg PO on alternate days for 10–15 doses
  - Option 3: nitazoxanide* 500 mg (child 1–4 years: 100 mg; 4–12 years: 200 mg) PO q12h for 3 days

For *Clonorchis sinensis* or *Opisthorchis viverrini*

  - Praziquantel (adult and child) 25 mg/kg PO (with food) q8h for 2 days

9. STRONGYLOIDIASIS (*STRONGYLOIDES STERCORALIS*)

- *Strongyloides stercoralis* not uncommon in northern Australia

Life cycle

Adult worms reside in upper small intestine → ova hatch and larvae are passed in faeces → in moist soil larvae moult into infectious filariform larvae → penetrate human skin and migrate to lungs and are swallowed → reach upper small intestine and mature into adult worms → (new cycle)

Clinical

- Cutaneous larva migrans—the site of skin penetration may be swollen and red
- Visceral larva migrans—larvae in lungs can cause pulmonary eosinophilia
- GI symptoms—vomiting, abdominal pain, diarrhoea and loss of appetite

---

*Available via Special Access Scheme <www.tga.gov.au/hp/access-sas.htm>

Diagnosis

- Faeces OCP or jejunal aspirate OCP—find motile larvae under microscope
- *Strongyloides* serology
- Filarial serology (positive in 15% patients)

Treatment

Immunocompetent patients

- Option 1: ivermectin (PO) st, repeat after 1–2 weeks (cure rate 83–100%)
- Option 2: albendazole (PO) q12h for 3 days, repeat after 1–2 weeks (cure rate 67–75%)

Immunocompromised patients

- Ivermectin (PO) daily on days 1, 2, 15 and 16

Complicated or disseminated infection

- Ivermectin (PO) daily (seek expert advice)

Dosage of above agents

- Ivermectin 200 mcg/kg (not for child under 15 kg) PO (with fatty food)
- Albendazole 400 mg (child ≤10 kg: 200 mg) PO q12h (with fatty food)

10.   WHIPWORM (*TRICHURIS TRICHIURA*)

Life cycle

Human ingests ova → ova hatch in small intestine → larvae penetrate small intestinal mucosa and mature → ova are passed in faeces → (new cycle)

Clinical

- Mild infection—asymptomatic
- Heavy infection—trichuris dysentery syndrome: bloody mucoid diarrhoea, tenesmus, anaemia, weight loss and growth retardation

Diagnosis

- Faeces OCP—find the ova
- Rectal biopsy—may reveal adult worms attached to the rectal mucosa

Treatment

To reduce worm burden but often not curative

- Option 1: albendazole 400 mg (child ≤10 kg: 200 mg) PO daily for 3 days
- Option 2: mebendazole 100 mg (child ≤10 kg: 50 mg) PO q12h for 3 days

11. SCHISTOSOMIASIS (BILHARZIASIS)

- Schistosomiasis may be seen in return travellers from endemic areas

Five species cause human disease:

- *Schistosoma haematobium*—in Egypt, sub-Saharan Africa and Middle East
- *Schistosoma japonicum*—in China and Southeast Asia
- *Schistosoma mansoni*—in sub-Saharan Africa, Middle East and South America
- *Schistosoma mekongi*—in Laos and Cambodia
- *Schistosoma intercalatum*—in West and Central Africa

Life cycle

Infected person passes ova from faeces or urine into fresh water → the ova hatch into miracidia (larvae) → enter into water snails and multiply into large amounts of cercariae → penetrate human skin → pass through lungs and liver and mature → migrate along portal vein to mesenteric or pelvic venules → mature and deposit enormous amounts of ova → ova penetrate intestinal/bladder wall and are passed in faeces or urine → (new cycle)

Clinical

- Cercarial penetration (lasts 1–2 days)—an urticarial rash at sites of penetration
- Larval migration (2–12 weeks)—cough may persist for months, eosinophilia pneumonitis, myositis, hepatitis and fever (Katayama syndrome)
- Egg deposition—can cause the following problems:
  - *S. haematobium*—recurrent cystitis, haematuria, fibrosis and calcification of ureters and bladder, chronic pyelonephritis, renal failure and bladder cancer
  - *S. japonicum*—liver fibrosis, hepatosplenomegaly and oesophageal varices; ectopic deposition of ova may cause pulmonary hypertension and paralysis
  - *S. mansoni*—colonic ulceration and polyposis, hepatosplenomegaly and oesophageal varicose

Diagnosis

- Schistosomiasis serology—for presumptive diagnosis in travellers from endemic areas (become positive 6–8 weeks after exposure to contaminated water)
- Faeces OCP, urine OCP—find the ova
- Rectal biopsy, cystoscopy and biopsy

Treatment

- Praziquantel (adult and child) 20 mg/kg PO 2 doses 4 hours apart (with food)

Repeat the course if inadequate response

- Recently infected patients may need a second treatment several weeks later
- Follow-up faeces/urine microscopy in 3 months after treatment to ensure cure

Advice to travellers to endemic areas

- Avoid swimming or wading in fresh water
- Drink boiled water (for at least 1 minute) or filtered water
- Bath water should be heated for 5 minutes at 65°C
- Vigorous towel drying after accidental and very brief water exposure may help prevent *Schistosoma* parasite from penetrating the skin

Community worm programs

In some Indigenous communities where intestinal helminth infections are endemic, regularly treating all children between 6 months and 12 years of age can improve children's nutrition and growth; use:

- Albendazole 400 mg (child ≤10 kg: 200 mg) PO st, every 6 months

WOUND INFECTION

1. POST-TRAUMATIC WOUND INFECTION

Pathogens

- *Staphylococcus aureus*
- *Streptococcus pyogenes*
- *Clostridium perfringens*
- Aerobic gram-negative bacilli
- *Pseudomonas aeruginosa* (common in penetrating injury through footwear)

Treatment

- Take a wound swab for culture
- Tetanus immunisation status must be assessed (see Tetanus, p. 393)
- Careful cleaning and debridement
- Delayed primary wound closure if indicated

Antibiotic treatment

Antibiotic is indicated for:

- Clean wounds but treatment/closure is delayed by ≥8 hours or debridement is difficult
- Contaminated wounds with muscle, soft-tissue and skeletal trauma
- Crush injuries
- Penetrating injuries
- Stab wounds

Mild wounds

- Option 1: amoxicillin/clavulanate (PO) for at least 5 days
- Option 2: cefalexin (PO) **plus** metronidazole (PO) for at least 5 days

If immediate penicillin allergy or water exposure of the wound

- Ciprofloxacin (PO) **plus** clindamycin (PO) for at least 5 days

Modify antibiotics according to culture and susceptibility results

Severe wounds

- Option 1: cefazolin (IV) **plus** metronidazole (IV)
  Once improved, change to oral therapy
  Cefalexin (PO) **plus** metronidazole (PO) for total 5–7 days
- Option 2: piperacillin/tazobactam (IV)
- Option 3: ticarcillin/clavulanate (IV)
  Once improved, change to oral therapy
  Amoxicillin/clavulanate (PO) for total 5–7 days

If immediate penicillin allergy or water exposure of the wound

- Ciprofloxacin (IV then PO) **plus** clindamycin (IV then PO) for total 5–7 days

Pseudomonas aeruginosa infection

- Option 1: piperacillin/tazobactam (IV) (higher dose)
- Option 2: ciprofloxacin (iv then PO) (higher dose)

Modify antibiotics according to Gram stain and culture results

Duration of treatment

- For usual wounds—total of 5–7 days (IV + PO)
- For injuries involving bones, joints or tendons—longer therapy

Dosage of above antibiotics

Mild wounds

- Amoxicillin/clavulanate 875 mg (child: 22.5 mg/kg up to 875 mg) PO q12h
- Cefalexin 500 mg (child: 12.5 mg/kg up to 500 mg) PO q6h
  or Cefalexin 1 g (child: 25 mg/kg up to 1 g) PO q12h (for mild skin infection)
- Metronidazole 400 mg (child: 10 mg/kg up to 400 mg) PO q12h
- Ciprofloxacin 500 mg (child: 12.5 mg/kg up to 500 mg) PO q12h
- Clindamycin 450 mg (child: 10 mg/kg up to 450 mg) PO q8h

Severe wounds

- Cefazolin 2 g (child: 50 mg/kg up to 2 g) IV q8h
- Metronidazole 500 mg (child: 12.5 mg/kg up to 500 mg) IV q12h
- Piperacillin/tazobactam 4 g (child: 100 mg/kg up to 4 g) IV q8h
- Ticarcillin/clavulanate 3 g (child: 50 mg/kg up to 3 g) IV q6h
- Ciprofloxacin 400 mg (child: 10 mg/kg up to 400 mg) IV q12h, then 750 mg (child: 20 mg/kg up to 750 mg) PO q12h
- Clindamycin 450 mg (child: 10 mg/kg up to 450 mg) IV q8h, then 450 mg (child: 10 mg/kg up to 450 mg) PO q8h

Pseudomonas aeruginosa infection
- Piperacillin/tazobactam 4 g (child: 100 mg/kg up to 4 g) IV q6h
- Ciprofloxacin 400 mg (child: 10 mg/kg up to 400 mg) IV q8h

2. SURGICAL WOUND INFECTION

- Take a wound swab for culture and sensitivity
- Drainage, irrigation and debridement (do not use topical antibiotics)
- Antimicrobial photodynamic therapy (a dye, e.g. indocyanine green, is activated by laser to produce a cytotoxic effect to kill the bacteria) may be considered for difficult wound infections (e.g. burn infection from multi-resistant *P. aeruginosa*)
- Maggot therapy has been reported faster and more effective in removal of dead tissue than surgical debridement; maggots also kill bacteria and stimulate wound healing—may be used for wounds infected by multi-resistant bacteria
- Antibiotic treatment

Mild to moderate infections (with surrounding cellulitis)

- Option 1: cefalexin (PO) for at least 5 days
- Option 2: flucloxacillin (PO) for at least 5 days
- Option 3: clindamycin (PO) for at least 5 days (if immediate penicillin allergy)

If gram-negative organisms are suspected
- Amoxicillin/clavulanate (PO) for at least 5 days

More severe infections (with systemic symptoms)

- Option 1: cefazolin (IV)
- Option 2: flucloxacillin (IV)
- Option 3: vancomycin (IV) (if immediate penicillin allergy)

If gram-negative organisms are suspected (e.g. post-GI or genital-tract surgery)
- Option 1: gentamicin (IV) (only for 72 hours)
- Option 2: piperacillin/tazobactam (IV)
- Option 3: ticarcillin/clavulanate (IV)

If MRSA is suspected
- Option 1: vancomycin (IV) **plus** cefazolin (**or** flucloxacillin) (IV)
- Option 2: vancomycin (IV) **plus** piperacillin/tazobactam (**or** ticarcillin/clavulanate) (IV)

Modify therapy according to culture and susceptibility testing
Change to oral (above) when significantly improved

Dosage of above antibiotics

- Cefalexin 500 mg (child: 12.5 mg/kg up to 500 mg) PO q6h
- Flucloxacillin 500 mg (child: 12.5 mg/kg up to 500 mg) PO q6h
- Clindamycin 450 mg (child: 10 mg/kg up to 450 mg) PO q8h
- Amoxicillin/clavulanate 875 mg (child: 22.5 mg up to 875 mg) PO q12h

- Cefazolin 2 g (child: 50 mg/kg up to 2 g) IV q8h
- Flucloxacillin 2 g (child: 50 mg/kg up to 2 g) IV q6h
- Vancomycin 25–30 mg/kg IV for the 1st dose (further dosing see p. 462)
- Gentamicin 4–7 mg/kg (child: 7.5 mg/kg up to 320 mg) IV for the 1st dose (further dosing see p. 459); if IV therapy is still required after 3 days, change to piperacillin/tazobactam or ticarcillin/clavulanate regimen
- Piperacillin/tazobactam 4 g (child: 100 mg/kg up to 4 g) IV q8h
- Ticarcillin/clavulanate 3 g (child: 50 mg/kg up to 3 g) IV q6h

WOUND INFECTION—WATER-RELATED

Wound infection with history of water (fresh, brackish or salty water) contact (e.g. in water activities, fishing, fish tank/aquarium cleaning, coral cuts or caving) may encounter special bacterial infections. Most of the infections are difficult to treat.

1. *AEROMONAS* SPP

Pathogen

- *Aeromonas hydrophila* (fresh or brackish water or mud exposure, infection through cuts and abrasions)

Clinical

- Can cause superficial skin infections, cellulitis, myositis or sepsis
- One in four cases has an underlying systemic illness

Antibiotic treatment

- Option 1: ciprofloxacin (IV or PO)
- Option 2: meropenem (**or** imipenem) (IV) (for multidrug-resistant organisms)

Duration of therapy

- 14 days
- Longer course for severe infection

Dosage of above antibiotics

- Ciprofloxacin 400 mg (child: 10 mg/kg up to 400 mg) IV q12h
- Ciprofloxacin 500 mg (child: 12.5 mg/kg up to 500 mg) PO q12h
- Meropenem 1 g (child: 20 mg/kg up to 1 g) IV q8h
- Imipenem 1 g (child: 25 mg/kg up to 1 g) IV q6h

2. SHEWANELLA PUTREFACIENS

Pathogen

- A gram-negative marine anaerobic bacterium (saltwater contact)

Risk factors

- Leg ulcers, diabetes, peripheral vascular disease or immunosuppression

Clinical

- Severe cellulitis with necrosis and bullae formation; may cause sepsis

Laboratory

- Wound swab or debrided tissue for culture
- Blood culture if septic

Treatment

- As *Aeromonas* infection (p. 451)
- Skin grafting may be required

3.   *VIBRIO* SPP

Pathogens

Salty or brackish water exposure

- *Vibrio velnificus*
- *Vibrio alginolyticus*
- Other non-cholera *Vibrio* spp

Clinical

- *Vibrio* spp should be suspected in skin infections in patients who have been exposed to saltwater
- Life-threatening infection can rapidly develop in patients with cirrhosis or iron overload (e.g. haemochromatosis)

Laboratory

- Wound swab for *Vibrio* culture
- If febrile and septic—blood culture for *Vibrio*

(Write '*Vibrio* culture' on the request forms for use of special culture medium)

Treatment

- Incision, drainage and debridement
- Antibiotic treatment
  - Doxycycline (PO or IV*)

For severe infection

  - Option 1: doxycycline (PO or IV*) **plus** ceftriaxone (**or** cefotaxime) (IV)
  - Option 2: doxycycline (PO or IV*) **plus** ciprofloxacin (PO or IV)

Duration of therapy

- Determined by clinical response, can exceed 2 weeks

---

*IV doxycycline is available via Special Access Scheme <www.tga.gov.au/hp/access-sas.htm>

Dosage of above antibiotics

- Doxycycline 200 mg (child >8 years: 4 mg/kg up to 200 mg) PO or IV for the 1st dose, then 100 mg (child >8 years: 2 mg/kg up to 100 mg) PO or IV q12h
- Ceftriaxone 1 g (child: 25 mg/kg up to 1 g) IV daily
- Cefotaxime 1 g (child: 25 mg/kg up to 1 g) IV q8h
- Ciprofloxacin 500 mg (child: 15 mg/kg up to 500 mg) PO q12h **or** Ciprofloxacin 400 mg (child: 10 mg/kg up to 400 mg) IV q12h

4. MYCOBACTERIUM MARINUM

Other names: fish-tank granuloma, swimming-pool granuloma

Source of infection

- Fish tank/swimming pool exposure

Clinical

- A localised papular or nodular skin lesion (fish-tank or swimming-pool granuloma)

Diagnosis

- Often made by biopsy (acid-fast bacilli) and culture

Differential diagnosis

- Sporotrichosis (*Sporothrix schenkii* infection)

Treatment

- Single lesion excision—antibiotic therapy may not be required
- Antibiotic therapy for more severe cases; surgical debridement may be required
  - Option 1: clarithromycin 500 mg (child: 12.5 mg/kg up to 500 mg) PO q12h
  - Option 2: doxycycline 100 mg (child >8 years: 2 mg/kg up to 100 mg) PO q12h
  - Option 3: cotrimoxazole 160/800 mg (child: 4/20 mg/kg up to 160/800 mg) PO q12h

For severe or unresponsive cases (susceptibility testing should be done)
  - Clarithromycin (PO) **plus** rifampicin (**or** ethambutol) (PO)

Duration of therapy

- 1–2 months after resolution of all lesions (total 3–4 months)

Dosage of above agents

- Rifampicin 600 mg (child: 10 mg/kg up to 600 mg; adult <50 kg: 450 mg) PO daily
- Ethambutol adult and child: 15 mg/kg PO daily

Y

YAWS

The infection may be seen in northern Australia.

Pathogen

- *Treponema pertenue*

Transmission

- Direct non-sexual contact, usually within the family
- The organism enters through damaged skin

Clinical

- **Early yaws**—inflammatory skin reaction at the inoculation site
  - Dissemination of the organism causes multiple papular lesions involving the palms, soles and bones
- **Late yaws**—10% of cases progress to late yaws
  - Single or multiple nodules or ulcers on the skin, hyperkeratotic lesions on the palms and soles, bony gummatous lesions may cause gross destruction and deformity, particularly skull, facial and hand bones
  - Unlike syphilis, usually no cardiovascular and neurological involvement

Diagnosis

- Detection of spirochaetes in exudate of lesions by dark-ground microscopy
- Syphilis serology—positive in both yaws and syphilis
- PCR for *Treponema pertenue* (swab of lesions, biopsy)—distinguish from syphilis

Treatment

- Most cases of early yaws will eventually subside
- Antibiotic treatment may shorten the course of disease
  - Option 1: azithromycin 2 g (child: 30 mg/kg up to 2 g) PO st
  - Option 2: benzathine penicillin 900 mg IM st

YELLOW FEVER

Pathogen

- Yellow fever virus—an arbovirus, classified as a flavivirus

Transmission

- **Jungle yellow fever**—a zoonosis transmitted among non-human hosts (mainly monkeys) by a variety of forest mosquitoes, which may also bite and infect humans; such infected humans may, if subsequently bitten

by *Aedes aegypti* mosquitoes, become the source of outbreaks of the urban form of the disease
- **Urban yellow fever**—transmitted from person to person by *A. aegypti* mosquitoes

Incubation

- 2–5 days

Distribution

- African and Central and South American countries

Clinical

- Acute viral haemorrhagic fever—sudden onset of fever, vomiting and prostration that may progress to haemorrhagic symptoms and jaundice
- Fatality rate—5% in Indigenous people in endemic areas; up to 50% in non-Indigenous individuals, or during epidemics

Preventive measures

For urban yellow fever
- Eradication of *A. aegypti* mosquitoes
- Protection from mosquito bites
- Vaccination

For jungle yellow fever
- Vaccination

Vaccination

Yellow fever vaccination is recommended for:

- Travellers ≥9 months of age who plan to visit endemic areas (a valid vaccination certificate is required for entry from infected areas into non-infected countries)
- Laboratory personnel who routinely work with yellow fever virus

Yellow fever vaccination is contraindicated for (in order not to vaccinate travellers unnecessarily):

- Egg anaphylaxis or previous yellow fever vaccination allergy
- Infants <9 months (risk of vaccine-related encephalitis)
- Elderly >65 years of age (risk of adverse reactions)
- Immunosuppressed or past history of thymus gland problems

Vaccination must be given in an approved yellow fever vaccination centre

- Yellow fever vaccine (e.g. Stamaril, Arilvax) adult, child ≥9 months: 0.5 mL IM or SC st, 10 yearly boosters if at ongoing risk

Provides yellow fever protection for 10 years

YERSINIA ENTEROCOLITIS

Other names: yersiniosis

Pathogens

- *Yersinia enterocolitica*
- *Yersinia pseudotuberculosis*

Transmission

- Direct contact with infected animals
- Ingestion of contaminated meats (pork, beef, lamb, etc), oysters, fish and unpasteurised milk

Incubation

- 24–48 hours

Clinical

- Enterocolitis—diarrhoea (watery or bloody), abdominal pain, fever, cervical or mesenteric adenitis and terminal ileitis
- It may be a cause of traveller's diarrhoea

Complications

- Mesenteric adenitis—unnecessary appendicectomy
- Post-enteritis arthritis and erythema nodosum
- Bacteraemia (rare)

Laboratory

- Culture of faeces, blood or vomit
- Faecal multiplex PCR testing—sensitivity 98–100%, result available in 24 hours
- *Yersinia* serology (acute and convalescent sera)

Treatment

- Most acute infections are self-limiting; antibiotics are not indicated
- Antibiotics are indicated for:
    - Immunocompromised patients
    - Prolonged disease
    - Extra-intestinal disease and systemic disease
  - Option 1: ciprofloxacin (PO) for 5 days
  - Option 2: norfloxacin (PO) for 5 days
  - Option 3: cotrimoxazole 160/800 mg (PO) for 5 days

For bacteraemia
  - Ciprofloxacin (IV then PO) for 3 weeks

Dosage of above agents

- Ciprofloxacin 500 mg (child: 12.5 mg/kg up to 500 mg) PO q12h
- Norfloxacin 400 mg (child: 10 mg/kg up to 400 mg) PO q12h
- Cotrimoxazole 160/800 mg (child: 4/20 mg/kg up to 160/800 mg) PO q12h
- Ciprofloxacin 400 mg (child: 10 mg/kg up to 400 mg) IV q12h

ZIKA

Zika is the first mosquito-borne virus to be associated with human birth defects and may be sexually transmitted.

Pathogen

- Zika virus—a flavivirus

Distribution

- Circulates in tropical Africa and the Americas
- Western Pacific region (Southeast Asia, the Pacific Islands, Australia and China) is the second most affected region

Transmission

- Spread mostly by the bite of an infected *Aedes* spp mosquito (*Aedes aegypti* and *Aedes albopictus*)
- Can be passed from pregnant woman to fetus (infection during pregnancy)
- Sexual transmission
- Through blood transfusion

Incubation

- 3–7 days

Clinical

- Many patients are asymptomatic or have mild symptoms: fever, rash, muscle and joint pain, conjunctivitis and headache; the symptoms usually last for 2–7 days
- Infection during pregnancy can cause fetal congenital Zika syndrome: microcephaly, ventriculomegaly, cerebellar hypoplasia, lissencephaly with hydrocephalus, fetal akinesia deformation sequence (FADS), etc
- It may cause Guillain-Barré syndrome (GBS) in some patients
- Once infected with Zika, the patient is likely to be protected from future infections; there is no evidence that the infection poses an increased risk of birth defects in future pregnancies

Laboratory

- Zika virus serology
- Zika virus PCR testing (blood, urine or spinal fluid)
- Test to exclude dengue and chikungunya: *Coxiella burnetii* PCR testing, chikungunya virus PCR testing

Treatment

- Symptomatic treatment: rest, drink fluids, paracetamol (do not take aspirin or NSAIDs)

- Recovery usually occurs within a week
- Admit to hospital if severe complication develops
- There is no specific treatment for the virus currently available

Prevention

- Protection against mosquito bites (e.g. long-sleeved shirts and long pants, insect repellent, mosquito net to cover babies)
- Prevent sexual transmission of Zika by using condoms or abstaining from sexual activity
- Pregnant women should not travel to areas with Zika
- Women should wait at least 8 weeks after travel (or 8 weeks after symptoms started if they get sick) before trying to get pregnant
- Men should wait at least 6 months after travel (or 6 months after symptoms started if they get sick) before trying to conceive (Zika virus stays in semen longer than in other body fluids)
- There is no vaccine to prevent Zika

Appendix 1

Aminoglycosides initial dosing and level monitoring

1. AMINOGLYCOSIDES INITIAL DOSE AND FURTHER DOSE INTERVAL

Step 1: Check serum creatinine and calculate creatinine clearance (CrCl)

Age group	CrCl (mL/min)
1 month~<2 years	40 x height (cm) ÷ serum Cr
2~12 years	49 x height (cm) ÷ serum Cr
12~20 years (female)	49 x height (cm) ÷ serum Cr
12~20 years (male)	62 x height (cm) ÷ serum Cr
Adult male	([140-age] x ideal weight [kg]*) ÷ (serum Cr x 0.814)
Adult female	Adult male's CrCl x 0.85

*Ideal weight = 50 kg (45.5 kg for female) + 0.9 kg/each cm over 152 cm

Step 2: Determine initial dose based on age and renal function

Age/renal impairment	CrCl (mL/min)	Starting dose (gentamicin/tobramycin)*
Once daily dosing		
Preterm <34 weeks	>60	3 mg/kg
Neonate 34–44 weeks	>60	3.5 mg/kg
Child <10 years	>60	7.5 mg/kg up to 320 mg
10–29 years	>60	6 mg/kg up to 560 mg
30–60 years	>60	5 mg/kg up to 480 mg
>60 years	>60	4 mg/kg up to 400 mg
>10 years with sepsis	>60	7 mg/kg up to 640 mg
8–12 hourly dosing	>60	3 mg/kg/day (divided)
(for endocarditis only)		(gentamicin only)
Mild renal impairment	40–60	70% of above dose
Moderate renal impairment	30–40	55% of above dose
Severe renal impairment	20–30	40% of above dose
End-stage renal failure	<20	Seek expert advice

*Initial dose for amikacin = above starting dose × 4

Step 3: Determine further empirical dosing intervals

CrCl (mL/min)	Dosing interval	Maximum empirical doses
>60	q24h	3 (at 0, 24, 48 hours)
40–60	q36h	2 (at 0, 36 hours)
<40	N/A	Once, then seek expert advice

2. AMINOGLYCOSIDE BLOOD LEVEL MONITORING

Once-daily or less frequent dosing monitor (computerised AUC method)

For aminoglycoside direct therapy

Indication:

- Infection from the pathogen that has shown resistance to other safer antibiotics
- Combination therapy for serious *Pseudomonas aeruginosa* infections and brucellosis

Method (start blood level check from the 1st day of direct therapy):

Step 1: Take 1st blood sample 5 minutes after completion of infusion

Step 2: Take 2nd blood sample 6–8 hours later

Step 3: The AUC (area under the curve) is calculated by computer program and the recommendation of subsequent dosage adjustment is given by comparing the actual AUC to the target AUC (80–100 mg/hour/L)

Frequency of monitoring

- Every 48 hours (repeat Steps 1–3)
- More frequently if renal function is changing rapidly or substantially (e.g. critically ill patients with severe sepsis or acute renal failure)

Multiple daily dosing monitor (trough level monitor)

For aminoglycoside synergistic treatment (e.g. endocarditis)

Indication:

- Low-dose treatment for streptococcal and enterococcal endocarditis

Step 1: Take blood just before the next dose to measure patient's trough level

Step 2: Compare the patient's trough level against the ideal trough level in the table below:

Antibiotic	Ideal trough level
Gentamicin—8 hourly dosing*	0.5–1 mg/L
Tobramycin—8 hourly dosing*	1–2 mg/L
Amikacin—8 hourly dosing*	4–8 mg/L

*If renal function is impaired, 12 hourly dosing

Step 3: Adjust dosage or dosing interval:

If patient's trough level < ideal trough level

- Increase dosage or decrease dosing interval

If patient's trough level > ideal trough level
- Reduce dosage or increase dosing interval

Frequency of monitoring

- Twice weekly (repeat Steps 1–3)
- More frequently if renal function is changing rapidly or substantially (e.g. critically ill patients with severe sepsis or acute renal failure)

Appendix 2

Vancomycin loading dose and blood level monitoring

Vancomycin blood level monitoring is recommended for all patients treated with vancomycin for longer than 48 hours.

1. INTERMITTENT INFUSION

Step 1: Give loading dose: 25–30 mg/kg (infusion rate: <10 mg/min)

Step 2: Give maintenance dose: 15–20 mg/kg and determine frequency of infusion

CrCl (mL/min)	Frequency
>60	q12h
20–60	q24h
<20	q48h

Step 3: Start blood level monitor after 48 hours (on the third day) of vancomycin treatment; take blood just before the next dose to measure patient's trough level

Step 4: Adjust dosage by comparing patient's trough level to the ideal trough level (15–20 mg/L or 20–25 mg/L for CNS infection)

If patient's trough level < ideal trough level
- Increase dose or decrease dosing interval

If patient's trough level > ideal trough level
- Reduce dose or increase dosing interval

If patient's trough level >25 mg/L (or >30 mg/L in CNS infection)
- Withhold next dose until trough level <20 mg/L (or <25 mg/L in CNS infection)

Frequency of monitoring
- Monitor blood trough levels every 3–5 days (or every 1–2 days for older patients or patients with renal impairment)

2. CONTINUOUS INFUSION

Continuous infusion is used for:

- Patients who require higher or more frequent doses (e.g. overweight patients with good renal function or CNS infection)
- Infections by a pathogen with a high vancomycin MIC
- Outpatient IV therapy

Step 1: Give loading dose infusion: 25–30 mg/kg (infusion rate: <10 mg/min)

Step 2: Give maintenance dose infusion: 15–20 mg/kg

Step 3: Check 'spot' blood level within 24 hours of vancomycin treatment, then at least once weekly (or more frequently if renal function or clinical condition changes)

Step 4: Adjust dosage by comparing patient's trough level against the target trough level (20 mg/L or 25 mg/L for CNS infection)

If patient's trough level < target trough level
- Increase infusion dose

If patient's trough level > target trough level
- Reduce infusion dose

Appendix 3

National Immunisation Program Schedule

Age	Disease	Vaccine choice
Birth	Hepatitis B (hep B)	H-B-Vax II
6 w to 2 m	Diphtheria/tetanus/pertussis (DTPa)	
	Haemophilus influenzae type b (Hib)	Infanrix Hexa
	Hepatitis B (hep B)	
	Poliomyelitis (IPV)	
	Pneumococcal (13vPCV)	Prevenar 13®
	Rotavirus	Rotarix or RotaTeq®
4 m	Diphtheria/tetanus/pertussis (DTPa)	
	Haemophilus influenzae type b (Hib)	Infanrix Hexa
	Hepatitis B (hep B)	
	Poliomyelitis (IPV)	
	Pneumococcal (13vPCV)	Prevenar 13®
	Rotavirus	Rotarix or RotaTeq®
6 m	Diphtheria/tetanus/pertussis (DTPa)	
	Haemophilus influenzae type b (Hib)	Infanrix Hexa
	Hepatitis B (hep B)	
	Poliomyelitis (IPV)	
	Pneumococcal (13vPCV)	Prevenar 13®
	Rotavirus	RotaTeq® (not for Rotarix)
12 m	Measles/mumps/rubella (MMR)	Priorix
	Haemophilus influenzae type b/ Meningococcal C (Hib-MenCCV)	Menitorix
18 m	Measles/mumps/rubella/varicella (MMRV)	Priorix Tetra® or Proquad
	Diphtheria/tetanus/pertussis (DTPa)	Infanrix or Tripacel
4 y	Diphtheria/tetanus/pertussis/poliomyelitis (DTPa-IPV)	Infanrix-IPV
School programs		
10–13 y	Hepatitis B (hep B) (if not past vaccinated)	H-B-VAX II or Engerix-B
10–13 y	Varicella (chickenpox) (VZV) (catch-up only)	Varilrix® or Varivax®
12–13 y	Human papillomavirus (HPV)	Gardasil9®
15–17 y	Diphtheria/tetanus/pertussis (dTpa)	Boostrix
17–18 y	Meningococcal ACWY (4vMenCV)	Menactra

Age	Disease	Vaccine choice
Aboriginal Australians and Torres Strait Islanders		
12–18 m	Pneumococcal (13vPPV) (high-risk areas*)	Prevenar 13®
12–24 m	Hepatitis A (hep A) (high-risk areas*)	VAQTA® Paed/Adolescent
6 m to 5 y	Influenza (annually)	Influenza vaccine
15–49 y	Influenza (annually)	Influenza vaccine
	Pneumococcal (23vPPV) (at-risk, 5 yearly)	Pneumovax® 23
≥50 y	Influenza (annually)	Influenza vaccine
	Pneumococcal (23vPPV) (5 yrly)	Pneumovax® 23
Other at-risk groups		
≥6 m	Influenza (at risk, annually)	Influenza vaccine
12 m	Pneumococcal (13vPPV) (at risk)	Prevenar 13®
4 y	Pneumococcal (23vPPV) (at risk)	Pneumovax® 23
Pregnancy	Influenza (at any time)	Influenza vaccine
Pregnancy	Diphtheria/tetanus/pertussis (dTpa) (3rd trimester)	Boostrix
≥65 y	Influenza (all people, annually)	Influenza vaccine
	Pneumococcal (23vPPV) (all people, 5 yearly)	Pneumovax® 23
70–80 y	Varicella zoster (once only)	Zostavax

*Higher risk areas: Queensland, Northern Territory, Western Australia and South Australia.
Table adapted with permission from *The Australian Immunisation Handbook* © Commonwealth of Australia

IMMUNISATION PROGRAM SCHEDULE—INDIVIDUAL DISEASES

Diphtheria/tetanus/pertussis (DTPa)

- 3 doses at 6 weeks to 2 months, 4 months, 6 months; 3 boosters at 18 months (DTPa), 4 years (DTPa) and 15–17 years (dTpa)

Haemophilus influenzae type B (Hib)

- 4 doses at 6 weeks to 2 months, 4 months, 6 months, 12 months (when using PRP-T [Infanrix Hexa or Hiberix])
- Indigenous children in higher risk areas*: 3 doses at 6 weeks, 4 months, 12 months (when using PRP-OMP [Comvax or PedvaxHIB])

Hepatitis A (hep A)

- Indigenous children in higher risk areas*: 2 doses during 12–24 months

Hepatitis B (hep B)

- 1 dose after birth (within 7 days), then 3 doses at 6 weeks (or 2 months), 4 months, 6 months
- If not past vaccinated or infected: 2 doses at 0, 4–6 months during 10–13 years

---

*Higher risk areas include Queensland, Northern Territory, Western Australia and South Australia

Human papillomavirus (HPV)

- 2 doses at 0 and 6–12 months during 12–13 years

Influenza

- All people ≥ 65 years: 1 dose annually
- 6 months and over with medical risk conditions: 1 dose annually
- Indigenous 6 months to <5 years: 1 dose annually
- Indigenous ≥15 years: 1 dose annually
- Pregnant women: 1 dose

Measles/mumps/rubella (MMR)

- 1 dose of at 12 months (MMR), 1 dose at 18 months (MMRV)

Meningococcal C (MenCCV)

- 1 dose at 12 months
- age <6 months with high risk: additional 2 doses (8 weeks apart) before 12 months
- age 6–11 months with high risk: additional 1 dose before 12 months

Meningococcal ACWY (4vMenCV)

- 1 dose at 17–18 years

Pneumococcal

- 3 doses of 13vPCV (Prevenar 13®) at 6 weeks to 2 months, 4 months, 6 months (up to 2 years)
- Indigenous children in higher risk areas*: 3 doses of 13vPCV (Prevenar 13®) at 6 weeks to 2 months, 4 months, 6 months; a booster of 23vPPV (Pneumovax® 23) at 18–24 months
- Medical at-risk children: 4 doses of 13vPCV (Prevenar 13®) at 6 weeks to 2 months, 4 months, 6 months, 12 months; a booster of 23vPPV (Pneumovax 23®) between 4 and 5 years of age
- Medical at-risk Indigenous people 15–49 years: 1 dose of 23vPPV (Pneumovax 23®)
- Indigenous people ≥50 years: 1 dose of 23vPPV (Pneumovax 23®) every 5 years
- All people ≥65 years: 1 dose of 23vPPV (Pneumovax 23®) every 5 years

Poliomyelitis (IPV)

- 3 doses at 6 weeks to 2 months, 4 months, 6 months; a booster at 4 years

Rotavirus

- 2 doses of Rotarix at 6 weeks to 2 months, 4 months (**or** 3 doses of RotaTeq at 6 weeks to 2 months, 4 months, 6 months)

Varicella (chickenpox) (VZV)

- 1 dose of MMRV at 18 months

Varicella zoster (herpes zoster)

- 1 dose of Zostavax at 70 years

Appendix 4

Vaccines and immunoglobulins

AUSTRALIAN BAT LYSSAVIRUS

- Merieux
- Rabipur

Immunoglobulin

- Imogam Rabies (human rabies immunoglobulin, HRIG)

AVIAN INFLUENZA

- Panvax H5N1

CHOLERA

- Dukoral (oral inactivated vaccine)

DIPHTHERIA

Combination vaccines for children <8 years

- Infanrix Hexa (DTPa-hepB-IPV-Hib)
- Infanrix IPV (DTPa-IPV)
- Quadracel (DTPa-IPV)
- Tripacel (DTPa)
- Pediacel (DTPa-hepB-IPV-Hib)

Combination vaccines for people ≥8 years

- ADT Booster (dT)
- Adacel (dTpa)
- Adacel Polio (dTpa-IPV)
- Boostrix (dTpa)
- Boostrix-IPV (dTpa-IPV)

Immunoglobulin

- Diphtheria toxoid

HAEMOPHILUS INFLUENZAE TYPE B

- Liquid PedvaxHIB (PRP-OMP)
- Hiberix (PRP-T)

Combination vaccines

- Infanrix Hexa (DTPa-hepB-IPV-Hib) (PRP-T)
- Pediacel* (DTPa-hepB-IPV-Hib)

HEPATITIS A

- Avaxim
- Havrix 1440

---

*Not registered in Australia

- Havrix Junior
- VAQTA®

Combination vaccines

- Twinrix Junior (360/10) (hepA-hepB)
- Twinrix (720/20) (hepA-hepB)
- Vivaxim (hepA-typhoid)

HEPATITIS B

- Engerix B
- H-B-VAX II

Combination vaccines

- Infanrix Hexa (DTPa-hepB-IPV-Hib)
- Twinrix (720/20) (hepA-hepB)
- Twinrix Junior (360/10) (hepA-hepB)
- Pediacel* (DTPa-hepB-IPV-Hib)

Immunoglobulin

- Hepatitis B immunoglobulin (HBIg)

HUMAN PAPILLOMAVIRUS (HPV)

- Cervarix
- Gardasil
- Gardasil 9

INFLUENZA

- FluQuardri
- FluQuadri Junior
- Fluarix Tetra®
- Afluria Quad

JAPANESE ENCEPHALITIS

- Jespect® (inactivated)
- Imojev® (live attenuated)

MEASLES

Combination vaccines (live attenuated)

- Priorix (MMR)
- M-M-R II (MMR)
- Priorix Tetra (MMRV)
- ProQuad (MMRV)

MENINGOCOCCAL DISEASE

Meningococcal B vaccine (4CMenBV)

- Bexsero® (meningococcal B)

---

*Not registered in Australia

Meningococcal C vaccines (MenCCV)

- Meningitec (meningococcal C)
- Menjugate® (meningococcal C)
- NeisVac-C® (meningococcal C)

Combination meningococcal C Vaccine

- Menitorix (meningococcal C + Hib)

Quadrivalent conjugate vaccines (4vMenCV)

- Menactra (meningococcal A, C, W135 and Y)
- Menveo (meningococcal A, C, W135 and Y)
- Nimenrix (meningococcal A, C, W135 and Y)

Quadrivalent polysaccharide vaccines (4vMenPV)

- Mencevax ACWY (meningococcal A, C, W135 and Y)
- Menomune (meningococcal A, C, W135 and Y)

MUMPS

Combination vaccines (live attenuated)

- Priorix (MMR)
- M-M-R II (MMR)
- Priorix Tetra® (MMRV)
- ProQuad (MMRV)

PERTUSSIS

Combination vaccines for children <8 years

- Infanrix Hexa (DTPa-hepB-IPV-Hib)
- Infanrix IPV (DTPa-IPV)
- Quadracel (DTPa-IPV)
- Tripacel (DTPa)
- Pediacel* (DTPa-hepB-IPV-Hib)

Combination vaccines for people ≥8 years

- Adacel (dTpa)
- Adacel Polio (dTpa-polio)
- Boostrix (dTpa)
- Boostrix-IPV (dTpa-IPV)

PNEUMOCOCCAL DISEASE

- Pneumovax® 23 (23vPPV)
- Prevenar 13® (13vPCV)
- Synflorix (10vPCV)

POLIOMYELITIS

- IPOL (IPV)

---

*Not registered in Australia

Combination vaccines for children <8 years

- Infanrix Hexa (DTPa-hepB-IPV-Hib)
- Infanrix IPV (DTPa-IPV)
- Quadracel (DTPa-IPV)
- Pediacel* (DTPa-hepB-IPV-Hib)

Combination vaccines for people ≥8 years

- Adacel Polio (dTpa-IPV)
- Boostrix-IPV (dTpa-IPV)

Q FEVER

- Q-VAX

RABIES

- Merieux
- Rabipur
- Verorab*

ROTAVIRUS

- Rotarix (oral live attenuated)
- RotaTeq® (oral live attenuated)

RUBELLA

Combination vaccines (live attenuated)

- Priorix (MMR)
- M-M-R II (MMR)
- Priorix Tetra® (MMRV)
- ProQuad (MMRV)

SWINE INFLUENZA

- Panvax H1N1
- Panvax H1N1 Junior

TETANUS

Combination vaccines for children <8 years

- Infanrix Hexa (DTPa-hepB-IPV-Hib)
- Infanrix IPV (DTPa-IPV)
- Quadracel (DTPa-IPV)
- Tripacel (DTPa)
- Pediacel* (DTPa-hepB-IPV-Hib)

Combination vaccines for people ≥8 years

- ADT Booster (dT)
- Adacel (dTpa)

*Not registered in Australia

- Adacel Polio (dTpa-IPV)
- Boostrix (dTpa)
- Boostrix-IPV (dTpa-IPV)

Immunoglobulin

- Tetanus immunoglobulin (TIG)

TUBERCULOSIS

- BCG vaccine

TYPHOID

- Vivotif Oral (oral live attenuated)
- Typherix
- Typhim Vi

Combination vaccine

- Vivaxim (typhoid-hep A)

VARICELLA (CHICKENPOX)

- Varilrix® (live attenuated)
- Varivax® (live attenuated)

Combination vaccine (live attenuated)

- Priorix Tetra® (MMRV)
- ProQuad (MMRV)

VARICELLA ZOSTER (HERPES ZOSTER)

- Zostavax (live attenuated)
- Shingrix (HZ/su)* (live attenuated)

Immunoglobulin

- Zoster immunoglobulin (ZIG)

YELLOW FEVER

- Stamaril (live attenuated)
- Arilvax* (live attenuated)

---

*Not registered in Australia

Appendix 5

Travel vaccination

CHOLERA

Routine vaccination is not recommended, as risk to travellers is very low
Indication for vaccination:

- Travellers with reduced gastric acidity entering rural areas of highly endemic countries
- Health or aid workers or water scientists going to work in disaster areas where cholera is possible
- Where traveller's diarrhoea is unacceptable (as a vaccine for traveller's diarrhoea)

Provides cholera protection for 2–3 years for adults

- Dukoral® adult, child >6 years: 1 sachet PO, 2 doses at intervals of 1–6 week, booster after 2 years; child 2–6 years: ½ sachet PO, 3 doses at intervals of 1–6 weeks, booster after 6 months

Note: avoid oral typhoid vaccine for 8 hours

DIPHTHERIA/TETANUS/PERTUSSIS

Indication for vaccination:

- Travellers who had last dose 10 years ago
- Travellers who had last dose 5 years ago and are undertaking prolonged travel overseas

Provides protection for 10 years

Vaccine choice:

- ADT (tetanus/diphtheria) adult 0.5 mL IM st
- Boostrix (tetanus/diphtheria/pertussis) adult, child ≥10 years: 0.5 mL IM st
- Adacel (tetanus/diphtheria/pertussis) adult, child ≥10 years: 0.5 mL IM st

Note: DTPa (Boostrix and Adacel) also covers pertussis and is suitable for adults who have close contact with children

HEPATITIS A

Indication for vaccination:

- All travellers ≥1 year of age travelling to developing countries
Provides lifetime protection for hepatitis A and B (combination vaccine) and 3 years' protection for typhoid (combination vaccine)

Vaccine choice:

- Avaxim ≥16 years: 0.5 mL IM, 2 doses at 0, 6–12 months
- Avaxim Paediatric 2–16 years: 0.5 mL IM, 2 doses at 0, 6–12 months
- Havrix 1440 ≥16 years: 1 mL IM, 2 doses at 0, 6–12 months
- Havrix Junior 2–15 years: 0.5 mL IM, 2 doses at 0, 6–12 months
- VAQTA® ≥18 years: 1 mL IM, 2 doses at 0, 6–12 months
- VAQTA® Paediatric/Adolescent 1–17 years: 0.5 mL IM, 2 doses at 0, 6–18 months
- Vivaxim (Hep A/typhoid) 1 mL IM, 2 doses at 0, 6–12 months
- Twinrix 720/20 (Hep A + B) ≥16 years: 1 mL IM, 3 doses at 0, 1, 6 months
- Twinrix Junior 360/10 1–15 years: 0.5 mL IM, 3 doses at 0, 1, 6 months

Rapid schedule—if very limited time before departure:

- Twinrix 720/20 (Hep A + B) ≥16 years: 1 mL IM, 4 doses on days 0, 7, 21 and at 12 months

If there is insufficient time for vaccination, a single injection of normal immunoglobulin can give protection for 3–4 months

HEPATITIS B

Indication for vaccination:

- All travellers intending to spend ≥1 month in Asia, Africa and South America

Provides lifetime protection for hepatitis B and A (combined vaccines)

Vaccine choice:

- Engerix B ≥20 years: 1 mL (<20 years and infants: 0.5 ml) IM, 3 doses at 0, 1, 6 months
- H-B-VAX II ≥20 years: 1 mL (<20 years and infants: 0.5 ml) IM, 3 doses at 0, 1, 6 months
- Twinrix 720/20 (Hep A + B) ≥16 years: 1 mL IM, 3 doses at 0, 1, 6 months

Rapid schedule if very limited time before departure:

- H-B-VAX II ≥20 years: 1.0 mL IM, 4 doses at 0, 7, 21 days and 12 months
- Twinrix 720/20 ≥16 years: 1 mL IM, 3 doses on days 0, 7, 21 and a booster at 12 months

INFLUENZA

Indication for vaccination:

- Should be offered to all international travellers
Provides protection for 1 year (pick at 3–4 months)

Vaccine choice:

Child 6 months to 3 years
- FluQuadri Junior—0.5 mL IM, 2 doses at least 4 weeks apart, then 1 dose annually

Child 3 years and older
- FluQuardri—0.5 mL IM annually

People aged 18 years and older
- Afluria Quad—0.5 mL IM annually

JAPANESE ENCEPHALITIS

Indication for vaccination:

- Travellers spending ≥1 month in rural areas of Asia or the Western Province of Papua New Guinea, particularly during the wet season
- Travellers spending ≥1 year in urban areas of Asia (except for Singapore)
- Consider vaccination for shorter term travellers in wet season where there is considerable outdoor activity or the accommodation is not mosquito-proof

Provides protection for 2–3 years

- Jespect® ≥2 months: 0.5 mL IM, 2 doses on days 0, 28 (the last dose is best given at least 35 days before travelling)

MEASLES/MUMPS/RUBELLA

Indication for vaccination:

- For those born after 1966 and before 1986, who have not received a second dose of MMR vaccine or 'catch-up' dose during the 1998 campaign (if unsure, check measles antibody levels for guide)

Provides protection for 10 years

- Priorix (measles/mumps/rubella) 0.5 mL IM st before travelling, or ideally 2 doses at 1 month interval

MENINGOCOCCAL VACCINE

Indication for vaccination:

- Travel to an area with increased risk of meningococcal disease
  - The 'meningitis belt' of sub-Saharan Africa
  - Pilgrims on the Hajj
  - Remote trekking or working in refugee camps
  - Entering areas of existing outbreaks

Provides protection for 3–5 years

Vaccine choice:

- Preferably, 4vMenPV at least 2 weeks before departure
  - Menactra adult, child >9 months: 0.5 mL IM st, 2 weeks before departure

- Menveo adult, child ≥9 months: 0.5 mL IM st, 2 weeks before departure

Revaccinate 3–5 yearly if at continuing risk

PNEUMOCOCCAL VACCINE

Indication for vaccination:

- For high-risk travellers (aged over 5 years) who have had no pneumococcal vaccine over the last 5 years
  - Asplenia, functional (including sickle-cell disease) or anatomical
  - Immunocompromised
  - Chronic illness
  - Tobacco smokers

Provides protection for 5 years

- Pneumovax 23 0.5 mL IM st, at least 2 weeks before travelling

POLIOMYELITIS

Indication for vaccination:

- Travellers to affected countries (see www.polioeradication.org) whose last polio vaccination was 10 years ago

Booster in previously immunised adults confers lifetime protection

Vaccine choice:

- IPOL 0.5 mL SC st
- Boostrix-IPV (tetanus/diphtheria/pertussis/polio) 0.5 mL IM st
- Adacel Polio (tetanus/diphtheria/pertussis/polio) 0.5 mL IM st

RABIES

Indication for vaccination:

- Overseas travellers who plan to handle any unvaccinated mammal that can bite and scratch
- Overseas travellers who will be spending prolonged periods in rabies-endemic rural areas (children are at greater risk of disease than adults)

Provides protection for 2 years

Vaccine choice:

- Merieux 1.0 mL IM, 3 doses on days 0, 7 and 28, then single booster 2 yearly, if continue to be at risk
- Rabipur adult, child ≥1 years: 1.0 mL IM, 3 doses on days 0, 7 and 28, then single booster 2 yearly if continue to be at risk
- MIRV (HDCV)* child ≥1 year: 1.0 mL IM, 3 doses on days 0, 7 and 28

*Not registered in Australia

If previously (>2 years ago) vaccinated—single booster dose before departure

ROTAVIRUS

Indication for vaccination:

- Infants travelling to developing countries

Vaccine choice:

- RotaTeq® infant ≥2 months: 2 mL PO, 3 doses at 2, 4, 6 months (or 3 doses between 2 and 6 months with at least 4 weeks interval)
- Rotarix infant ≥2 months: 1 mL PO, 2 doses at 2, 4 months (or 2 doses between 2 and 6 months with at least 4 weeks interval)

TICK-BORNE ENCEPHALITIS

Indication for vaccination:

- Travellers to endemic areas

Provides protection for 3 years

- FSME-Immun* 0.5 mL IM, 3 doses at 0, 1–3 months, 9–12 months, booster 3 yearly

Rapid schedule if very limited time before departure:

- FSME-Immun* 0.5 mL IM, 3 doses on days 0, 7, 21 with a booster at 12–18 months

TUBERCULOSIS

Indication for BCG vaccination (tuberculin test negative):

- Children <5 years of age who will stay in countries with high TB risk for >3 months
- Children 5–16 years of age who will live in countries with high TB risk
- Adults with high tuberculosis risk (e.g. healthcare workers)
    - BCG vaccine 0.1 mL (infant <12 months: 0.05 ml) intradermal inj st (at an authorised travel or BCG vaccination clinic)

TYPHOID

Indication for vaccination:

- For all travellers ≥2 years old to endemic countries
- Should be completed at least 2 weeks before travel
- Do not take antibiotics when taking oral vaccine

Three oral doses protect for 3 years; four oral doses protect for 5 years
One injection protects for 3 years

---

*Not registered in Australia

Vaccine choice:

- Vivotif oral (typhoid live) adult, child ≥6 years: 1 capsule PO, 3 doses on days 1, 3 and 5, then 3 yearly; or 4 doses on days 1, 3, 5 and 7, then 5 yearly
- Typherix adult, child ≥2 years: 0.5 mL IM st, then 3 yearly
- Typhim Vi adult, child ≥2 years: 0.5 mL IM st, then 3 yearly
- Vivaxim (typhoid/hepatitis A) 1 mL IM st, then 3 yearly

VARICELLA

Indication for vaccination:

- Travellers who have had no history of chickenpox or varicella vaccination and would like to have the protection.

Possible lifetime protection

- Varilrix (varicella live) 0.5 mL SC, 2 doses at 0, 6 weeks or later
- Varivax (varicella live) 0.5 mL SC, 2 doses at 0, 4–8 weeks

YELLOW FEVER

Indication for vaccination:

- Travellers ≥9 months of age who plan to go to infected areas and then go to other non-infected countries or return to Australia (a valid vaccination certificate is required for entry from infected areas into non-infected countries)

Contraindications:

- Egg anaphylaxis or previous yellow fever vaccination allergy
- Infants <9 months (risk of vaccine-related encephalitis)
- Elderly >65 years of age (risk of adverse reactions)
- Immune suppressed or past history of thymus gland problems

Do not vaccinate travellers unnecessarily
Vaccination must be given in an approved yellow fever vaccination centre
Provides protection for 10 years

- Stamaril (yellow fever live) adult, child ≥9 months: 0.5 mL IM or SC st, 10 yearly boosters if at ongoing risk
- Arilvax* (yellow fever live) adult, child ≥9 months: 0.5 mL IM or SC st, 10 yearly boosters if at ongoing risk

---

*Not registered in Australia

Appendix 6

Organism susceptibility to antibiotics

These tables will assist empirical selection of antibiotics when laboratory susceptibility is not available or only limited antibiotics are tested. The designation of susceptibility used in the tables is 75%.

How to use

To find an antibiotic that an organism is sensitive to
1. Find the organism in the left-hand column of the table.
2. Follow the organism row to find an S.
3. Find the number at the top of the S column.
4. Match the number with the antibiotic list above the table.
Repeat Steps 2–4 to find other sensitive antibiotics.

To check whether an organism is sensitive to an antibiotic
1. Find the organism in the left-hand column of the table.
2. Find the antibiotic in the antibiotic list above the table.
3. Find the number of the antibiotic in the top row of the table.
4. Cross-match the organism row with the column of the antibiotic number.
If the cross-match is an S, the organism is sensitive to the antibiotic.

To learn how many antibiotics an organism is sensitive to
1. Find the organism in the left-hand column of the table.
2. Follow the organism row to find an S.
3. Find the number at the top of the S column.
4. Match the number with the antibiotic list above the table.
Repeat Steps 2–4 until all sensitive antibiotics have been found.

To learn an antibiotic's spectrum
1. Find the antibiotic in the list above the table.
2. Find the antibiotic number in the top row of the table.
3. Follow this column down to find an S.
4. Follow this row to the left to find the organism that is sensitive to the antibiotic.
Repeat Steps 1–4 until all organisms have been found, known as the spectrum.

S = sensitive for that organism
? = no data or the antibiotic is not recommended for that organism
C = sensitive to some community-acquired MRSA
* = CSF and eye infections only

Penicillins

1. Benzylpenicillin
2. Penicillin V/procaine penicillin
3. Flucloxacillin/dicloxacillin
4. Amoxicillin/ampicillin
5. Amoxicillin + clavulate
6. Piperacillin + tazobactam
7. Ticacillin + clavulate

Cefalosporins

8. Cefalexin/cefalotin/cefazolin
9. Cefaclor/cefuroxime
10. Cefoxitin

Gram-negative organism	1	2	3	4	5	6	7	8	9	10
Acinetobacter spp										
Aeromonas spp						S	S			
Burkholderia cepacia										
Burkholderia pseudomallei					S	S	S			
Campylobacter jejuni and *coli*					?	?	?			
Citrobacter freundii						S	S			
Escherichia coli					S	S	S	S	S	S
Enterobacter spp						S	S			
Haemophilus influenzae	S			S	S	S	S		S	S
Klebsiella spp					S	S	S	S	S	S
Moraxella catarrhalis					S	S	S	S	S	S
Morganella spp						S	S			
Neisseria gonorrhoeae					S	S	S		S	S
Neisseria meningitidis	S	S		S	S	?	?		S	S
Pasteurella multocida	S	S		S	S	S	S		?	S
Proteus mirabilis				S	S	S	S	S	S	S
Proteus vulgaris						S	S			
Providencia spp						S	S			
Pseudomonas aeruginosa						S	S			
Salmonella spp				S	S	?	?	?	?	?
Serratia spp						S	S			
Shigella spp					S	S	S	S	S	S
Stenotrophomonas maltophilia							S			
Yersinia spp					S	S	S			

Adapted from AMH 2012, Australian Medicines Handbook Pty Ltd, Adelaide, SA. Note that AMH content is updated 6-monthly, see www.amh.net.au.

Cefalosporins

11 Cefotaxime/ceftriaxone
12 Cefepime
13 Ceftazidime

Aminoglycosides

14 Amikacin
15 Gentamicin
16 Tobramycin

Carbapenems

17 Doripenem/meropenem
18 Ertapenem
19 Imipenem

Glycopeptides

20 Vancomycin/teicoplanin
21 Clindamycin/lincomycin

Gram-negative organism	11	12	13	14	15	16	17	18	19	20	21
Acinetobacter spp				S	S	S	S		S		
Aeromonas spp	S	S	S	S	S	S	S	S	S		
Burkholderia cepacia							S	?	S		
Burkholderia pseudomallei		S	S				S	?	S		
Campylobacter jejuni and coli				S	S	S	S	S	S		?
Citrobacter freundii	S	S	S	S	S	S	S	S	S		
Escherichia coli	S	S	S	S	S	S	S	S	S		
Enterobacter spp		S	S	S	S	S	S	S	S		
Haemophilus influenzae	S	S	S	S	S	S	S	S	S		
Klebsiella spp	S	S	S	S	S	S	S	S	S		
Moraxella catarrhalis	S	S	S	?	?	?	S	S	S		
Morganella spp	S	S	S	S	S	S	S	S	S		
Neisseria gonorrhoeae	S	S	S	?	?	?	?	?	?		
Neisseria meningitidis	S	S	S	?	?	?	?	?	?		
Pasteurella multocida	S	S	S	?	?	?	S	S	S		
Proteus mirabilis	S	S	S	S	S	S	S	S	S		
Proteus vulgaris	S	S	S	S	S	S	S	S	S		
Providencia spp				S	S	S	S	S	S		
Pseudomonas aeruginosa		S	S	S	S	S	S		S		
Salmonella spp	S	S	S	?	?	?	?	?	?		
Serratia spp	S	S	S	S	S	S	S	S	S		
Shigella spp	S	S	S	S	S	S	S	S	S		
Stenotrophomonas maltophilia											
Yersinia spp	S	S	S	S	S	S	S	S	S		

Adapted from AMH 2012, Australian Medicines Handbook Pty Ltd, Adelaide, SA. Note that AMH content is updated 6-monthly, see www.amh.net.au.

Macrolides

22 Azithromycin
23 Clarithromycin
24 Roxithromycin
25 Erythromycin

Tetracyclines

26 Doxycycline
27 Minocycline
28 Tigecycline

Quinolones

29 Norfloxacin
30 Ciprofloxacin
31 Moxifloxacin

Gram-negative organism	22	23	24	25	26	27	28	29	30	31
Acinetobacter spp							S	S	S	S
Aeromonas spp					S	S	S	S	S	S
Burkholderia cepacia							?			
Burkholderia pseudomallei	?	?	?	?	S	S	?			
Campylobacter jejuni and coli	S	S	S	S	S	S	?	?	?	?
Citrobacter freundii					?	?	S	S	S	S
Escherichia coli					?	?	S	S	S	S
Enterobacter spp					?	?	S	S	S	S
Haemophilus influenzae	S	S	S	?	S	S	S	?	S	S
Klebsiella spp					?	?	S	S	S	S
Moraxella catarrhalis	S	S	S	S	S	S	S	?	S	S
Morganella spp								S	S	S
Neisseria gonorrhoeae	S	?	?	?	S	S	?			
Neisseria meningitidis	?	?	?	?	?	?	?	?	S	S
Pasteurella multocida					S	S	S	?	S	S
Proteus mirabilis								S	S	S
Proteus vulgaris								S	S	S
Providencia spp								S	S	S
Pseudomonas aeruginosa								S	S	S
Salmonella spp	S				S	S	S	?	S	S
Serratia spp							S	S	S	S
Shigella spp							S	?	S	S
Stenotrophomonas maltophilia							S			
Yersinia spp	?	?	?	?	S	S	?	?	S	S

Adapted from AMH 2012, Australian Medicines Handbook Pty Ltd, Adelaide, SA. Note that AMH content is updated 6-monthly, see www.amh.net.au.

Others

32	Aztreonam
33	Chloramphenicol
34	Daptomycin
35	Linezolid
36	Metronidazole/tinidazole

37	Nitrofurantoin
38	Quinupristin + dalfopristin
39	Rifampicin/rifabutin
40	Sodium fusidate
41	Trimethoprim
42	Trimethoprim + sulfamethoxazole

Gram-negative organism	32	33	34	35	36	37	38	39	40	41	42
Acinetobacter spp											
Aeromonas spp	S	S				?				S	S
Burkholderia cepacia											S
Burkholderia pseudomallei	?	?				?		?			S
Campylobacter jejuni and *coli*	?	S				?		?			?
Citrobacter freundii	S					S				S	S
Escherichia coli	S	S				S				S	S
Enterobacter spp	S	S								S	S
Haemophilus influenzae	S	S						S		S	S
Klebsiella spp	S	S				S				S	S
Moraxella catarrhalis	?	?				?	?	?	?		S
Morganella spp	S	S				S				S	S
Neisseria gonorrhoeae	?	S				?	?	?	?	?	?
Neisseria meningitidis	?	S				?		S	S		?
Pasteurella multocida	S	S				?		?	?	?	S
Proteus mirabilis	S	S								S	S
Proteus vulgaris	S	S								S	S
Providencia spp	S	S								S	S
Pseudomonas aeruginosa	S										
Salmonella spp	?	S				?				S	S
Serratia spp	S									S	S
Shigella spp	S	S				?					S
Stenotrophomonas maltophilia											S
Yersinia spp	S	S			?	?				S	S

Adapted from AMH 2012, Australian Medicines Handbook Pty Ltd, Adelaide, SA. Note that AMH content is updated 6-monthly, see www.amh.net.au.

Penicillins

1. Benzylpenicillin
2. Penicillin V/procaine penicillin
3. Flucloxacillin/dicloxacillin
4. Amoxicillin/ampicillin
5. Amoxicillin + clavulate
6. Piperacillin + tazobactam
7. Ticacillin + clavulate

Cefalosporins

8. Cefalexin/cefalotin/cefazolin
9. Cefaclor/cefuroxime
10. Cefoxitin

Gram-positive organism	1	2	3	4	5	6	7	8	9	10
Corynebacterium jeikeium										
Enterococcus faecalis	S			S	?	S				
Enterococcus faecium										
Listeria spp	S			S	?	S	S			
Staphylococcus aureus			S		S	S	S	S	?	?
Staphylococcus aureus (MRSA)										
Staphylococcus saprophyticus	S	S	S	S	S	S	S	S	S	S
Coagulase-negative staph			S		S	S	S			
Streptococcus group A, B, C, D	S	S	S	S	S	S	S	S	S	S
Streptococcus milleri group	S	S	S	S	S	S	S	S	S	S
Streptococcus pneumoniae	S	S	?	S	S	S	S	S	S	S
Viridans streptococcus group	S	S	?	S	S	S	S	S	S	S
Anaerobes										
Actinomyces	S	S		S	S	S	S	?	?	?
Bacteroides fragilis group					S	S	S			S
Clostridium perfringens	S	S		S	S	S	S	S	S	S
Clostridium difficile										
Fusobacteria spp	S	S		S	S	S	S	S	S	S
Peptostreptococcus spp	S	S	?	S	S	S	S		S	S
Prevotella melaninogenica					S	S	S	S	S	S
Propionibacterium	S	S	?	S	S	S	S	S	S	S
Miscellaneous										
Clamydophila Chlamydia spp										
Legionella spp										
Mycobacterium avium complex										
Mycobacterium tuberculosis										
Mycoplasma pneumoniae										
Nocardia spp										

Adapted from AMH 2012, Australian Medicines Handbook Pty Ltd, Adelaide, SA. Note that AMH content is updated 6-monthly, see www.amh.net.au.

Cefalosporins
11 Cefotaxime/ceftriaxone
12 Cefepime
13 Ceftazidime

Aminoglycosides
14 Amikacin
15 Gentamicin
16 Tobramycin

Carbapenems
17 Doripenem/meropenem
18 Ertapenem
19 Imipenem

Glycopeptides
20 Vancomycin/teicoplanin
21 Clindamycin/lincomycin

Gram-positive organism	11	12	13	14	15	16	17	18	19	20	21
Corynebacterium jeikeium										S	
Enterococcus faecalis							S		S	S	
Enterococcus faecium										S	
Listeria spp				S	S	S	S	?	S	S	
Staphylococcus aureus	?	S	?	S	S	S	S	S	S	S	S
Staphylococcus aureus (MRSA)										S	C
Staphylococcus saprophyticus	S	S	S	S	S	S	S	S	S	S	S
Coagulase-negative staph										S	S
Streptococcus group A, B, C, D	S	S	S				S	S	S	S	S
Streptococcus milleri group	S	S	S				S	S	S	S	S
Streptococcus pneumoniae	S	S	S				S	S	S	S	S
Viridans streptococcus group	S	S	S				S	S	S	S	S
Anaerobes											
Actinomyces	?	?	?				S	?	S	S	S
Bacteroides fragilis group							S	S	S		S
Clostridium perfringens	S	S	S				?	S	?	S	S
Clostridium difficile										S	
Fusobacteria spp	S	S	S				S	S	S		S
Peptostreptococcus spp	S	S	S				S	S	S	S	S
Prevotella melaninogenica	S	S	S				S	S	S		S
Propionibacterium	S	S	S				S	?	S	?	S
Miscellaneous											
Clamydophila Chlamydia spp											?
Legionella spp										?	?
Mycobacterium avium complex				S							
Mycobacterium tuberculosis				S							
Mycoplasma pneumoniae											?
Nocardia spp				S		?	?	?	S	?	?

Adapted from AMH 2012, Australian Medicines Handbook Pty Ltd, Adelaide, SA. Note that AMH content is updated 6-monthly, see www.amh.net.au.

Macrolides

22 Azithromycin
23 Clarithromycin
24 Roxithromycin
25 Erythromycin

Tetracyclines

26 Doxycycline
27 Minocycline
28 Tigecycline

Quinolones

29 Norfloxacin
30 Ciprofloxacin
31 Moxifloxacin

Gram-positive organism	22	23	24	25	26	27	28	29	30	31
Corynebacterium jeikeium							?			
Enterococcus faecalis							S			S
Enterococcus faecium							S			S
Listeria spp	?	?	?	?	?	?	S			S
Staphylococcus aureus	S	S	S	S	S	S	S	?	?	S
Staphylococcus aureus (MRSA)							S			
Staphylococcus saprophyticus	S	S	S	S	S	S	?	?	?	?
Coagulase-negative staphylococci								?	?	
Streptococcus group A, B, C, D	S	S	S	S	S	S	S			S
Streptococcus milleri group	S	S	S	S	S	S	S			
Streptococcus pneumoniae	S	S	S	S	S	S	S			S
Viridans streptococcus group	S	S	S	S	?	?	S			S
Anaerobes										
Actinomyces	S	S	S	S	S	S	?			S
Bacteroides fragilis group							S			S
Clostridium perfringens	S	S	S	S			S			S
Clostridium difficile							S			
Fusobacteria spp	S	S	S	S	?	?	S			S
Peptostreptococcus spp	S	S	S	S			S			S
Prevotella melaninogenica	S	S	S	S	?	?	S			S
Propionibacterium	S	S	S	S	S	S	?			S
Miscellaneous										
Clamydophila Chlamydia spp	S	S	S	S	S	S	?			S
Legionella spp	S	S	S	S	?	?	?	?	S	S
Mycobacterium avium complex	S	S		?			?			S
Mycobacterium tuberculosis	?	?					?		S	S
Mycoplasma pneumoniae	S	S	S	S	S	S	?	?	?	S
Nocardia spp					?	S	S		?	S

Adapted from AMH 2012, Australian Medicines Handbook Pty Ltd, Adelaide, SA. Note that AMH content is updated 6-monthly, see www.amh.net.au.

Others

32 Aztreonam
33 Chloramphenicol
34 Daptomycin
35 Linezolid

36 Metronidazole/tinidazole
37 Nitrofurantoin
38 Quinupristin + dalfopristin
39 Rifampicin/rifabutin
40 Sodium fusidate
41 Trimethoprim
42 Trimethoprim +
   sulfamethoxazole

Gram-positive organism	32	33	34	35	36	37	38	39	40	41	42
Corynebacterium jeikeium			S	S			?	S	S		
Enterococcus faecalis			S	S		S				S	S
Enterococcus faecium			S	S		S	S			S	S
Listeria spp		*	?	S		?	S	?		?	S
Staphylococcus aureus	S		S	S		S	S	S	S	?	?
Staphylococcus aureus (MRSA)			S	S			S	S	S	?	C
Staphylococcus saprophyticus	S	S	?			S	?	S	?	S	S
Coagulase-negative staphylococci			S	S		S	S	S	S	S	S
Streptococcus group A, B, C, D	S	S	S			S	S	?		S	S
Streptococcus milleri group	S	S	S			S	S	?		?	?
Streptococcus pneumoniae	S	S	S			S	S	?			
Viridans streptococcus group	S	S	S			S	S	?			
Anaerobes											
Actinomyces		S	?	?		?		?	?	?	?
Bacteroides fragilis group		S	?	S	S	?		?	?	?	?
Clostridium perfringens		S	?	?	S	?	S	?	?	?	?
Clostridium difficile			?	?	S	?		?	?	?	?
Fusobacteria spp		S	?	?	S	?		?	?	?	?
Peptostreptococcus spp		S	S	?	S	?		?	?	?	?
Prevotella melaninogenica		S	?	?	S	?		?	?	?	?
Propionibacterium		S	S	?		?		?	?	?	?
Miscellaneous											
Clamydophila Chlamydia spp		S		S				?		?	?
Legionella spp		?		S		?	S	S	?	?	?
Mycobacterium avium complex				S				S		?	?
Mycobacterium tuberculosis				S				S		?	?
Mycoplasma pneumoniae		S		S		?	S	?		?	?
Nocardia spp		?		S		?		?	?	?	S

Adapted from AMH 2012, Australian Medicines Handbook Pty Ltd, Adelaide, SA. Note that AMH content is updated 6-monthly, see www.amh.net.au.

Appendix 7

School exclusion

Disease	Incubation	School exclusion
Amoebiasis	2–4 weeks	Until diarrhoea has stopped
Campylobacter enteritis	2–5 days	Until diarrhoea has stopped
Chickenpox	2–3 weeks	For 5 days after rash first appears (until all blisters scabbed over)
Conjunctivitis	1–3 days	Until eye discharge has stopped
Diarrhoea	Hours to days	Until 24 hours after diarrhoea has stopped
Diphtheria	2–5 days	Until 2 negative throat swabs and doctor signs a recovery certificate
Erythema infectiosum	1–2 weeks	No need (infectious before rash)
Glandular fever	4–6 weeks	No need, unless sick
Haemophilus influenzae type b (Hib)	A few days	Until doctor signs recovery certificate
Hand, foot and mouth disease	3–7 days	Until blisters have dried
Head lice	5–7 days	No need, as long as on treatment
Hepatitis A	2–6 weeks	For 2 weeks after first symptoms or for 1 week after onset of jaundice
Hepatitis B	4–20 months	No need
Hepatitis C	2–26 weeks	No need
Herpes labialis (cold sores)	1 week	Until it has healed (cover cold sores with dressings if possible)
Impetigo (school sores)	1–3 days	Until treatment starts (sores should be covered with dressing)
Influenza	1–3 days	Until the child feels better
Lice		After treatment has started
Measles	10–14 days	Until 5 days after rash appears
Meningitis (bacterial)	Days to months to years	Until treatment has finished
Molluscum contagiosum	2–7 weeks	No need
Mumps	12–25 days	For 9 days after onset of swelling or until the swelling goes down
Poliomyelitis	7–21 days	Until 14 days from onset and doctor signs a recovery certificate
Ringworm	Several days	After fungal treatment has started
Rubella	2–3 weeks	For 5 days after rash appears
Salmonella enteritis	8–48 hours	Until diarrhoea has stopped
Scabies	2–6 weeks	After treatment has started, reinfection: 1–4 days
Scarlet fever	1–3 days	Until ≥24 hours of antibiotic treatment and gets better

Disease	Incubation	School exclusion
Shigellosis	12–50 hours	Until diarrhoea has stopped
Swine flu	3–7 days	Until 7 days after onset of symptoms
Trachoma (eye infection)	1 week	After treatment has started
Tuberculosis	2–10 weeks	Until doctor signs recovery certificate
Typhoid/paratyphoid fever	10–14 days	Until doctor signs recovery certificate
Whooping cough (pertussis)	4–21 days	Until 5 days of antibiotic treatment or 3 weeks after the onset of cough

Appendix 8

Abbreviations

A–a	alveolar–arterial gradient
ABLV	Australian bat lyssavirus
ABPA	allergic bronchopulmonary aspergillosis
AE	Australian encephalitis
AHD	alveolar hydrated disease
AIDS	acquired immunodeficiency syndrome
ALT	alanine aminotransferase
ANP	acute necrotising pancreatitis
APRI	AST to platelet ratio index
ARF	acute rheumatic fever
ARV	antiretroviral
ASAP	as soon as possible
AST	aspartate aminotransferase
ATLL	adult T-cell leukaemia/lymphoma
BAL	bronchoalveolar lavage
BCG	Bacillus Calmette-Guerin
BFV	Barmah Forest virus
bid	two times a day
BIG	botulinum immune globulin
BP	blood pressure
BSE	bovine spongiform encephalopathy
BSL	biosafety level
BV	bacterial vaginosis
CA-MRSA	community-acquired methicillin-resistant staphylococci
CAP	community-acquired pneumonia
CCHF	Crimean-Congo haemorrhagic fever
CDT	*Clostridium difficile* toxins
CF	cystic fibrosis
CHIKV	Chikungunya virus
CIN	cervical intraepithelial neoplasia
CJD	Creutzfeldt-Jakob disease
CMV	cytomegalovirus
COPD	chronic obstructive pulmonary disease
CRP	C-reactive protein
CRS	congenital rubella syndrome
CSD	cat-scratch disease
CSF	cerebrospinal fluid
CSOM	chronic suppurative otitis media

CXR	chest x-ray
DAA	direct-acting antiviral
DAIR	debridement and implant retention
DCR	dacryocystorhinostomy
DDA	direct-acting antivirals
DIC	disseminated intravascular coagulation
DOT	direct observed therapy
DSO	distal subungual onychomycosis
DVT	deep vein thrombosis
EBV	Epstein-Barr virus
ED	emergency department
eGFR	estimated glomerular filtration rate
EHEC	enterohaemorrhagic *E. coli*
EIEC	enteroinvasive *E. coli*
ELISA	enzyme-linked immunosorbent assay
ENT	ear, nose and throat
ERCP	endoscopic retrograde cholangiopancreatography
ESR	erythrocyte sedimentation rate
ETEC	enterotoxigenic *E. coli*
EUC	electrolytes, urea and creatine
EUS-FNA	endoscopic ultrasound-guided fine-needle aspiration
FAD	flea allergy dermatitis
FBC	full blood count
FEV	forced expiratory volume
FMT	faecal microbiota transplantation
G6PD	glucose-6-phosphate dehydrogenase
GBS	group B streptococcus
G-CSF	granulocyte colony-stimulating factor
GI	gastrointestinal
GIT	gastrointestinal tract
GSS	Gerstmann–Sträussler–Scheinker syndrome
HAP	hospital-acquired pneumonia
HAV	hepatitis A virus
HBIg	hepatitis B immunoglobulin
HCAP	healthcare-associated pneumonia
HCV	hepatitis C virus
HDV	hepatitis D virus
HeV	hendra virus
HEV	hepatitis E virus
HFMD	hand, foot and mouth disease
HHV	human herpesvirus

Hib	*haemophilus influenzae* type b
HIV	human immunodeficiency virus
HPC	high-prevalence country
HPV	human papillomavirus
HRT	hormone replacement therapy
HS	hidradenitis suppurativa
HSCT	haematopoietic stem cell transplantation
HSE	herpes simplex encephalitis
HSV	herpes simplex virus
HUS	haemolytic uraemic syndrome
ICP	intracranial pressure
ICU	intensive care unit
id	intradermally
IgA	immunoglobulin A
IgE	immunoglobulin E
IgG	immunoglobulin G
IgM	immunoglobulin M
IGRA	interferon-gamma release assay
IM	intramuscularly
inh	inhalation
inj	injection
IP	intraperitoneally
IPD	invasive pneumococcal disease
IPV	inactivated poliovirus vaccine
IUCD	intrauterine contraceptive device
IV	intravenously
IVI	intravenous infusion
JE	Japanese encephalitis
KOH	potassium hydroxide
KUB	kidney, ureter, bladder
KUNV	Kunjin virus
LCM	lymphocytic choriomeningitis
LFT	liver function test
LGV	lymphogranuloma venereum
LMWH	low-molecular-weight heparin
MAC	mycobacterium avium complex
MAH	mycobacterium avium hominis
mane	in the morning
MAP	mycobacterium avium paratuberculosis
M/C/S	microscopy, culture and sensitivity
MDR	multiple antibiotic resistance

MDT	multi-drug therapy
MIC	minimum inhibitory concentration
MMRV	measles, mumps, rubella vaccine
MOE	malignant otitis externa
MR-CNS	methicillin-resistant, coagulase-negative staphylococci
MRSA	methicillin-resistant *Staphylococcus aureus*
MRSE	methicillin-resistant *Staphylococcus* epidermidis
MS-CNS	methicillin-sensitive, coagulase-negative staphylococci
MSM	men who have sex with men
MSSA	methicillin-susceptible *Staphylococcus aureus*
MSU	midstream urine
MTCT	mother-to-child transmission
MVE	Murray Valley encephalitis
neb	nebulise
NGT	nasogastric tube
NHIG	normal human immunoglobulin
NNRTI	non-nucleoside reverse transcriptase inhibitor
nocte	at night
NPA	nasopharyngeal aspirate
NRTI	nucleoside/nucleotide reverse transcriptase inhibitor
NTM	non-tuberculous mycobacteria
OCP	oral contraceptive pill
OCP	ova cysts parasites
oint	ointment
OME	otitis media with effusion
PAM	primary amoebic meningoencephalitis
PCR	polymerase chain reaction
PCSI	pneumonia comorbidity and severity indicators
PI	protease inhibitor
PID	pelvic inflammatory disease
PNS	pilonidal sinus
PO	orally
PPI	proton-pump inhibitor
PPROM	pre-term pre-labour rupture of membranes
PR	per rectal
PRN	as needed
PV	per vaginam
q12h	12 hourly
q2h	2 hourly
q4h	4 hourly
q6h	6 hourly

q8h	8 hourly
qid	four times a day
RBC	red blood count
RR	respiratory rate
RSV	respiratory syncytial virus
RUQ	right upper quadrant
SARS	severe acute respiratory syndrome
SBP	spontaneous bacterial peritonitis
SC	subcutaneously
SIL	squamous intraepithelial lesion
SIRS	systemic inflammatory response syndrome
SOB	short of breath
SSPE	subacute sclerosing panencephalitis
st	single dose
STI	sexually transmitted infection
STSS	staphylococcal toxic shock syndrome
tab	tablet
TB	tuberculosis
tds	three times a day
TIG	tetanus immunoglobulin
TNF	tumor necrosis factor
top	topically
TORCH	toxoplasmosis, rubella, CMV and herpes simplex infections
TSLS	toxic shock-like syndrome
TURP	transurethral resection of the prostate
UAT	urinary antigen test
URTI	upper respiratory tract infection
UTI	urinary tract infection
VAP	ventilator-associated pneumonia
VHFs	viral haemorrhagic fevers
VISA	vancomycin-intermediate *Staphylococcus aureus*
VRE	vancomycin-resistant enterococci
VUR	vesicoureteral reflux
VVC	vulvovaginal candidiasis
VZV	varicella zoster virus
WBC	white cell count
WNV	West Nile virus
WSO	white superficial onychomycosis
XDR	extensively drug-resistant
ZIG	zoster immunoglobulin

Index

Page numbers followed by *f* indicate figures, *t* indicate tables and *b* indicate boxes.